T0141063

Rix's Expert Psychiatric Evidence

Professor Rix has assembled an A-team of experts to guide novice and experienced practitioner alike through the perils and pitfalls of working as an expert witness. The reader benefits not just from the authors' combined years of experience in psychiatric evaluation and courtroom practice but also from the wealth of historical detail used to illustrate dilemmas that ensnare the unwary. Those seeking to avoid a similar fate will have reason to be grateful.

Alec Buchanan, Professor of Psychiatry, Yale School of Medicine, USA

This erudite, comprehensive textbook is an essential acquisition to the library of anyone who gives expert evidence in the field of psychiatry in the United Kingdom. Experts in other fields will also find it useful for its general guidance on the duties of experts and their approach to the writing of reports and the giving of evidence. Whether you practise in the criminal, family or civil courts, this is a book to which you will turn time and again for the answers to questions that always arise in the life of any expert witness.

Sir Martin Spencer, High Court Judge and Chair of the Expert Witness Institute

There is often confusion about the precise role of the medical expert witness and the different types of evidence that may be provided. This is clearly dealt with in this book (chapter 1). Professor Rix has a wonderful conversational style as seen in the chapter 'Going to Court'. For many nowadays an infrequent experience, so this is essential reading. Having a clear resource outlining the legal systems within the British Isles will be useful for all witnesses (not just psychiatrists).

Dr Margaret M Stark, President, Faculty of Forensic & Legal Medicine of the Royal College of Physicians, UK

Prof Keith Rix and his collaborators have put together an extremely comprehensive, engaging and practical guide. Experts play a crucial role in our justice system and their evidence is often key in determining the right outcome. The pitfalls that could trip up, embarrass or be potentially catastrophic for the uninitiated expert are set out and often illustrated with real world examples to make them all the more memorable. Summaries of the key points are usefully interspersed at appropriate points throughout the book.

Although written for psychiatrists, the many legal principles, procedures and general recommended approaches will no doubt transfer to other disciplines.

As a criminal and professional discipline lawyer, I found the book to be immensely instructive. It will assist in finding an appropriate expert, asking the right questions and maximising the benefit of instructing an expert. It will also assist when perusing expert reports to identify areas of potential weakness that could be exploited.

I was heartened by the suggested approach to the structure of reports to ensure that the reasoning for the expert's conclusions is given due prominence. There is so much more to recommend in this book.

Ms Sue Swan, Associate Solicitor, Cartwright King Solicitors

Praise for the first edition

An excellent guide for those coming into psychiatric medico-legal work but also a first class refresher for the expert … a well-written, well-rounded and well-produced book.

BMA Medical Book Awards 2012 – "Highly commended"

I wish I had a book like this to help me during my initial stages of forensic training. I am sure most of the forensic trainees would treasure a book like this. I would certainly recommend that this book be read by anyone who wishes to do some court work … It answers most of the questions that I have had during my training so far and for which I have looked far and wide for answers.

Dr Sajid Muzaffar, (then) Specialty Registrar in Forensic Psychiatry

This really is a *tour de force* … Real practical advice in all chapters against a background of legal and medical analysis, which is just what young practitioners need.

His Honour Judge Simon Lawler QC

This is an excellent read and of value both to those starting out and those already with some experience as an expert.

Dr Mike Ventress, Consultant Forensic Psychiatrist

An admirable manual for psychiatrists, indeed for all medical practitioners who choose, or (as often happens) are obliged to do forensic work and for the lawyers who enlist them … in short I consider this a masterwork.

James Badenoch QC, 1 Crown Office Row

This book will appeal to experienced and inexperienced expert psychiatric witnesses and I recommend it unreservedly.

Dr Mike Isaac in the Journal of Legal and Forensic Medicine

Expert Psychiatric Evidence should be read by every mental health practitioner who is required to or chooses to offer an opinion on people involved in legal proceedings.

Richard Latham in The Journal of Forensic Psychiatry and Psychology

The greatest recommendation is that the book had a tendency to disappear repeatedly from my desk in the brief time that I have had a review copy, as many colleagues have borrowed it for a few hours to look up particular points of interest.

Dr Cosmo Hallstrom in The Psychiatrist

I wish I had access to (this book) a few years ago, when inadvertently, unwillingly, with legal ignorance and naivety, I became an expert witness in a case …. It is extremely detailed but readable, at times even amusing …. This book will help psychiatrists, perhaps also lawyers, avoid major mistakes.

Dr Jane Garner in The Advocate

Overall, this is an excellent book, and it would be a foolish trainee or new consultant in psychiatry who did not possess, read and inwardly digest it. The book deserves a place in the personal library of any expert witness, however experienced he or she is …. Rix's book provides a solid foundation for expert witness practice, and I wholeheartedly recommend it

Dr Michael Isaac in the Academy of Experts The Expert and Dispute Resolver

Psychiatric experts learn from their teachers, their mentors and specific courses they may attend. Up until now the totality of what they need to know has not been summarised in any one place. It is now .... This is undoubtedly an extremely useful textbook

Dr Fiona Mason in Medicine, Science and the Law

The author of this book brilliantly enmeshes psychiatry and the law – this is, after all, what expert witnesses in this field need to do to be most helpful to the court.

Professor Penny Cooper in the Expert Witness Institute Newsletter

Keith Rix ... writes here with authority and detail ... The book is written with a refreshing frankness ... for a book on a technical area of forensic psychiatry *Expert Psychiatric Evidence* is an unusually easy read. It also has a very good index.

Dr Alec Buchanan in Journal of the American Academy of Psychiatry and Law

This handbook provides invaluable guidance on a wide variety of topics

Dr Maurice Lipsedge in Clinical Risk

Rix's Expert Psychiatric Evidence

Second edition

Editors in Chief

Dr Michael Powers, QC, BSc, MB, BS, Hon LLD, DA, FFFLM
Professor Keith Rix, MPhil, LLM, MD, FRCPsych, Hon FFFLM

Editors

Professor Keith Rix, MPhil, LLM, MD, FRCPsych, Hon FFFLM
Dr Laurence Mynors-Wallis, MA, DM, MRCP, FRCPsych
Dr Ciarán Craven, SC, MB, BCh, BAO, BSc, MFFLM

Consulting Editors

Alderney, Guernsey and Sark

Mr Richard McMahon QC

Ireland

Dr Ciarán Craven SC

Isle of Man

Mr Paul Rodgers
Dr Ignacy Ziajka

Northern Ireland

Dr David Sharpe QC

Scotland

Mr Andrew Brown QC
Mr Douglas Fairley QC
Dr Marian Gilmore QC

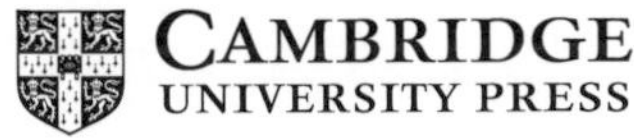

CAMBRIDGE
UNIVERSITY PRESS

University Printing House, Cambridge CB2 8BS, United Kingdom

One Liberty Plaza, 20th Floor, New York, NY 10006, USA

477 Williamstown Road, Port Melbourne, VIC 3207, Australia

314–321, 3rd Floor, Plot 3, Splendor Forum, Jasola District Centre, New Delhi – 110025, India

79 Anson Road, #06–04/06, Singapore 079906

Cambridge University Press is part of the University of Cambridge.

It furthers the University's mission by disseminating knowledge in the pursuit of education, learning, and research at the highest international levels of excellence.

www.cambridge.org
Information on this title: www.cambridge.org/9781911623687
DOI: 10.1017/9781911623670

First published 2011
Second edition 2021

Printed in the United Kingdom by TJ Books Limited, Padstow Cornwall

A catalogue record for this publication is available from the British Library.

ISBN 978-1-911-62366-3 Hardback
ISBN 978-1-911-62367-0 Cambridge Core
ISBN 978-1-911-62368-7 Print-online Bundle

Every effort has been made in preparing this book to provide accurate and up-to-date information that is in accord with accepted standards and practice at the time of publication. Although case histories are drawn from actual cases, every effort has been made to disguise the identities of the individuals involved. Nevertheless, the authors, editors and publishers can make no warranties that the information contained herein is totally free from error, not least because clinical standards are constantly changing through research and regulation. The authors, editors and publishers therefore disclaim all liability for direct or consequential damages resulting from the use of material contained in this book. Readers are strongly advised to pay careful attention to information provided by the manufacturer of any drugs or equipment that they plan to use.

Contents

Online Appendices – See Inside Cover for Access

1 Letter of Response to Request for a Report
2 Time Sheet
3 Cost Estimates
4 Sample Contract for Litigants-in-Person Soliciting Reports
5 File Front Sheet
6 Appointment Letter
7 Information to Accompany Appointment Letter
8 Consent Form for Medicolegal Report
9 General Data Protection Regulation Consent Form
10 Privacy Notice
11 Notes of History and Examination Findings for Appendix B
12 Declaration for an Expert Report in the Republic of Ireland
13 Additional Declaration for Experts in England and Wales Instructed by the Prosecution Only
14 Expert Witness Self-Certificate for Experts in England and Wales Instructed by the Prosecution Only
15 Report Covering Letter
16 Report Template (Criminal)
17 Report Template (Personal Injury)

Contributors

Dr Danny Allen, MB, BS, LLM, MRCGP, MFFLM, FRCPsych
Consultant Psychiatrist, Oxford Health NHS Foundation Trust & Phoenix Mental Health Services

Dr James Briscoe, MB, ChB, MMedSci, MRCPsych
Consultant Psychiatrist, Midlands Partnership NHS Foundation Trust; Director, James Briscoe Ltd; Trustee of the Grange Annual Medico-Legal Conference

Mr Andrew Brown, QC, LLB, DLP
Convener, Mental Health Tribunal for Scotland; Former Senior Advocate Depute, Crown Office

Dr Ciarán Craven, SC, MB, BCh, BAO, BSc, MFFLM
Barrister at Law, King's Inns and Gray's Inn

Mr Douglas Fairley, QC, LLB, DipLP
Westwater Advocates; Member, Police Appeals Tribunal

Dr Marian Gilmore, QC, LLB, Dr de l'Univ
Arnot Manderson Advocates; Chair Police, Appeals Tribunal; Convenor, Mental Health Tribunal for Scotland

Dr Anthony Howard, LLB, MB, ChB, MSc (Ortho Eng), PhD, PGC (Med Ed), MRCSEd
Barrister at Law, 9 St John Street, Manchester; NIHR Clinical Lecturer in Trauma & Orthopaedic Surgery; Assistant Coroner for West Yorkshire

Dr Chris Jones, BMedSci, LLB, BSc, MD, MRCPsych
Member of the Mental Health Tribunal; Member of the Parole Board; Retired Consultant Forensic Psychiatrist

Mr David Rhys Jones, LLB
Legal Officer, Helen Bamber Foundation; Co-Director Forrest Medico-Legal Services CIC

Professor Cornelius Katona, MD, FRCPsych
Medical and Research Director, Helen Bamber Foundation; Honorary Professor, Division of Psychiatry, University College London

Mr Andrew Leak, BA, LLM
Senior Protection Associate, UNHCR; Director ASL (Medico-Legal Services) Ltd; Former Medico-Legal Services Lead, Helen Bamber Foundation

Mr Richard McMahon, QC, LLB, LLM
The Deputy Bailiff of Guernsey

Dr Laurence Mynors-Wallis, MA, DM, MRCP, FRCPsych
Consultant Adult Psychiatrist, Dorset HealthCare University NHS Foundation Trust; Visiting Professor Bournemouth University

Dr Srikanth Nimmagadda, MB, BS, MA, MSc, MMedSci, LLM, DPM, MRCPsych, MFFLM, FIIOPM
Consultant Forensic Psychiatrist; Professor of Organisational Psychological Medicine; Director of Academic Unit, Institute of Organisational Psychological Medicine

Professor Rajan (Taj) Nathan, MSc, MD, MRCPsych
Consultant Forensic Psychiatrist & Director of Research, Development &

Clinical Effectiveness, Cheshire and Wirral Partnership NHS Foundation Trust; Senior Research Fellow, University of Liverpool; Visiting Professor, University of Chester

Dr Michael Powers, QC, BSc, MB, BS, Hon LLD, DA, FFFLM
Master of the Bench of Lincoln's Inn

Professor Keith J. B. Rix, MPhil, LLM, MD, FRCPsych Hon, FFFLM
Honorary Consultant Forensic Psychiatrist, Norfolk and Suffolk NHS Foundation Trust; Visiting Professor of Medical Jurisprudence, University of Chester; Mental Health and Intellectual Disability Lead, Faculty of Forensic and Legal Medicine of the Royal College of Physicians

Mr P. T. Rodgers, LLB, MEng, ACGI
Advocate, Isle of Man

Mr Karl Rowley, QC, MA (Oxon)
Head of the Family Group, St John's Buildings, Manchester

Dr David R. K. Sharpe, QC, MB, BCh, BAO, LLM, DPH, MFFLM, FRCP, FRCS, FIMC, FFSEM, FCIArb
Barrister at Law – Northern Ireland, England & Wales and the Republic of Ireland

Dr G. E. P. Vincenti, MB, BS, LLB, DOccMed, FRCPsych
Consultant Psychiatrist in independent practice; formerly Medical Director, Cygnet Hospital, Harrogate

Dr Ignacy Ziajka, MD
Specialist Associate Royal College of Psychiatrists; Consultant Adult Psychiatrist, Community Mental Health Team for Adults, Isle of Man

Foreword to the Second Edition

The Rt Hon. Lord Hodge,
Deputy President and Justice of the Supreme Court

In legal actions concerning many fields of human activity, courts and tribunals rely on the evidence of experts to deliver justice. The complexity of our society and of the judgments, which laws and regulations call on judges to make, mean that judges often depend on experts in reaching their decisions. They may depend on experts not only to explain technical facts underlying the dispute which is being adjudicated, but also to give an independent professional opinion on matters which require professional judgement and which will inform the decision to be made. This gives considerable power to the expert witness and with that power goes a responsibility to perform the task to the best of his or her ability. Any failure to do so can cause serious damage not only to justice, but also to the expert's professional reputation if the failure is exposed by cross-examination and if the judge comments adversely on the witness's performance of that task.

In *Kennedy v Cordia (Services) LLP* [2016] UKSC 6, the UK Supreme Court listed circumstances in which expert evidence is admissible. Such evidence is admissible if: (1) it will assist the court in its task; (2) the witness has the necessary knowledge and experience; (3) the witness is impartial in his or her presentation and assessment of the evidence; and (4) there is a reliable body of knowledge or experience to underpin the expert's opinion.

While, as the various chapters of this book show, there are different formulations in different contexts about what is expected of the expert witness, the fundamental requirements are the same across the board.

It is unlikely that a lawyer will call as a witness an expert unless something which he or she says in a report or in oral evidence is to some extent helpful to the lawyer's client. But the primary duty of the expert witness is to the court. The expert's opinion is valuable only if it is objective and independent of the exigencies of the litigation. The evidence which he or she gives must be impartial and the expert must avoid advocacy on behalf of the party from whom his or her instructions came. That does not mean that an expert has no duties to his or her instructing party. As this book shows, the expert may have duties, for example, to advise the instructing party's legal team on the evidence needed to present the case properly and on how to address the evidence of another expert which is adverse to that case.

It is important that an expert does not venture supposedly expert opinions on matters which are beyond his or her field of expertise. The expert must stay within the area of his or her competence and be self-critical in assessing what that area is. Similarly, the expert witness must consider whether there is a reliable body of scientific knowledge or experience to back the opinions which he or she advances. Otherwise, in each case, he or she may be embarrassed in cross-examination and by adverse comments in the judge's judgment.

The summary of the duties of experts which is quoted in Box 1.4 in Chapter 1 of this book is a useful thumbnail sketch. But, as the advice set out more fully in this book demonstrates, there is so much to be learned from experience, both one's own and that of others. People who decide to take up the task of becoming an expert witness need assistance if they are to perform their important task well. One needs not only a thorough awareness of the nature and scope of one's professional duties, but also an understanding of the forensic context in which the evidence will be prepared and delivered. Professor Rix and the other contributors to this book explain court proceedings and discuss the differing requirements as to the subject matter of expert evidence of different tribunals. The advice covers the procedures to be followed principally in England and Wales, but reference is also made to procedures in other jurisdictions or to sources of knowledge of such procedures. There is practical advice on establishing a business as a medico-legal expert, on how to conduct a medico-legal consultation and an experts' meeting. Of note is the straightforward advice, based on practical experience, of how an expert should conduct himself or herself in court, in examination in chief, on cross-examination and on re-examination. Obtaining appropriate training as an expert witness from a professional body is a valuable support to taking on the role and keeping up to date with both clinical practice and the developing requirements of the law in the area of expertise is essential.

I commend the advice on the structure of an expert medical report with its emphasis on brevity and the importance of (1) distinguishing fact within the expert's knowledge from asserted or assumed fact and (2) separating factual narrative from opinion. Clarity in presenting expert evidence greatly assists the task of the judge. I am pleased that Professor Rix has quoted the pithy observation of the late Lord Prosser: '[W]hat carries weight is the reasoning, not the conclusion' (*Dingley v Chief Constable of Strathclyde Police (No. 1)*, 1998 SC 548).

I congratulate Professor Rix and the other editors of and contributors to this informed and practical book. Service as an expert witness is the service of justice. The final chapter of the book concludes with the words, 'It matters not "which side has won". Has your testimony assisted in the delivery of justice?' I agree.

Patrick S. Hodge
Deputy President and Justice of the Supreme
Court of the United Kingdom
October 2019

Foreword to the First Edition

The Rt Hon. The Baroness Hale of Richmond,
Past President and Justice of the Supreme Court

Judges and juries need the help of experts of many kinds in order to understand matters which are not within their ordinary knowledge and experience. But they also need to know that the experts to whom they turn for help are reliable, not quacks, not hired guns, but independent professionals who understand that their principal duty is to the court and not to the person who is paying them. Nowhere is this more so than in psychiatry, which is 'not an exact science' (*R (B) v Ashworth Hospital Authority* [2005] 2 AC 278, para. 31), and unfortunately liable to be treated with even more suspicion by the non-expert than many other disciplines which regularly come before the courts.

The reliable expert is one who is not only on top of her subject, both in the books and on the ground, but also has a thorough understanding of the role and the issues which arise in the particular case in which she has been asked to advise. The reliable expert psychiatrist, therefore, is one who has read and absorbed this book. It is a mine of useful information. It is full of practical tips and do's and don'ts. It explains the difference between a witness of fact, a professional witness who has played a part in the relevant events, and an expert witness who provides an independent evaluation of the situation. It contains an extraordinarily comprehensive discussion of the many different legal contexts in which expert psychiatric evidence may become relevant. It is peppered with delightful anecdotes which show that it is the product of the real experiences of a real human being. There cannot be many psychiatrists who have appeared before an agricultural land tribunal but this one has.

In short, this book ought to increase the confidence of the court in the reliability of the expert evidence which it is hearing. But, just as important, it ought to increase the confidence of the psychiatrist who is setting out upon or developing a practice as an expert witness. We want and need psychiatrists to be prepared to do this important but challenging work. We hope that they will not be put off doing so by the recent decision of the Supreme Court, in *Jones v Kaney* [2011] UKSC 13, that a paid expert witness can be liable in negligence to her client. There is little risk that a psychiatrist who follows the wise guidance in this book (including the need to keep continually up to date) will find herself in that unfortunate position.

Acknowledgements and Preface to the Second Edition

It is nearly a decade since the publication of the first edition of RCPsych Publications' *Expert Psychiatric Evidence*. This second edition has taken longer to prepare than we would have wished and in part the delay has been the result of trying to ensure that it is of assistance to experts preparing reports throughout the British Isles and not just those preparing reports in England and Wales. The chapter 'Reports for the Channel Islands, the Republic of Ireland, the Isle of Man, Northern Ireland and Scotland' has been abandoned and we have sought to integrate the laws and procedures of those jurisdictions throughout the book. To this end, we have been assisted by consulting editors for all of those jurisdictions apart from Jersey. We are conscious of the fact that our treatment of these jurisdictions may yet be uneven and if some readers identify gaps or think that we could do better in explaining how psychiatric expertise is applied to a particular issue in a particular jurisdiction, we would be pleased to hear from them, and especially if they would like to be the third edition's consulting editor for Jersey.

This edition also differs from the first edition in that it is now an edited text and it is no longer a single author volume. Dr Laurence Mynors-Wallis brings to the text considerable experience of personal injury litigation, especially clinical negligence, and coronial cases. Dr Ciarán Craven SC is our legal co-editor, as well as being the consulting editor for his own jurisdiction of Ireland. A member of both the Bar of Ireland and the Bar of England and Wales, he has wide experience of inquests, mental health, capacity and medical law cases informed by clinical practice. Editorial oversight has also been provided by Dr Michael Powers QC, who is also qualified both in medicine and in law. We are pleased to have contributions to a number of chapters from leading expert psychiatric witnesses.

The greater length of this edition is a reflection not only of the deeper treatment of the jurisdictions outside England and Wales, but also of the many relevant cases that have been heard in the courts since 2011, especially the criminal courts, greater attention to vulnerable witnesses and defendants that is reflected in both statute and guidance, and many more procedural rules that affect expert witnesses. We have attempted to state and explain the relevant principal case law, statutory provisions and professional guidance affecting expert witnesses as of 1 September 2019. However, as the law and guidance can and will change over time, in any case the expert should not hesitate to seek clarification from, and be guided by, their instructing lawyers. Where we refer to particular sets of rules, we encourage readers to check the latest version online. There will have been changes by the time this edition is published. It is not uncommon to read an expert report and deduce from it that the expert has not read the relevant rules for a number of years.

This edition includes two specimen reports. Both illustrate a suggested change in the format of the expert psychiatric report. The traditional approach has been for the central factual section of the report to set out the subject's full history and mental state at some length and in a format that resembles the traditional psychiatric case history. Not only does this often make for an unacceptably long report, but it requires the reader to assimilate an often quite considerable amount of information that is not relevant to the issues in question and the opinions that will be derived from this factual information. We hope that the two specimen reports illustrate an attempt to produce shorter reports with a more succinct and relevant factual section to which the full case history can be appended (Appendix A) or not even appended at all (Appendix B). The full history and mental state examination on which the Charles Dickens report (Appendix B) is based is not appended to the report, but is available as online Appendix 11.

The first edition included a number of appendices in the form of letters and forms for adaptation by readers for their own use. These are listed in the Table of Contents, but they are not included in the printed version of the text. They are available on the Cambridge University Press website, along with report templates for criminal and civil personal injury cases, and all in a form which permits easy editing and adaptation to readers' own uses.

The dissolution of the Northern Ireland Assembly has caused us some difficulty. Although the Mental Capacity Act (Northern Ireland) 2016 received Royal Assent in May 2016, because the Assembly has not sat for over two years, implementation has been delayed. It is uncertain to what extent the Act will have been implemented by the time this book is published. But what this illustrates is the importance of checking statute law online. The online versions of Acts of Parliament are being constantly updated to include changes brought into force since enactment.

When K. R. used a particular set of consulting rooms for his medicolegal assessments, a receptionist would telephone him to inform him that his next 'patient' had arrived. Although he tried, perhaps not very successfully, to explain that the person was not his 'patient', it was difficult to know what to suggest to the receptionist regarding how she should refer to them. Although they became the 'subjects' of his expert reports, it did not seem wise to tell the receptionist that they were his 'subjects' as that would probably have resulted in comments behind his back about his adoption of royal airs and graces. But unless the context has required otherwise, we have used the term 'subject' throughout this book and to distinguish the subjects of expert reports from patients and also from clients. We consider this an important distinction, particularly insofar as the doctor's duty of care to the subject of an expert report is not the same as their duty of care to a patient.

As we were preparing to go to press, the Academy of Medical Royal Colleges published *Acting as a Professional or Expert Witness*. It was published too late to cross-reference its many recommendations in the way that we have referred to General Medical Council and Medical Council guidance. However, as one of us (K. R.) contributed to its drafting, there is a close correspondence between the Academy's recommendations and the content of this edition, so psychiatrists who act on the recommendations in this book should also be achieving the standards that the Academy expects of doctors who act as expert medical witnesses. Nevertheless, we urge readers to read *Acting as a Professional or Expert Witness* and ensure that they do follow its guidance. However, we do need to point out that, in contrast to the classification in the first edition of this book, we have abandoned the term 'professional witness' because what the Academy, the General Medical Council and the courts term a 'professional witness' is, according to the law of evidence, an 'expert witness' in that the evidence they give is 'evidence of fact, given by an expert, the observation, comprehension and description of which require expertise' (Hodgkinson and James 2015, p. 10). The courts in particular are unlikely to abandon the term lest they are required to pay 'professional witnesses' the same as they pay 'expert witnesses'.

We are grateful to the following for permission to reproduce copyright material or for granting licences to do so: The Advocate's Gateway (Box 7.29); Cambridge University Press

(Boxes 3.1, 3.2, 3.3, 7.19, 7.21 and 8.5 from *BJPsych Advances* articles); Churchill Livingstone (Box 7.23 based on, and a quotation from, R. Bluglass and P. Bowden (eds), *Principles and Practice of Forensic Psychiatry* (1990)); the General Medical Council (quotations from *Good Medical Practice* and *Acting as a Witness in Legal Proceedings*); Law Brief Publishing (quotations from D. Boyle, *On Experts: CPR35 for Lawyers and Experts* (2016)); the Law Society (quotations from C. Taylor and J. Krish, *Advising Mentally Disordered Offenders: A Practical Guide and Assessment of Mental Capacity; A Practical Guide for Doctors and Lawyers*, 3rd edn (2010)); SEAK Inc. (Box 17.2 based on S. Babitsky, J. J. Mangravati, Jr and C. J. Todd, *The Comprehensive Forensic Services Manual: The Essential Resources For All Experts* (2000)); and Sweet & Maxwell (Box 1.1, Box 6.5 and other quotations based on, or taken from, T. Hodgkinson and M. James, *Expert Evidence: Law and Practice*, 4th edn (2015)). The online appendices 9 (GDPR consent form) and 10 (privacy notice) reflect the advice of Mr Michael Deacon, 1 Crown Office Row, obtained through the Medical and Dental Defence Union of Scotland.

We are also grateful to the following for their comments on parts of the draft: Dr James Briscoe; Dr Nicholas Hallett; Ms Diana Kloss MBE, St Johns Buildings Chambers; Dr Linda Montague; Dr Asif Ramzan; and HHJ Adèle Williams.

K.R. acknowledges with thanks the resources made available to him by the University of Chester and its Law Library and similar assistance afforded by Shaun Kennedy and his colleagues in Information Services at the Royal College of Psychiatrists.

Last but not least, we are grateful to Anna Whiting, Jessica Papworth, Saskia Weaver-Pronk, Sophie Rosinke and Rajeswari Azayecoche at Cambridge University Press for all of their assistance.

Although we have also been assisted in this edition by a number of consulting editors, it is inevitable that there will be some mistakes of omission and commission. As this is *Rix's Expert Psychiatric Evidence*, the only one of us who should be blamed for such mistakes is K. R. If readers will kindly point them out, we will endeavour to correct them in the next edition.

Ciarán Craven SC
Laurence Mynors-Wallis
Michael Powers QC
Keith Rix
October 2019

Acknowledgements and Preface to the First Edition

I prepared my first criminal report, for a defendant's solicitors, when I was an honorary senior registrar in about 1981. It was a salutary experience. The solicitors sent the report to their client. He was remanded in custody. Notwithstanding the confidentiality that attaches to communications between prisoners and their solicitors, the prison authorities read my report. They contacted my consultant to ask him if he thought that it was a good idea for the prisoner to read my opinion about him. Needless to say, in trying to uphold the ethical principle of doing justice, I had fallen foul of the principle of doing no harm.

It was the beginning of a steep learning curve. Since then I have had 30 more years of preparing expert psychiatric reports and giving evidence in various courts. I use the term 'court' for any court of law, tribunal or body concerned with the process of arbitration or dispute resolution or professional conduct committee or panel.

I have given evidence to an agricultural land tribunal. It was convened in the lounge bar of a Yorkshire Dales country hotel. The tribunal sat in a raised area, usually occupied by the band. The parties, the witnesses and experts sat at small tables but without the customary pint. We were surrounded by pictures of sheep-shearing and cattle markets, including *Sheep Shearing at Hawes*. I purchased this as a leaving present for a colleague who kept his own sheep.

I have given evidence in the panelled court rooms at the Royal Courts of Justice. There, enticingly for me, if no one else, the side walls are lined from floor to ceiling with bookshelves teeming with the law reports of the last two centuries. The most conspicuous signs of the 21st century are the laptop computers of the judges and counsel.

At the beginning I was fortunate to be trained by Dr Angus Campbell. I owe an enormous debt to many more psychiatrists, and lawyers, than I will go on to acknowledge by name. In the early 1980s, training as a psychiatric expert witness was very much on the apprenticeship model, if you were fortunate, as I was, to begin preparing reports as a trainee. If not, and as it was for me once I became a consultant, it was a case of learning on the job.

This meant learning from other experts and from lawyers, and learning from one's mistakes. I continue to make mistakes. For as long as I go on learning from them, I hope to continue as an expert witness.

My acquisition of experience has not been a smooth process. I learned a lot and changed my practice a lot after going on a two-day course run by Bond Solon, a legal training consultancy based in London. The first day was on report writing and the second day on witness skills. So Chapters 4 ('The structure, organisation and content of the generic report') and 11 ('Going to court') particularly bear the Bond Solon stamp. The same two chapters are also particularly influenced by Babitsky *et al.* (2000), *The Comprehensive Forensic Services Manual: The Essential Resources For All Experts*, albeit that it is written for an American audience, and Lord Justice Wall's *A Handbook for Expert Witnesses in Children Act Cases* (2007).

When I entered the final stage of my transition from general psychiatry to forensic psychiatry I was fortunate to join the dynamic and stimulating group of then young consultants and trainee forensic psychiatrists at the Yorkshire Regional Centre for Forensic Psychiatry (Newton Lodge). I still value its study days, to which I occasionally return.

At this time, I was responding to frequent requests from senior registrars for teaching and training. They stimulated me to publish many of my case reports and papers on medico-legal subjects. I also learned a lot from them. They confirmed the view I already had, that when you stop learning from your junior doctors it is time to stop being a consultant.

For the last few years, I have been attending courses on risk assessment run by Northern Networking Events Ltd in Edinburgh. These have influenced the way in which I carry out risk assessments and incorporate them into expert reports.

Over the last ten years the annual residential conference organised by my consulting rooms, The Grange, has provided rich fare in terms of teaching and training by other experts and by solicitors, judges, barristers and coroners. As this text took its final shape at the time of the last conference I can specifically acknowledge the influence of Mr Andrew Axon, Park Lane Plowden Chambers, Mr Bill Braithwaite QC, Exchange Chambers, Ms Bridget Dolan, 3 Serjeants' Inn, and Ms Diana Kloss MBE, St John's Buildings. I owe no lesser a debt to contributors to previous Grange conferences. If they recognise some of their pearls of wisdom, I hope that they will forgive me for not remembering their source sufficiently to acknowledge them by name. I am also indebted to those who have attended the conferences and shared knowledge, experience and ideas. In 2010 we spent a lot of time looking at how medico-legal reports can be part of the case-based discussions that are going to inform our annual appraisals and the General Medical Council's revalidation process.

This text was also nearing completion when I attended Professor Penny Cooper's inaugural lecture at the City Law School and this is reflected in what I have written about cross-examination.

The Grange itself, where psychiatrists and psychologists have consulting rooms for medico-legal work, established by Dr Peter Wood in 1998, and with its roots in the Bradford consulting rooms of the late Dr Hugo Milne, a pioneer of forensic psychiatry in Yorkshire, has been a means of achieving my continuing professional development. This is particularly through its regular educational meetings as well as the annual residential conference. Equally importantly, it has provided a support group, which is essential for psychiatrists in an area of practice where disgruntled, disappointed and sometimes vexatious litigants are only too ready to fire off complaints to the General Medical Council and are now able to sue experts.

Over the last few years I have had the opportunity to study the law, and the development of this text has also been influenced by my teachers and fellow students on the LLM in Medical Law and Ethics at De Montfort University, Leicester.

The purpose of this book is to provide assistance to trainee psychiatrists and relatively inexperienced consultants who are at, or near, the bottom of their learning curve. It is also intended to provide a resource to experts who are approaching the plateau of the learning curve. However, the law is constantly changing, as are the needs and expectations of society, so the psychiatric expert will probably never reach a plateau of expertise. I hope that parts of the book will also be of use to other medical experts and psychologists.

This book is heavily referenced to both statute and case law. They define the role of the psychiatric expert witness in a particular case. However, given the dynamic nature of the law, a book like this will never be up to date. It was meant to represent the law up to about November 2010 but I have made brief reference to the Family Procedure Rules, which came into effect on 6 April 2011, the Law Commission's report *Expert Evidence in Criminal Proceedings in England and Wales*, laid before Parliament on 21 March 2011, and the case of *Jones v Kaney* [2011] UKSC 13, which has the effect of removing expert witnesses' immunity from suit. Significant updates as to the law and other developments will be posted on my website (http://www.drkeithrix.co.uk).

I encourage readers to study carefully relevant law reports. When I was a boy, I thought that the law was 'black and white'. Of course it is not. There is no better way of trying to understand the law, in particular the interpretation of statutes and the precedents established in case law, than to study judicial thinking and reasoning, particularly those of the Appeal Court judges and the judges of the Supreme Court. Many law reports also tell a story, which I know psychiatrists find appealing, and some record, probably for posterity, the virtues, but also the failings, of expert psychiatric witnesses.

This book is intended for readership in the British Isles but the British Isles are made up of a number of legal 'jurisdictions'. There are substantial differences between the laws of these various jurisdictions. Scots law is now based on the Roman law that applied in the reign of the Emperor Justinian but in Orkney and Shetland Udal law, a remnant of Old Norse law, is still of limited application. The Viking influence also remains to this day in the Isle of Man, where the Viking term 'deemster' is used for the three permanent, full-time judges of the High Court. The inquisitorial legal systems of the Channel Islands have greater affinity with the legal systems of mainland Europe than with the adversarial systems of the rest of the British Isles.

It would have made the 'central' chapters of this book, by which I mean the chapters relating to reports for different forms of court proceedings and court cases, unnecessarily complicated, and their reading very difficult, if I had tried to weave together the laws of these various jurisdictions. It has not been an easy decision, but I have decided to build the central chapters mainly on the laws of England and Wales, but have added where appropriate 'good practice' points from other jurisdictions, and I have included a chapter in which I have set out some of the particular requirements or important features of the other jurisdictions within the British Isles (Chapter 10). Unless otherwise indicated, but not entirely so, the opening and closing 'generic' chapters should be applicable at least to a very large extent in all these jurisdictions.

It is customary in the preface to a book to deal with the issue of gender. This is particularly important for the psychiatrist who travels to what Professor Nigel Eastman terms 'Legalland'. This is where 'the reasonable man' lives, where one of the most influential figures is 'the man on the Clapham omnibus' and where, if you read only the statute law, you would be surprised that the population had not gone into extinction because all the inhabitants seem to be male. I have not followed the convention of using the male personal pronoun and asking readers to give it the meaning of male or female but have instead opted for the most part to use the plural personal pronoun.

As far as I am aware, the law does not recognise the term 'service user' and nor did it recognise the term 'client', which this term replaced, or perhaps there were some others in between which I have forgotten. 'Client', I thought, was particularly unfortunate, as it emphasises dependency, being derived from the Latin word for someone dependent on a patron, and it sits uncomfortably with the autonomy of today's patient. So, at the risk of being very old-fashioned, where appropriate I have used the term 'patient'. There are three reasons: (1) by the time this book is published, 'service user' will probably be obsolete; (2) judges continue to use the term 'patient'; and (3) the term 'patient' comes closest to the central role of the doctor, in that it derives from the Latin intransitive verb '*patior*', which means simply 'I suffer'. It has the connotation of one who bears or endures suffering and, if doctors cannot cure, they should at least help their patients bear or endure suffering, and that includes the suffering of going to law or being on the receiving end of legal proceedings.

Also on the subject of terminology, although I have used the term 'intellectual disability' wherever possible, the meaning of some judgments would be misrepresented if I had not used the terminology of the statute or judgment where 'mental handicap' is the term used. In any event, even the *ICD-10 Classification of Mental and Behavioural Disorders* (World Health Organization, 1992) uses the term 'mental retardation' and it is only a few years since the law ceased to use the term 'mental defective'.

I have referred to Daniel McNaughtan as the person. This is on the basis that 'McNaughtan' was the spelling of the family name. I have followed the legal convention of referring to 'the M'Naghten rules'. My specimen criminal report (Appendix 11) on Daniel McNaughtan relies heavily on West & Walk's *Daniel McNaughton: His Trial and the Aftermath* (1977). However, I have been unable to find an account of a mental state examination of Daniel McNaughtan, so I am particularly indebted to Siân Busby, the author of the novel *McNaughten* (2009), for providing me with an account of his mental state based on her study of the historical materials and elaborated with a novelist's appropriate literary licence.

Insofar as this book does not include model terms and conditions of engagement, it is incomplete. The reason for this is that mine have been drawn up and are updated by a firm of solicitors. The conditions of the licence under which I use them preclude me from publishing them. Appendix 1, which is a generic letter of response to a request for a report, does, though, cover some of the relevant points, and I am grateful to Mr James Wood of Schofield Sweeney, Solicitors, Bradford, for advice on its construction.

This book bears some similarity to one that I started to plan many years ago with Dr Rajan (Taj) Nathan. I am pleased to acknowledge my valuable discussions with him at the time. It also includes material on the reliability of admissions in police interviews which I prepared with Dr John Kent and Dr Mike Ventress and which we intended to publish as a companion to our paper on fitness to be interviewed by the police (Ventress *et al.* 2008).

I am grateful to the following publishers for permission to reproduce copyright material: the British Medical Association ('Capacity to engage in sexual activity' and 'Capacity to make a gift'); Churchill Livingstone (Professor Bluglass's case of infanticide and Box 28); the Scottish Executive (Box 11), and SEAK Inc. (Box 46). Over the course of 30 years I have made notes following discussions with solicitors and counsel, I have kept extracts from the advices of counsel and I have kept extracts from letters of instruction. I apologise if any of these are based on copyright material about which I am unaware. I will be pleased to rectify any such omissions in a second edition.

I am grateful to the following for their comments on my first draft or parts of it: Mr James Badenoch QC, 1 Crown Office Row; Mr Bill Braithwaite QC, Exchange Chambers; Dr James Briscoe; Dr Ian Bronks; Professor Patricia Casey; Mr Michael Carlin; Her Honour Judge E. A. Carr QC; His Honour Judge John Cockroft; Mr Alan Gough and Ms Helen Gough, Gough Advocates, Isle of Man; Mr David Hinchcliff, HM Coroner for West Yorkshire Eastern District; Mr Robert Holt, Mental Health Tribunal Judge; Dr Rob Kehoe; Ms Diana Kloss MBE, St Johns Buildings Chambers; His Honour Judge Simon Lawler QC; Dr Sajid Muzaffar; Mr Ben Nolan QC, Broad Chare Chambers; Dr Mike Ventress; and Dr Peter Wood.

I am grateful to my daughter, Rowena Rix, Kingsley Napley LLP, for proofreading, to Dr Digby Jess, Exchange Chambers, for assistance with legal referencing, and to my personal assistant, Debbie Small, for all manner of general assistance. I am also indebted to my son-in-law, Chris Burgess, who built my website, from which some of the material in this book is taken.

I am also grateful to Dave Jago and his colleagues at RCPsych Publications for helping me deliver the finished product, to Ralph Footring, copy-editor, and to Shaun Kennedy in the College Library. Nevertheless, I am ultimately responsible for any mistakes, from which I intend to learn.

Keith J. B. Rix

Table of Cases

As is common legal practice, in the listing below, 'Re' is transposed such that, for example, Re IA (A Child) (Fact Finding; Welfare; Single Hearing; Experts' Reports) [2013] EWHC 2499 (Fam) appears as IA (A Child) (Fact Finding; Welfare; Single Hearing; Experts' Reports), Re [2013] EWHC 2499 (Fam).

Irish criminal cases, such as The People (DPP) v Higgins [2015] IECA 200, are listed in this table under DPP (or Attorney General as appropriate).

Table of Statutes and Directives

Europe and European Union

England and Wales

Ireland

Isle of Man

Jersey

Northern Ireland

Scotland

Table of Statutory Instruments and Regulations

European Union

England and Wales

Ireland

Guernsey

Isle of Man

Northern Ireland

Table of Practice Directions

England and Wales

Ireland

Table of Codes of Conduct, Guidance, Conventions and Protocols

United Nations

England and Wales

Ireland

Isle of Man

Northern Ireland

Scotland

Abbreviations

ADHD	attention deficit hyperactivity disorder
ADM(C)A	Assisted Decision-Making (Capacity) Act 2015
AI(S)A	Adults with Incapacity (Scotland) Act 2000
ALT	agricultural land tribunal
AMO	approved medical officer
AMP	approved medical practitioner
AWLP	*Acting as a Witness in Legal Proceedings*
BAILII	British and Irish Legal Information Institute
BMA	British Medical Association
BWS	battered woman syndrome
CAFCASS	Children and Family Court Advisory and Support Service
CBT	cognitive behavioural therapy
CCA	Child Care Act 1991
CEA	Criminal Evidence Act 2019
CFA	Child and Family Agency
CFA 2014	Children and Families Act 2014
CJA 1991	Criminal Justice Act 1991
CJA 2003	Criminal Justice Act 2003
CJA 2009	Coroners and Justice Act 2009
CJA(NI)	Criminal Justice Act (Northern Ireland) 1966
CJC	Civil Justice Council
CJPOA	Criminal Justice and Public Order Act 1994
CLCA	Civil Liability and Courts Act 2004
CL(I)A	Criminal Law (Insanity) Act 2006
CMH	Central Mental Hospital
CPD	continuing professional development
CPIA	Criminal Procedure and Investigations Act 1996
CP(I)A	Criminal Procedure (Insanity) Act 1964
CP(IUP)A	Criminal Procedure (Insanity and Unfitness to Plead) Act 1991
CPR	Civil Procedure Rules
CPS	Crown Prosecution Service
CP(S)A	Criminal Procedure (Scotland) Act 1995
CrPR	Criminal Procedure Rules
CSD(J)L	Capacity and Self-Determination (Jersey) Law 2016
CV	curriculum vitae
CYCT	Child Youth and Community Tribunal
DDA	Disability Discrimination Act 1995
DLS	Directorate of Legal Services
DPA	Data Protection Act 2018
DSM5	*Diagnostic and Statistical Manual of Mental Disorders* (5th edn)
DVCVA	Domestic Violence, Crime and Victims Act 2004
DWP	Department for Work and Pensions
DX	Document Exchange
ECHR	European Convention on Human Rights
FOM	Faculty of Occupational Medicine
FPR	Family Procedure Rules
FTBI	fitness to be interviewed
FTP	fitness to plead and stand trial
GDPR	General Data Protection Regulation
GMC	General Medical Council
GMP	*Good Medical Practice*

GRH	ground rules hearing
HCA	historical child abuse
HCP	healthcare professional
HHJ	His Honour Judge
HMRC	Her Majesty's Revenue & Customs
ICD-10	ICD-10 *Classification of Mental and Behavioural Disorders* (10th revision)
IME	independent medical examination
IQ	intelligence quotient
IT	information technology
J	Mr/Mrs Justice
LAA	Legal Aid Agency
LCJ	Lord Chief Justice
LIP	litigant in person
LJ	Lord/Lady Justice
LPA	lasting power of attorney
LSD	lysergic acid diethylamide
MAEP	*Multi-Source Assessment Tool for Expert Psychiatric Witnesses*
MC	Medical Council
MCA	Mental Capacity Act 2005
MCA(NI)	Mental Capacity Act (Northern Ireland) 2016
MDO	medical defence organisation
MHA	Mental Health Act
MHT	mental health tribunal
MPT	Medical Practitioners Tribunal
MR	Master of the Rolls
NFOAPA	Non-Fatal Offences Against the Person Act 1997
NGRI	not guilty by reason of insanity
NHS	National Health Service
NICE	National Institute of Health and Clinical Excellence
OAPA	Offences Against the Person Act 1861
OHP	occupational health physician
OPL	over the prescribed limit
P	President
PACE	Police and Criminal Evidence Act 1984
PCE(NI)O	Police and Criminal Evidence (Northern Ireland) Order 1989
PDP	personal development plan
PHA	Protection from Harassment Act 1997
PIABA	Personal Injuries Assessment Board Act 2003
PNB	Police Negotiating Board
PO	Post Office
PPD	paranoid personality disorder
PPO	public protection order
PPOR	public protection order with restrictions
PTSD	post-traumatic stress disorder
QC	Queen's Counsel
RCJ	Rules of the Court of Judicature (Northern Ireland) 1980
RMP	registered medical practitioner
RTA	Road Traffic Act 1988
RSC	Rules of the Superior Courts
SGC	Sentencing Guidelines Council
SJE	single joint expert
SMP	selected medical practitioner
SOA	Sexual Offences Act 2003
TP(FTT)(HESCC)R	Tribunals Procedure (First-tier Tribunal) (Health, Education and Social Care Chamber) Rules 2008
UK	United Kingdom

UKVI	United Kingdom Visas & Immigration
UN	United Nations
US	United States
VAT	value added tax
YJCEA	Youth Justice and Criminal Evidence Act 1999

The Expert Medical Witness

Keith Rix

These Courts rely on the professionalism and rigor of the experts who come before them.
Eleanor King J in *Local Authority v S* [2009] EWHC 2115 (Fam)

At least since 1282, when a coroner called a surgeon to advise whether an arrow injury to the chest could be fatal (Sayles 1936), doctors have been needed to assist the administration of justice. Dr Andrew Duncan, Senior, recognised this in 1795 in his University of Edinburgh lectures on forensic medicine: 'Many questions come before the Courts ... where the opinion of medical practitioners is necessary either for the exculpation of innocence or the detection of guilt ... an opinion consistent with truth and with justice.' This duty was identified by Percival (1803, p. 120): 'It is a complaint made by coroners, magistrates and judges, that medical gentlemen are often reluctant in the performance of the offices, required from them as citizens qualified by professional knowledge, to aid the execution of public justice.'

The Role of the Medical Expert Witness

Expert evidence is only admissible if it is 'information which is likely to be outside of the experience of a judge or jury' because '[i]f, on the proven facts, a judge or jury can form their own conclusions without help, then the opinion of an expert is unnecessary' (*R v Turner* [1975] QB 834). So, '[i]f matters arise in our law which concern other sciences or faculties we commonly apply for the aid of that science or faculty' (*Buckley v Rice-Thomas* (1554) 1 Plowd 118) and '[i]n matters of science no other witnesses can be called' (*Folkes v Chadd* (1782) 3 Doug KB 157). Medicine is such a science.

Hodgkinson and James (2015, p. 10) divide expert evidence into five categories (Box 1.1).

Whether an injury was caused by a hammer or a knife is a matter of opinion (Category 1). To understand this opinion, expert medical evidence is necessary to explain terms such as 'laceration', 'incision' and 'abrasion' (Category 2). Expert evidence of fact (Category 3) falls into two sub-categories: (a) what 'he or she has observed', where the judge or jury is unlikely to appreciate the facts due to their technical nature; and (b) 'his or her knowledge and experience of a subject matter, drawing on the work of others, such as the findings of published research or the pooled knowledge of a team of people with whom he or she works' (*Kennedy v Cordia (Services) LLP* [2016] UKSC 6). This includes:

> ... evidence ... which is used to support or contradict the opinion evidence. This is evidence which is commonly given by experts, because ... they rely upon their expertise and experience ... So an expert may say what he has observed in other cases and what they have taught him for the evaluation for the facts of the particular case. (*Aktieselskabet de Danske Sukkerfabrikker v Bajamar Compania Naviera SA* [1983] 2 Ll R 210)

Box 1.1 The Five Categories of Evidence Given by Expert Witnesses

1. Expert evidence of opinion, on facts adduced before the court
2. Expert evidence to explain technical subjects or the meaning of technical words
3. Evidence of fact, given by an expert, the observation, comprehension or description of which require expertise
4. Evidence of fact given by an expert, which does not require expertise for its observation, comprehension and description, but which is a necessary preliminary to the giving of evidence in the other four categories
5. Admissible hearsay of a specialist nature

Hodgkinson and James 2015, p. 10

It is a matter of fact (Category 3a) whether a wound is a laceration, an incised wound or an abrasion, but medical expertise is needed to describe it. The medical expert may also rely on a study of knife wounds (Category 3b). No medical expertise is necessary to describe the garment overlying the wound (Category 4).

Whereas at common law hearsay statements are inadmissible as evidence of the truth of what was said, one exception, *other than in Ireland*, is hearsay of a specialist nature (Category 5), such as an extract from the victim's hospital records. However, a statement from the records as to who the victim said caused the injury will be inadmissible hearsay.

In Ireland, medical records are still, strictly speaking, hearsay. Although they may be accepted 'as *prima facie* giving a reasonably accurate account of the events which they purport to record and of the opinion of the doctors from whom they emanate . . . [i]f in any particular they are contradicted by sworn testimony I shall reject such documentary record unless it is supported by other sworn testimony which I prefer' (*Hughes v Staunton* Prof Neg LR 244 (Irish High Court, unreported, 16 February 1990)). The records must be admitted or proved in the usual way (*McGregor v HSE* [2017] IEHC 504).

The Law of Expert Evidence

Until the court accepts you as an expert witness, it does not matter how well-qualified and experienced you are and how expert you think you are. Understanding this requires an understanding of several interrelated aspects of the law on expert evidence.

Admissibility

In *Kennedy*, relying in part on *R v Bonython* (1984) 38 SASR 45, Lord Reed and Lord Hodge identified four considerations which govern the admissibility of what in Scotland is termed 'skilled' evidence (Box 1.2).

Assistance

Lord Reed and Lord Hodge said that these considerations apply to skilled evidence of fact as well as opinion, although, when the first consideration, assistance, is applied to opinion evidence, the threshold is *necessity* as expert evidence is unnecessary if the matters are within the experience or knowledge of the judge or jury. As Lawton LJ held in *Turner*: 'Jurors do not need psychiatrists to tell them how ordinary folk who are not suffering from

Box 1.2 **Lord Reed's and Lord Hodge's Four Considerations Governing the Admissibility of Expert or Skilled Evidence**

(i) whether the proposed skilled evidence will assist the court in its task;
(ii) whether the witness has the necessary knowledge and experience;
(iii) whether the witness is impartial in his or her presentation and assessment of the evidence; and
(iv) whether there is a reliable body of knowledge or experience to underpin the expert's opinion.

Kennedy v Cordia (Services) LLP [2016] UKSC 6

any mental illness are likely to react to the stresses and strains of life.' This is for the ordinary folk on the jury.

To assist, evidence also has to be *relevant* to a matter in issue. Relevance has a strict legal meaning derived from the sixteenth-century Scots legal term meaning 'legally pertinent'. It must be logically probative or disprobative of something which requires proof; evidence which makes the matter requiring proof more or less probable (*DPP v Kilbourne* [1973] AC 729). If it leaves the court no more certain as to the probability of the matter, it is not relevant and should not be admitted (*Bonython*). Expert opinion of uncertainty or inability to assist on the balance of probability may nevertheless assist a court when faced with opposing evidence.

Finally, the evidence has to be *reasoned*: 'Proper evaluation of the opinion can only be undertaken if the process of reasoning which led to the conclusion, including the premises from which the reasoning proceeds, are disclosed by the expert' (*Coopers (South Africa) (Pty) Ltd v Deutsche Gesellschaft für Schädlingsbekämpfung mbH*, 1976 (3) SA 352).

Lord Reed and Lord Hodge quoted approvingly Lord Prosser: '[W]hat carries weight is the reasoning, not the conclusion' (*Dingley v Chief Constable of Strathclyde Police (No. 1)*, 1998 SC 548). Informing the court of the factors which made up the opinion allows the court, as appropriate, to take a different view (*Flynn v Bus Átha Cliath* [2012] IEHC 398).

Knowledge and Experience

Having the necessary knowledge and experience means being competent to assist: a '"skilled person" ... who has by dint of training and practice, acquired a good knowledge of the science or art concerning which his opinion is sought' (*R v Bunnis* (1964) 50 WWR 422). It is possible to 'acquire expert knowledge in a particular sphere through repeated contact with it in the course of one's work, notwithstanding that the expertise is derived from experience and not formal training' (Malek 2013, p. 1189).

Lord Reed and Lord Hodge summarised this, relying on *Myers v The Queen* [2015] UKPC 40:

> The skilled witness must demonstrate ... that he or she has relevant knowledge and experience to give either factual evidence, which is not based exclusively on personal observation or sensation, or opinion evidence. Where the skilled witness establishes such knowledge and experience, he or she can draw on the general body of knowledge and understanding of the relevant expertise.

An early example is that of a solicitor whose expertise in handwriting was acquired studying church registers (*R v Silverlock* (1894) 2 QB 766).

So, the expertise necessary to assist is defined legally by sufficient skill, acquired through education, training or experience. This should reassure doctors concerned that the 'status-based tests' of expertise set out by the General Medical Council's (GMC) expert in *Pool v General Medical Council* [2014] EWHC 3791 (Admin) represented a change in the law. The expert's tests are too restrictive and wrong in law (Rix, Haycroft and Eastman 2017).

What *Pool* illustrates, like Sir Roy Meadow's statistical evidence about sudden infant death syndrome (*General Medical Council v Meadow* [2006] EWCA Civ 1390), and the neuropathologist Dr Waney Squier's evidence about non-accidental head injury (*Squier v General Medical Council* [2016] EWHC 2739 (Admin)), is that the expert should not express opinions outside their field of expertise. This includes not questioning the validity of experts in other fields. In *Ali v Caton* [2013] EWHC 1730 (QB), the judge criticised a neuropsychologist for 'his mistaken questioning ... of (the claimant's psychiatrist's) views about J's hearing of voices'. The GMC's *Good Medical Practice* (GMP) (2019) states: 'You must recognise and work within the limits of your competence' and, in its *Acting as a Witness in Legal Proceedings* (AWLP), it states:

> You must only give expert testimony and opinions about issues that are within your professional competence or about which you have relevant knowledge of the standards and nature of practice at the time of the incident or events that are the subject of the proceedings. If a particular question or issue falls outside your area of expertise, you should either refuse to answer or answer to the best of your ability but make it clear that you consider the matter to be outside your competence.

It is permissible for an expert to research a topic to enhance their existing expertise by obtaining 'the views of others, including work colleagues, so long as he records where he went for that advice' (*R v Pabon* [2018] EWCA Crim 420).

Impartiality

In setting out the requirement for impartiality, Lord Reed and Lord Hodge relied on the guidance in *National Justice Compania Naviera SA v Prudential Assurance Co. Ltd (The Ikarian Reefer) (No. 1)* [1993] 2 Lloyd's Rep 68, which includes the duty and responsibility of the expert to present to the court evidence that is, and can be seen to be, the independent product of the expert uninfluenced as to form and content by the exigencies of the litigation and to provide assistance by way of objective, unbiased opinion on matters within their expertise. 'The duty of the expert is to be objective and wholly free from bias in favour of one party or the other' (*County Council v SB* [2010] EWHC 2528 (Fam)), which can be difficult as 'there is a natural bias to do something serviceable for those who employ you and adequately remunerate you' (*Lord Abinger v Ashton* (1873–74) LR 17 Eq 358) and 'whether consciously or unconsciously ... expert witnesses ... often tend ... to espouse the cause of those instructing them to a greater or lesser extent, on occasion becoming more partisan than the parties' (*Abbey National Mortgages plc v Key Surveyors Nationwide Ltd* [1996] 1 WLR 1534). In *Re M (Adoption: Leave to Oppose)* [2009] EWHC 3643 (Fam), an expert who only gave evidence on behalf of parents accused of child abuse was found to lack the expected detached objectivity.

One of the findings made against Dr Squier was that she failed to be objective and unbiased. In *Ali*, the judge criticised a neuropsychologist 'who lost the objectivity that is essential for a witness who is requested to provide independent expert evidence to the court'. In *Williams v Jervis* [2009] EWHC 1837 (QB), the judge criticised a neurologist who 'approached the case with a set view of the claimant and looked at the claimant and her claimed symptomatology through the prism of his own disbelief . . . From that unsatisfactory standpoint he unfortunately lost the focus of an expert witness and sought to argue a case'. In *Poole v Wright* [2013] EWHC 2375 (Civ), the court concluded that the evidence of the defendant's expert, who 'seems to have adopted the role of private investigator into the claimant's case', was not of a quality to assist the court.

As the expert's 'primary duty is always owed to the court and not to their client or the person who retains them' (*O'Leary v Mercy University Hospital Cork Ltd* [2019] IESC 48), it overrides any obligation to those instructing them. This duty is to provide unbiased opinion, not 'a partisan report which backs up his client at every turn' (*Nicholls v Ladbrokes Betting & Gaming Ltd* [2013] EWCA Civ 1963). In *Newman v Laver* [2006] EWCA Civ 1135, one of the reasons for not preferring a neuropsychiatrist's evidence was that he gave the impression of trying too hard to support a particular conclusion without sufficient independence. In *Vernon v Bosley (No. 2)* [1999] QB 18, a psychiatrist was criticised as irresponsible for expressing views at the end of lengthy personal injury litigation which were not easy to reconcile with his recent examination of the plaintiff for family proceedings, where he indicated that the plaintiff's health had dramatically improved. I once witnessed the cross-examination of a psychiatrist who had prepared his first report in the mistaken belief that he was being instructed by the defendant's solicitors. His second report was very different; by this time, he had realised that he was instructed by the claimant's solicitors. At trial, it was too late to avoid what the defendant's counsel described as 'the iron fist in the velvet glove'.

In *Vernon v Bosley (No. 1)* [1997] 1 All ER 577 CA, Thorpe LJ recognised the difficulty:

> The area of expertise . . . may be likened to a broad street with the plaintiff walking on one pavement and the defendant on the opposite one. Somehow the expert must be ever mindful of the need to walk straight down the middle of the road and resist the temptation to join the party from whom his instructions come on the pavement . . . [T]he expert's difficulty . . . is much increased if he attends the trial for days on end as a member of the litigation team. Some sort of seduction into shared attitudes, assumptions and goals seems to me almost inevitable.

This can happen in conferences with counsel. So, attach a note to your file: 'I must remember, and perhaps point out, that I am not part of this team. I am providing independent assistance to the court.'

Such 'unconscious partisanship' has been described by Langbein (1985): '[An expert witness] experienced the subtle pressures to join the team – to shade one's views, to conceal doubt, to overstate nuance, to downplay weak aspects of the case.' The risk is of exaggerating your opinion and misleading 'the team' only to have to retreat at the experts' meeting or, worse, under cross-examination. By then, the costs of the litigation, and the potential damage to your reputation, will have increased. As Lewis (2006) put it in the context of clinical negligence:

> It is worth emphasising that claimants' lawyers do not want to be given a case simply to please them, whether out of sympathy, or a natural inclination to oblige, or because that is perceived as the way to more cases and fees. It is easy enough to offer a finding of substandard treatment at a distance and in writing; but it is quite another to defend it under cross-examination. It does the patient no favours if a case initially supported by the expert has to be discontinued at a later stage when he realises what he is up against.

There is also a risk of bias where the treating doctor becomes the medical expert. In *Vernon v Bosley (No. 1)*, Thorpe LJ observed that '[i]n the field of psychiatry it may be more difficult for those who have treated the plaintiff (claimant) to approach the case with true objectivity'. In *A London Borough Council v K* [2009] EWHC 850 (Fam), the judge criticised a general practitioner who 'had an unconditional loyalty to the mother repeatedly demonstrated during the investigations leading up to [the] hearing and in his evidence, [who] was irredeemably under her influence, speaking more than once of a "bond of trust" between them'. In *Re B (A Child) (Sexual Abuse: Expert's Report)* [2000] 2 WLUK 784, the court held it to be 'elementary' that a psychiatrist who was treating the children should not give evidence as an expert in care proceedings on behalf of one of the parents. Former Supreme Court Judge Lord Hughes of Ombersley, in guidance for advocates (Inns of Court College of Advocacy 2019), states: 'The necessary relationship of trust between treating clinicians and their patients may be inconsistent with a duty to the court to provide truly independent evidence.' However, Braithwaite and Waldron (2010) point out that 'the treating doctor is likely to know far more about the patient than an outsider who has seen the patient for a few minutes or an hour or two'.

In Ireland, it is normal practice for the treating doctor to prepare the report for litigation, but such reports are invariably confined to condition, prognosis and factual causation. Indeed, if a treating doctor is *not* called to give evidence, the court may look askance at what it will often consider is an omission. In *Dardis v Poplovka* [2017] IEHC 149, while the judge considered that he could not draw a specific inference from the failure to call the treating doctor, it could not 'just be ignored as if he had been airbrushed out of the story. Where a plaintiff elects not to call one of his treating doctors . . . this places a question mark over this aspect of the plaintiff's case'. Furthermore:

> It may be said that in general where it is necessary to resolve a conflict between the expert medical evidence given by treating physicians on behalf of a plaintiff, applicant or claimant . . . and medical evidence given by those physicians examining and advising on behalf of the defendant or respondent . . . unless there is compelling evidence or other good and sufficient reason to do otherwise, the court is entitled to prefer the evidence of the treating physicians in relation the provision of advice and treatment afforded to their patient having due regard to the professional duty of care owed in the provision of such services. (*Flanagan v Minister for Public Expenditure and Reform* [2018] IEHC 208)

As Hodgkinson and James (2015, p. 185) comment:

> The issue is always one of fact, degree and proportionality but, in general, the more serious and prolonged the symptoms and the treatment regime, the greater the faith that the patient puts in his treating doctors, the more central the doctor is in the treatment regime and the more psychological/psychiatric injuries involved, the less likely the court is to permit a treating doctor to give expert evidence.

Reliability

As Lord Reed and Lord Hodge observed in *Kennedy*, what amounts to a reliable body of knowledge or experience depends on the subject matter of the proposed expert evidence. As observed in *R v Dlugosz* [2013] EWCA Crim 2: '[I]n determining the issue of admissibility, the court must be satisfied that there is a sufficiently scientific basis for the evidence to be admitted.'

Lord Reed and Lord Hodge recognised in *Kennedy* that 'where the subject matter . . . is within a recognised scientific discipline' it would be easy for the court to be satisfied as to reliability. Most doctors should be confident that their subject matter is within the recognised scientific discipline of medicine. However, some psychiatrists should note the advised wariness of the Canadian courts 'in accepting evidence of experts in the behavioural sciences' (*R v McIntosh* [1997] OJ No. 3172, 117 CCC (3d) 385 (Ont. CA)) and their conclusion that 'the testimony of experts in the behavioural or "soft" sciences is not amenable to assessment with the criteria established for weighing scientific evidence' (*R v Orr* [2015] BCJ No. 366 (CA)). Experts offering such evidence should be prepared to be tested on 'the evidence, research or studies on which [the] opinions were based' (*Orr*).

The Criminal Procedure Rules (CrPR) set out factors which the court may take into account in assessing whether there is a sufficiently reliable basis for expert opinion, especially expert scientific opinion, to be admitted (Box 1.3). This mirrors an obligation on the part of the expert to provide such information as the court may need to decide on the reliability of their opinion. So, anticipate 'a new and more rigorous approach on the part of advocates and the court to the handling of expert evidence' (*R v H* [2014] EWCA Crim 1555).

In *R v Gilfoyle* [2001] 2 Cr App R 5, expert evidence on 'psychological autopsy' was ruled inadmissible partly because there were no criteria by which the court could test the quality of the opinions and no substantial body of academic writing approving the methodology. Piper and Merskey (2004) have cogently argued that it is impossible to make a diagnosis of dissociative identity disorder reliably and have suggested that the US and Canadian courts cannot responsibly accept testimony in its favour.

Box 1.3 **Factors which May Be Taken into Account in Determining the Reliability of Expert Opinion**

(a) extent and quality of data, validity of methods by which obtained;
(b) if relying on inference, proper explanation of its safety;
(c) if relying on method, proper account of matters, such as degree of precision or margin of uncertainty, affecting accuracy or reliability;
(d) extent to which others have reviewed material on which expert relies and their views;
(e) extent to which opinion based on material outside field of expertise;
(f) completeness of information available to expert and whether took account of all relevant information (including its context);
(g) if there is a range of expert opinion, where the expert's opinion lies and whether their preference has been properly explained;
(h) whether methods followed established practice and, if not, whether the reason for divergence properly explained.

Criminal Procedure Rules CPD V Evidence 19A: Expert Evidence 19A.5

Credibility

The expert witness has to be credible. This is a judgement based on such matters as impartiality, independence, plausibility, believability, trustworthiness, conviction, reputation and demeanour. The court reaches this judgement on the basis of the expert's performance in court, particularly in the witness box. It may take into account judicial comment in other cases and findings of regulatory bodies. Furthermore, CrPR 19.3(3)(c) requires the party serving an expert report to serve with it notice of anything of which it is aware which might reasonably be thought capable of undermining the reliability of the expert's opinion or detracting from the expert's credibility or impartiality. But mere complaint to a regulator or even an allegation of professional negligence may have no relevance or bearing on the expert's credibility (*Everard v Health Service Executive* [2015] IEHC 592).

Do not be afraid of providing an opinion which those instructing you wish that they had not obtained. Your report may go to the back of the file, but not your credibility. When the solicitor or counsel wants an opinion upon which she knows she can rely, she will come back to you.

Some counsel file expert reports under the name of the expert. If your opinion has been 'black' when instructed by the claimant's solicitors and 'white' when instructed by the defendant's solicitors in similar cases, expect a tough cross-examination.

Weight

The court has regard to the weight of the expert's evidence, that is its cogency or probative worth in relation to the disputed facts. Weight is itself a question of fact; a matter of common sense and experience that the judge or jury decides. 'Expert testimony, like all other evidence, must be given only appropriate weight. It must be as influential in the overall decision-making process as it deserves: no more, no less' (Bell 2010). In practice, expert evidence is regulated 'by way of weight rather than admissibility' (*Re M & R (Minors)* [1996] 4 All ER 239). In the brain damage case of *Dixon v Were* [2004] EWHC 2273 (QB), instead of ruling the evidence of a general psychiatrist inadmissible, the court decided the issue on weight: '[A]s neuropsychiatry deals with problems arising or appearing to arise after brain damage, whereas general psychiatry is principally concerned with illness, [the neuropsychiatrist's] evidence is entitled to particular weight.'

As Hodgkinson and James (2015, p. 31) comment:

> . . . the most effective way of assessing expertise is, rather than conducting a difficult exercise based almost entirely upon the limited evidence as to qualification, experience and skill at the admissibility stage, to hear the witness's substantive evidence and use this as the basis upon which to judge not only the quality of his evidence, but his competence to give it.

The Duties and Responsibilities of the Medical Expert

The doctor's duty 'to aid the execution of public justice' (Percival 1803) gives justice a pre-eminent position for medical experts among the four basic principles of medical ethics: respect for autonomy, beneficence, non-maleficence and justice. There is also a role for virtue ethics which inform such characteristics as would be identified in the credible expert witness (see 'Credibility' above). They include honesty and trustworthiness: 'You must be honest and trustworthy when giving evidence to courts or tribunals' (GMP). The duties of the medical expert witness are the duties of an expert witness and the duties of a doctor.

The Duties of the Expert Witness

The duties of an expert witness have been refined over the years by judges. *The Ikarian Reefer* remains a landmark case. Guidance therein has become increasingly embodied in rules made, and guidance issued, or endorsed, by the courts and tribunals: in England and Wales, the Civil Procedure Rules (CPR), the CrPR and the Family Procedure Rules (FPR) (collectively, 'the Rules'). Similar rules exist in specialist tribunals. There are also specific rules for other jurisdictions, so it is important to ascertain what rules apply in a particular case. Practice in one jurisdiction can influence practice in another jurisdiction.

The Rules may be supplemented by further guidance such as the *Guidance for the instruction of experts in civil claims* (Civil Justice Council 2014) ('the Guidance'), although much of its core guidance is generally applicable, and *Standards for Expert Witnesses in Children Proceedings in the Family Court* (Annex to FPR 25BPD). In Scotland, there is similar guidance in the Law Society of Scotland's *Expert witness code of practice*. Medical experts must also adhere to AWLP and to any guidelines specific to their speciality.

The Rules make it clear that:

- the paramount or overriding duty of the expert is to assist the court on matters within their own area or areas of expertise; and
- this overrides any obligation to the person from whom the expert has received instructions or is paid.

The expert also has a duty to those instructing her. In *Stanley v Rawlinson* [2011] EWCA Civ 405, where a trial judge had criticised an expert who appeared 'to go beyond the usual role of an expert witness by advising them on the evidence they needed to meet the opposing case', it was held on appeal that 'it is often likely to be the professional duty of the expert to proffer just such advice'.

Medical experts therefore owe a responsibility to those who instruct them and to the subject of their report to:

- identify weaknesses as well as strengths in their case;
- recommend any further treatment that is advisable;
- suggest any other expertise that may be required; and
- advise on evidence that may be needed to meet the opposing case.

There is no incompatibility between the expert's overriding duty to the court and his duty to those instructing him:

> His duty to the client is to perform his function as an expert with the reasonable skill and care of an expert drawn from the relevant discipline [including] a duty to perform the overriding duty of assisting the court . . . If the expert gives an independent and unbiased opinion which is within the range of reasonable expert opinions, he will have discharged his duty both to the court and his client. (*Jones v Kaney* [2011] UKSC 13)

This book incorporates as much as possible of this overlapping guidance. Box 1.4 details the seven duties of experts as set out in the Guidance.

Box 1.4 **Summary of the 'Duties of Experts' Set Out in *Guidance for the instruction of experts in civil claims***

1. A duty to exercise reasonable skill and care to those instructing them and to comply with any relevant professional code. Overriding duty to help the court on matters within their expertise.
2. Be aware of the overriding objective that courts deal with cases justly. This includes dealing with cases proportionately, expeditiously and fairly. Assist the court so to do.
3. Provide opinions which are independent, regardless of the pressures of the litigation. Useful test: the expert would express the same opinion if given the same instructions by another party. Do not promote the point of view of the instructing party or engage in the role of advocate or mediator.
4. Confine opinions to matters material to the disputes between the parties and only in relation to matters within their expertise. Advise without delay if questions or issues fall outside their expertise.
5. Take into account all material facts, set out those facts and any literature relied upon, indicate if opinion is provisional or qualified or if further information is needed before giving final and unqualified opinion.
6. Inform those instructing them without delay of any change in their opinions on any material matter and the reasons.
7. Be aware that failure to comply with rules or court orders, or any excessive delay for which they are responsible, may result in a financial penalty to those instructing them and may lead to their evidence being debarred.

Civil Justice Council 2014, paras 9–15

It is not enough for the expert to set out a declaration to the effect that they have complied with their duties. It is necessary to comply. The psychologist in *Re F (A Child: Failings of Expert)* [2016] EWHC 2149 (Fam) (see also Chapter 2, 'Compliance and Truth') declared his compliance and made the appropriate statement of truth, but when the judge considered the transcripts of the mother's covert recordings of the psychologist's assessment of her and her child, he concluded that:

> The overall impression is of an expert who is overreaching his material . . . it is represented in such a way that it is designed to give it its maximum forensic impact . . . a manipulation of material which is wholly unacceptable and, at very least, falls far below the standard that any Court is entitled to expect of any expert witness ... his disregard for the conventional principles of professional method and analysis displays a zealotry which he should recognise as a danger to him as a professional.

The case had to be re-heard with a different expert.

The Duties of the Doctor

The GMC does not distinguish between the doctor's duty of care to an 'ordinary patient' and to a person with whom they are not in a traditional therapeutic relationship, although, for people who are the subject of expert reports, some of the medical expert's duties can be deduced from AWLP. However, Ireland's Medical Council (MC) is more specific. The MC

(2019, para. 40.5) provides that, if asked to conduct an examination and give the results to a third party, such as an insurance company, employer or legal representative, it should be explained that there is a 'duty to the third party as well as to the patient' and that relevant information cannot be excluded from the report. It cautions that the same standards of professionalism in conducting such examinations and preparing reports apply as in the case of care and treatment of patients.

The nature of the doctor's duty to the subject of an expert report has been elucidated by two Canadian cases. In *Rubens v Sansome*, 2017 NLCA 32, involving an independent medical examination (IME) based on review of medical records, it was held that a psychiatrist, Dr Rubens, who had reviewed the records, owed the claimant a duty of care in the same way as a physician conducting a face-to-face IME. On appeal, the court concluded that the relationship between Dr Rubens and Mr Sansome was 'sufficiently proximate to give rise to a duty of care' and that there were no relevant policy considerations to negate that duty. As the decision in *Parslow v Masters* [1993] 6 WR 273 (Sask QB) indicates, '[t]here is at best only a difference of degree and not of substance in the situation where the patient attends a physician for a third party medical rather than for professional services'.

The expert medical witness occupies a position of privilege which may bring professional and financial rewards; but with privilege goes responsibility in the form of a duty properly to assist in the administration of justice. To fulfil this duty, it is necessary to be properly trained at the 'frontier' between medicine and law and this chapter should assist. For the ethical medical expert, the rewards should far outweigh the costs. Next, we set out what the medical expert needs to know about courts, law and procedure in the British Isles.

Further Reading

Hodgkinson, T. and James, M. (2015) *Expert Evidence: Law and Practice*, 4th edn (Sweet & Maxwell).

Tottenham, M., Prendergast, E. J., Joyce, C. and Madden, H. (2019) *A Guide to Expert Witness Evidence* (Bloomsbury).

Courts, Laws and Procedures

Keith Rix

Expert witnesses are a crucial resource. Without them we [the judges] could not do our job.
Dame Elizabeth Butler-Sloss in Butler-Sloss and Hall (2002)

There is a world of difference between an agricultural land tribunal (ALT) held in the bar of a country hotel and an Old Bailey murder trial (Rix 1997).

The ALT panel comprises a solicitor or barrister as chair, a 'landlord's representative', nominated by the Country Landowners' Association, and a 'tenant's representative', nominated by the National Farmers' Union. The chair is addressed as 'Sir' or 'Madam'. Oral evidence may require the oath or an affirmation. Rules of evidence are relaxed; the ALT may admit evidence even if inadmissible in a court of law. The parties are the applicant and the respondent. The applicant bears the burden of proving their case, such as suitability to succeed to a farm tenancy, on the balance of probabilities (the 'civil standard' of proof, which means 'more probable than not'). The panel decides the case unanimously or by a majority. Where appropriate, the ALT seeks to avoid formality and inflexibility.

An Old Bailey murder trial takes place before a judge and jury. The judge is addressed as 'My Lord' or 'My Lady'. Oral evidence requires an oath or affirmation. Rules of evidence are strict. Proceedings are far from informal. The parties are the Queen, whose case is put by the prosecution, and the defendant. The prosecution bears the burden of proving its case beyond reasonable doubt (the 'criminal standard'). The defendant has to prove nothing unless raising a particular defence. The judge directs as to the law. The jury decides guilt by a unanimous verdict or, if permitted, by a majority verdict.

These proceedings have in common the delivery of justice. This may require medical expertise. In order to assist, medical experts need to understand the law and the procedural rules that govern the use of expert evidence. We now introduce the legal systems of the British Isles. AWLP states: 'You must understand and follow the law and codes of practice that affect your role as an expert witness.'

The Legal Systems of the British Isles

There are nine legal jurisdictions in the British Isles. We treat England and Wales as a combined jurisdiction. The others are Alderney, Guernsey, Ireland, the Isle of Man, Jersey, Northern Ireland, Sark and Scotland. They can be divided into common law jurisdictions and code or civil law jurisdictions, but this is a blurred distinction.

The common law means the law that was common throughout England in the Middle Ages. In common law jurisdictions precedential weight is given to the decisions of judges, courts and other tribunals and, although they have equal weight with the statutes passed by the legislature and regulations of the executive, judges interpret the statutes and decide, by reference to previous cases where possible, those cases that cannot be decided unambiguously by reference to statute or regulations. The decision in a single case is binding on the parties, unless successfully appealed, but not binding, however, on parties in other cases.

Civil or code law jurisdictions base their laws on the Napoleonic Code, which originates in the Roman *Corpus Juris Civilis*. Relying on codes or statutes which are meant to cover all matters that may be brought before a court of law, decisions in previous cases are only advisory and not binding unless a long series of cases has been decided similarly. Courts have no jurisdiction in matters not covered by code or statute. Judicial precedent has less weight. Judges have more freedom to act independently in interpreting statutes and codes and may interpret them less predictably. They rely more on scholarly literature, such as legal treatises and academic literature, which is no more than informative in common law jurisdictions, than on decisions in previous cases. Principle carries more weight than precedent.

England and Wales, Ireland, Northern Ireland and Scotland are all common law jurisdictions.

Irish law has its origins in British common law, which replaced the Gaelic Brehon law. It comprises statutes of the pre-Union Irish Parliament, Statutes of England and of Great Britain applied to Ireland, post-Union Statutes of the Parliament of Great Britain and Ireland, all pre-dating Irish independence, post-Independence Statutes up to 1937 and legislation that has been passed since 1937 when Ireland's last Constitution was adopted.

Manx law also has its origins in Brehon law, along with Norse Udal law, but is now heavily influenced by English common law, which operates alongside the Acts of Tynwald, the Manx parliament, and Acts of the Imperial Parliament at Westminster that apply to, or are adopted by, the Isle of Man.

Although Scotland is regarded as a common law jurisdiction, it has a unique legal system that mixes elements of common and civil law. Its common law originates in the 'customary law' of generally accepted usage and practice of the tribes that inhabited Scotland in the first millennium. Before the Union, Scotland adopted the continental civil law approach of favouring principle over precedent and applied Roman law or the 'Code of Justinian' where there was no native Scots law rule. There is still a greater attachment to principle than in Anglo-Saxon common law. One important principle in Scotland is corroboration. In a criminal trial, an accused may only exceptionally be convicted on the testimony of a single witness. That ceased to be the norm in civil cases, as the Civil Evidence (Scotland) Act 1988, s 1 provides that the court may find a crucial fact proved even if relevant evidence derives from a single source. In certain actions, such as divorce, the source must be someone other than a party to the case. Although lack of corroboration would not be fatal, the court's satisfaction as to proof would be a matter of weight, rather than sufficiency, of evidence.

Scotland's and Ireland's civil and criminal procedure rules are not codified as much as in England and Wales and their courts do not exercise the same control over the admission of expert evidence; the parties decide if it is needed and what type of evidence is required. It is, however, for the court to be satisfied that a witness has appropriate competency and expertise (*Hainey v Her Majesty's Advocate* [2013] HCJAC 47).

The Channel Isles comprise the Crown dependencies of the Bailiwick of Jersey and the Bailiwick of Guernsey. Alderney and Sark are independent Crown dependencies within the Bailiwick of Guernsey.

The laws of Jersey and Guernsey are rooted in Norman customary law, which has its origins in Roman law. Principles derived from English common law are applied and there are statutes passed by the legislatures, The States of Guernsey and The States of Jersey. However, in the Bailiwick of Guernsey, in the areas of legal practice where expert psychiatric evidence may be admitted, the law bears no resemblance to any old customary law and is derived from statute or common law principles. Furthermore, there is so little customary Norman law now used that there is no significant distinction between the Bailiwick and England and Wales as to the overall system of law. Jersey also relies on modern French civil law.

Proceedings in the Bailiwick of Guernsey are adversarial. Apart from the composition of the Royal Court of Guernsey trying a criminal matter on indictment, there is very little difference procedurally from the Crown Court in England and Wales and the courts use *Blackstone's Criminal Practice* or *Archbold* with no need to refer to any aspect of French law. Similarly, in a civil trial for damages, again apart from the court's constitution, procedure largely reflects what happens in England and Wales and in tort cases Guernsey law looks to the common law of England and Wales. Accordingly, the law of negligence develops along similar lines to England and Wales. Breach of statutory duty necessarily requires there to be some legislation creating the duty in the first place and health and safety legislation is not as full as that in England and Wales, but any gaps are likely to be resolved through having regard to how a particular provision would be viewed elsewhere. In children cases, legislation has drawn on the Scottish system; there are a Children's Convenor and a Child Youth and Community Tribunal (CYCT), which keeps some matters outside the court system.

Sark has its own laws based on Norman customary law, but Guernsey legislature, having developed out of the Royal Court of Guernsey, is applied in matters of criminal justice for the entirety of the Bailiwick without such laws having to be approved by the States of Alderney or the Chief Pleas of Sark. By contrast, in civil matters, each legislature has to approve a law before it can be sent for Royal Assent. That is why, for example, Guernsey and Alderney have the same Children Law, whereas Sark has a later, and edited, version appropriate to that jurisdiction, but its laws are no more and no less based on Norman customary law; it is just that certain elements of customary law have not been abrogated by primary legislation.

The relationship between Alderney and Guernsey is different because of its legislative framework, on the basis of which The States of Guernsey provides its major services. So, policing, healthcare, social security and childcare are transferred services. However, the court system in Alderney (and in Sark) is separate from the first instance courts in Guernsey and, although the Royal Court has concurrent jurisdiction in civil matters, someone could choose to commence proceedings in the Royal Court of Guernsey rather than in either Alderney or Sark. But, consequently, they then miss out on one stage of appeal because appeals from the Court of Alderney and the Court of the Seneschal of Sark lie to the Royal Court of Guernsey.

Proceedings in common law jurisdictions are adversarial and in code law jurisdictions they are inquisitorial.

In adversarial proceedings, opposing parties seek to defeat each other's case before a neutral fact-finder, a judge or jury, relying on rules, procedures and legitimate forensic and other techniques to present their own case in the best possible light and undermine their opponent's. Judges rely on the parties' counsel to elicit the evidence from witnesses upon which they base their decision and in theory rarely ask questions, but in practice some seem congenitally incapable of keeping quiet (perhaps itching because they are no longer in the pit?). This is the system in criminal cases described in *R v Criminal Cases Review Commission, ex p Pearson* [1999] 3 All ER 498 as:

> ... so familiar as to require no description. But we draw attention to two characteristic features of jury trial ... First, the procedure is adversarial. There is no duty on the trial judge, as in an inquisitorial proceeding, to investigate what defences might, if pursued, be open to a defendant, nor to interrogate or call witnesses. It is the function of the judge to direct the jury on the relevant law and to summarise ... the evidence, and to define the issues raised ... The judge need not, and should not, go further. Secondly, the decision on the defendant's guilt is made following a trial, continuous from day to day, by a jury assembled only for that trial, with no responsibility for the proceedings before the trial begins or after it ends. Thus the decision-making tribunal must reach its decision on the argument and evidence deployed before it at a final, once-for-all, trial.

Or, as 'The Secret Barrister' (2018) describes it: '*adversarialism* being a loose term for the model pitting the state against the accused in a lawyer-driven skirmish for victory played out before an impartial body of assessors – comprising a courtroom, judge, jury, accused, lawyers, witnesses, questions and speeches in some sort of configuration. And plenty of wigs'.

In inquisitorial proceedings, the parties' cases are investigated by a disinterested examining judge who can question witnesses, interrogate suspects and order investigations and who develops the legal arguments that the two sides can be expected to advance. Their dossier goes to a trial judge who can also examine witnesses, asking what are meant to be all relevant questions, thus leaving little questioning for the parties' advocates. However, some adversarial argument may take place.

Inquests and fatal accident inquiries are inquisitorial (see Chapter 15).

The Criminal Justice Process

When it is suspected that a crime has been committed, there may be a victim who may be the complainant who alleges that a crime has been committed, but not all complainants are victims. There may be witnesses who have seen or heard what happened. There may be a suspect who, if charged, becomes the detainee, then the accused (or defendant). Medical experts may be required to assess victims, complainants, witnesses, suspects/detainees and accused. They may also be instructed to give an opinion on findings made by other medical practitioners. The expert's findings and opinions deduced from them may then form the basis of expert evidence. Medical experts may be instructed by the prosecution, the defence or occasionally by the court.

The Criminal Courts of the British Isles

Where the trial takes place (Box 2.1) depends on a number of considerations.

There are special courts for children. In several jurisdictions, there are special arrangements for children and young people outside the court system. In Scotland, they take the form of children's hearings for children and young people. Where the grounds of referral to a children's hearing are disputed, the sheriff conducts a proof hearing at which medical evidence may be admitted. As the sheriff is exercising civil powers, the standard of proof is the civil standard. In Guernsey and Alderney, children can be dealt with outside the court system by the CYCT.

Box 2.1 Criminal Courts in the British Isles

	England and Wales, Northern Ireland	Ireland	Scotland	Isle of Man	Jersey	Guernsey	Alderney	Sark
Summary courts	Youth Court Magistrates' Court	District Court (Dublin Metropolitan Children Court) District Court	Justice of the Peace Court Sheriff Court	Juvenile Court Court of Summary Jurisdiction	Youth Court Magistrate's Court	Juvenile Court Magistrate's Court	Court of Alderney	Court of the Seneschal
Higher courts	Crown Court Central Criminal Court	Circuit Criminal Court Central Criminal Court Special Criminal Court	Sheriff and Jury Court High Court of Justiciary	Court of General Gaol Delivery	Royal Court	Royal Court	Royal Court (Guernsey)	Royal Court (Guernsey)

In general, summary courts deal with minor offences and the higher courts with more serious offences.

In summary courts, there is no jury. The emphasis is on speed, straightforwardness and economy. In most summary courts, cases are heard by one or more, but usually three, lay magistrates (England and Wales) or justices of the peace (Scotland). Some summary cases are heard by legally qualified judges known in England and Wales as district judges, in Ireland, Jersey and Guernsey as judges, in Scotland as sheriffs or summary sheriffs and in the Isle of Man as bailiffs. In Ireland, the only court of summary jurisdiction is the District Court (apart from a summary court-martial) presided over by a single, legally qualified judge, sitting alone. In Northern Ireland, magistrates' courts are presided over by a legally qualified district judge and the youth court by lay magistrates. In the Isle of Man, the terms magistrate and justice of the peace are both used. In the Court of Alderney, the Chairman sits with three to six jurats, who are lay people appointed by the Lieutenant-Governor of Guernsey, assisted by a legally qualified clerk, but there is a power to constitute the court by a single legally qualified person. In Sark, the court is constituted by a single person, usually the Seneschal or the Deputy Seneschal, neither of whom is legally qualified. The court can, however, be constituted by a Lieutenant-Seneschal, who must be legally qualified.

In most higher courts, judges sit with a lay jury or jurats. Jury sizes vary. In the Isle of Man, it is usually seven, but for offences of murder and treason it must be twelve and at the discretion of the judge, who is known as the Deemster, it can be twelve for other serious offences. In England and Wales and Northern Ireland, it is twelve and, in Scotland, it is fifteen. In Ireland, it is twelve to fifteen, but if there are more than twelve, immediately before the jury retires to consider its verdict, twelve are selected by ballot in open court and the non-selected jurors are discharged. In Ireland, there is a constitutional entitlement to a trial by jury in respect of all 'non-minor offences', but in the Irish Special Criminal Court, which hears terrorism and organised crime cases, three judges sit alone. In England and Wales and in Northern Ireland, the judge can sit alone where there has been or may be jury tampering. Also in Northern Ireland, the judge can sit alone to hear indictable cases where the criminal offence was committed either from a motive of 'religious or political hostility' or on behalf of a proscribed organisation connected with the 'affairs of Northern Ireland'. In jury trials, the jury decides the verdict and the judge decides the sentence. The Royal Court of Guernsey, sitting with a criminal matter on indictment, is constituted by the Bailiff, the Deputy Bailiff, the Judge of the Royal Court or a Lieutenant-Bailiff, who is legally qualified, and a minimum of seven jurats who are elected by a special electoral college known as the States of Election. Guilt (or a special verdict) is found by a simple majority of the jurats. If an equal number of jurats constitute the court, and are evenly split, the presiding judge gets a vote. The court is similarly constituted on sentencing. In Jersey, the jurats decide the verdict and, with the judge, the sentence, but there is also a provision for empanelling a lay jury.

There are special provisions for armed forces personnel. *In the UK*, they are tried in the court-martial where the judge advocate sits with officers and warrant officers. The judge advocate rules on the law and the officers decide the facts. Sentence is decided by the full court. *In Ireland*, offences against military law are tried by court-martial: a summary court-martial (presided over by a legally qualified military judge, sitting alone), a limited court-martial (a military judge and three members) or a general court-martial (a military judge and five members).

To secure a conviction, the burden is on the prosecution ('burden of proof') to establish the accused's guilt to the criminal standard of proof. The accused has to prove nothing.

There are exceptions, such as when the issues are unfitness to plead and stand trial, insanity or diminished responsibility manslaughter (see Chapter 7). The burden of proof is then on the defendant to prove their case to the civil standard of proof.

The following account of criminal procedure is based mainly on the England and Wales CrPR because these are the most highly developed rules and directions that affect medical experts involved in criminal proceedings. They take the form of Part 19 Expert Evidence and its accompanying Practice Direction. They may be influential in other jurisdictions. *Guernsey*, for example, does not have much by way of rules, and no equivalent of CrPR, but in dealing with procedural matters, if it is considered helpful, the court looks at what happens in the Crown Court in England and Wales, but otherwise does what seems right. *In the Isle of Man*, there are no analogous rules, but experts are encouraged to follow best practice in England and Wales or other jurisdictions.

In England and Wales, experts have to declare that they have read and complied with Part 19; such declarations 'are not matters of form but of substance' because the rules not only 'provide the structure for the admission of (expert) evidence but also ensure that expert opinion evidence is of the highest quality, that it is balanced and that it is well researched' (*R v Berberi* [2014] EWCA Crim 2961).

In Ireland, experts are not appointed by criminal courts. The Criminal Procedure Act 2010, s 34 prohibits an accused from calling an expert witness (a person who appears to the court to possess the appropriate qualifications or experience about the matter to which the witness's evidence relates) or adducing expert evidence (evidence of fact or opinion given by an expert witness) unless leave is granted. When leave is granted, the prosecution must be given a reasonable opportunity to consider the report or summary before the expert witness gives the evidence or the evidence is otherwise adduced.

Assistance with Case Management

The Criminal Procedure Rules 19.2(1)(b) obliges experts to assist with case management by complying with court directions and immediately informing the court of any significant failure to do so by the expert or another.

Disclosure Obligations

In England and Wales, in order to confirm compliance with the Criminal Procedure and Investigations Act 1996 (CPIA), as amended, experts instructed by the prosecution must include a declaration confirming that they have read and followed *Guidance for Experts on Disclosure, Unused Material and Case Management* (Crown Prosecution Service 2009) and recognise the continuing nature of their responsibilities of disclosure. This reflects CrPR 19.3(3)(d), which requires the expert to be prepared to make available for inspection by another party 'a record of any examination, test or experiment on which the expert's findings and opinion are based, or that were carried out in the course of reaching those findings and opinion, and . . . on which any such examination, measurement or test was carried out'.

In Scotland, similarly, the Crown Office and Procurator Fiscal Service *Guidance booklet for expert witnesses – The role of the expert and disclosure* states:

Box 2.2 A Quick Guide to Disclosure Obligations When Instructed by Prosecution

- Retain – you should retain everything, including physical, written and electronically captured material, until otherwise instructed.
- Record – you should keep records of all of the work you have carried out and any findings you make in relation to the investigation. The requirement to record begins at the time you receive instructions and continues until the end of your involvement in the case.
- Reveal – you must make the Crown aware of all relevant material you have in your statement or report, and your records should be made available to the defence if requested.
- Review – you should review your conclusions if any new information comes to light, both before and after a trial or appeal.

> The Crown is obliged to disclose any information that forms part of the prosecution case that the Crown intends to use at trial, and any information obtained or generated during the investigation that is for the accused, i.e. that materially weakens the Crown case or materially strengthens the defence case. It is important to remember that it is the nature of any information which is significant and not the format in which it is held. The Crown's disclosure duty may encompass a negative finding as such a finding may support the defence case or undermine the Crown case.

This means that the expert has to 'ensure that all relevant material from your investigations or examinations is revealed to the Crown in your report or witness statement. This includes all results or findings, regardless of whether the result is a negative one or assists the defence rather than the Crown.' As to what is 'relevant', the onus is on the expert because, having regard to the scientific and technical nature of some forensic evidence, the Crown 'is not best placed to determine the materiality of that information'.

Disclosure obligations have been summarised as 'the four R's' (Box 2.2).

In Ireland, there is a similar disclosure obligation on the prosecution.

The Isle of Man has recently enacted an analogous Criminal Procedure and Investigations Act 2016. As the Isle of Man has not yet issued any rules, there is no statutory obligation to make a declaration in the terms stated above. However, it is a recognised standard for analogous declarations to be provided.

Pre-Hearing Discussion of Expert Evidence

Where more than one party wants to introduce expert evidence, the parties may agree to (CrPR 19CPD1), or the court may direct (CrPR 19.6(2)(a)), a pre-hearing discussion of the issues by the experts. Following a discussion that has taken place without an order of the court, a joint statement has to be prepared dealing with (1) the extent of agreement, (2) the points of and short reasons for any disagreement, (3) action, if any, to resolve outstanding disagreement and (4) any further material issues not raised and the extent to which they are agreed. Providing 'short reasons' does not mean cutting and pasting vast sections from the reports. A statement prepared following a discussion ordered by the court may also have to include the reasons for agreement.

An expert's failure to comply with a direction for a pre-hearing discussion requires the expert's instructing party to seek the court's permission to introduce expert evidence (CrPR 19.6(4)).

If the parties consider it necessary, they may provide an agenda that 'helps the experts focus on the issues which need to be discussed'. It must not be in the form of leading questions or hostile in tone. There must be no requirement that the experts should avoid or defer reaching agreement on any matter within their competence. The discussion may be a meeting by telephone or live link and should be so where that will avoid unnecessary delay and expense. The content is confidential and must not be disclosed without the court's permission (CrPR 19.6(3)). Legal representatives of the parties may attend, but should not normally intervene, except to answer questions put to them by the experts or to advise on the law. The experts may hold part of their discussion in their absence. Individual copies of the statements must be signed or otherwise authenticated, in manuscript or electronically, at the end of the discussion or otherwise within five business days and copies provided to the parties within ten business days of signing.

If an expert significantly alters an opinion, the joint statement must include an explanatory note or addendum by that expert.

Single Joint Experts

In England and Wales, there is a power under CrPR 19.7 for the court to direct that evidence is given by a single joint expert (SJE) where more than one defendant wants to introduce expert evidence on an issue. This is not a provision for the prosecution and the defence to appoint an SJE. *In the Isle of Man*, there are no such directions in this regard, but it is possible that an SJE could be appointed.

The Civil Justice Process for Personal Injury Actions

In the civil courts (Box 2.3), the assistance of medical experts is most often required where claims are made for damages for personal injuries, particularly injuries resulting from road or industrial accidents, by patients who allege that they have been harmed by medical negligence and about diseases that have occurred in the workplace, through occupation of premises or the use of products. Personal injuries include 'any disease and any impairment of a person's physical or mental condition' (Limitation Act 1980, s 38). The use of 'includes' indicates that this is not meant to be an exhaustive definition. There is an identical definition in the *Isle of Man's* Limitation Act 1984 and a near identical definition in *Ireland's* Civil Liability Act 1961, s 2(1), Personal Injuries Assessment Board Act 2003 (PIABA) and Civil Liability and Courts Act 2004 (CLCA).

Medical evidence is necessary in order to quantify the injuries suffered and their consequences and to allow the parties to agree, or the court to decide, how much money ('quantum'), if any, to award the claimant. The medical expert's role usually involves identifying the nature of the injury and assisting with the investigation of any facts that require medical knowledge for their elucidation. Evidence is also needed to assist as to the validity of the claim. This means addressing 'causation': whether the injury sustained is an injury attributable to the accident or the allegedly negligent medical care. In an industrial disease claim, the medical expert may also have to give an opinion whether exposure to a substance made a 'material contribution' to the injury or condition, although in *Ireland*, 'material contribution' is not part of the law on causation – however compelling it might otherwise be (see below). The medical expert may also be asked to assist as to whether the injury was 'reasonably foreseeable', but this is ultimately a matter for the court. Evidence as to whether a disease is

Box 2.3 Civil Courts in the British Isles Dealing with Personal Injury Actions

	England and Wales	Northern Ireland	Scotland	Ireland	Isle of Man	Jersey	Guernsey	Alderney	Sark
Courts	County Court High Court	County Court High Court	Court of Session Sheriff Court All Scotland Sheriff Personal Injury Court Court of Session	District Court Circuit Court High Court	High Court	Royal Court	Royal Court	The Court of Alderney	The Court of the Seneschal
Parties	Claimant Defendant	Plaintiff Defendant	Pursuer Defender	Plaintiff Defendant	Claimant Defendant	Plaintiff Defendant	Plaintiff Defendant	Plaintiff Defendant	Plaintiff Defendant

associated with a particular exposure or process, and it is, or ought to have been, known that it was, and was, in fact, likely caused by or attributable to it is, of course, a different matter.

Usually, the expert is instructed by solicitors (or advocates in the Isle of Man) acting for one of the parties and is therefore a party, or party-appointed, expert. In England and Wales and the Isle of Man, the parties are the claimant and the defendant. Different terminology is used in other jurisdictions (Box 2.3). We use the terms claimant, defendant and solicitor as generic terms unless the context requires otherwise.

An expert may be jointly selected but instructed by only a single party as an agreed expert; they are still a party expert and will usually be paid by the instructing party. Sometimes the expert may be jointly instructed by the solicitors acting for two or more defendants. An expert so instructed is also a party expert. The party expert's duty is to provide his report to, and only communicate with, his instructing solicitors unless they agree, or the solicitors acting for the opposing party put questions to the expert under CPR 35.6 or the court orders it. Occasionally, the expert is instructed by the opposing parties on a joint basis as an SJE.

This section is based on the England and Wales CPR, taking into account the Guidance which the CPR expect experts to apply.

The CPR are mirrored by the Rules of the High Court 2009, as amended, of the Isle of Man and, in relation to expert evidence, the Evidence in Civil Proceedings (Guernsey and Alderney) Rules 2011. *Northern Ireland* relies on the Rules of the Court of Judicature (Northern Ireland) 1980 (RCJ), which are similar to the pre-CPR rules in England and Wales.

In Ireland, a paper-based system, the Personal Injuries Assessment Board (the Injuries Board) deals with many civil personal injury actions, including road traffic accident claims, but not clinical negligence claims, without court proceedings. There are no oral hearings. Awards are based on the consideration of medical reports, usually but not necessarily provided by the treating general practitioner, and its *General Guidelines as to the amounts that may be awarded in Personal Injury cases: Book of Quantum* (2016) (the *Book of Quantum*). If either party rejects the award, an authorisation can be issued permitting the bringing of proceedings. However, where the injury alleged is primarily or mainly psychological in nature, an authorisation issues as a matter of course. The same applies to claims in trespass (assault, battery, false imprisonment).

A personal injury case starts when someone believes that they have been wronged and they consider seeking a legal remedy. The wrong is called a 'tort' or, in Scotland, a 'delict'. The purpose of civil proceedings is to use financial compensation to 'put the party who has been injured, or who has suffered, in the same position as he would have been' but for the wrong (*Livingstone v Rawyards Coal Co.* (1880) 5 App Cas 25). This is the principle of the law of damages. This is the law's best response: a sum of money is given proportionate to the pain, suffering and loss of amenity caused by the injury. Loss of amenity is the effect on the claimant's enjoyment of life and effects on their special senses.

The categories of damage and the usual amounts of compensation are set out in the Judicial College's *Guidelines for the Assessment of General Damages in Personal Injury Cases* (2019) ('Judicial College Guidelines'), for Northern Ireland in the Judicial Studies Board for Northern Ireland's *Guidelines for the Assessment of Damage in Personal Injury Cases in Northern Ireland* (2019) and for Ireland in the *Book of Quantum*, but it does not deal with some injuries at all (e.g. any psychological injury), however described. The Judicial College

Guidelines are also used in Guernsey and Alderney. Medical experts should familiarise themselves with the categories of injuries in their field and if appropriate the approach to the assessment of severity.

Damages for pain, suffering and loss of amenity are known as 'general damages'. There may also be 'special damages' for future financial loss and expense such as 'loss of earnings' and 'care'. The size of a settlement or award can depend very much on the special damages. Medical evidence will be needed to persuade the court, or for the parties to agree, that the injury has restricted the claimant's ability to follow their employment or has resulted in a need for care.

The Pre-Action Stage

First, the potential claimant consults a solicitor. How the solicitor proceeds at this 'pre-action stage' may be governed by a pre-action protocol. They are intended to resolve as many disputes as possible without recourse to litigation through early but well-informed settlements. In England and Wales, there are protocols for personal injury, clinical disputes, disease and illness (including mesothelioma) and low value personal injury road traffic accident claims. There are similar pre-action protocols in Scotland and Northern Ireland. Although they do not exist in the Channel Isles, there is a similar emphasis on such alternative dispute resolution and practitioners look to England as a source of good practice. If litigation takes place, there may be penalties for non-compliance with the relevant pre-action protocol. The procedure in Injuries Board cases in Ireland is governed by the PIABA, the Personal Injuries Board Rules 2004 and the CLCA, which also makes provision for a pre-action protocol in clinical negligence cases, with objectives consistent with the equivalent in England and Wales, but yet to be commenced.

Clinical negligence cases are a more complex form of personal injury case, as expert evidence may be needed as to breach of duty. These are cases where the issue is of treatment having gone wrong by reasons of acts or as a result of omission or where the issue is of valid or informed consent not having been obtained. There are three elements in the tort of negligence: a duty of care must be owed by the defendant to the claimant; a breach of that duty; and damage resulting therefrom. The concept of a duty of care originates in the 'neighbour principle' expounded in 'the snail in the ginger beer case' (*Donoghue v Stevenson* [1932] AC 562): 'You must take reasonable care to avoid acts or omissions which you can reasonably foresee would be likely to injure your neighbour.' Thus, in a clinical negligence case, the solicitor will usually need, at an early stage, an advisory report dealing at least with liability, that is breach of duty and usually also causation, as the potential claimant will need to prove that the alleged negligence has contributed to his present condition, that is, prove causation. In many personal injury cases, an opinion will also be needed on condition and prognosis in order to know whether any significant injuries or damage can be attributed to the allegedly negligent care or the accident.

In England and Wales, the *Pre-Action Protocol for the Resolution of Clinical Disputes* (Vos 2019, C3A-001), and a similar protocol *in Northern Ireland*, allow for separate expert opinions on breach of duty, causation, condition and prognosis and the value of the claim. In short, the role of the medical expert is to assist the solicitor to decide whether their client appears to have a case and whether it should be pursued. *In Ireland*, adequate supportive expert evidence is required in order to justify the institution and prosecution of proceedings claiming damages against a medical practitioner or hospital and to do so without such evidence is an abuse of the process of court and, for the practitioners involved, professional misconduct.

A report at the pre-action stage is not governed by the CPR because these only apply to cases that are subject to civil proceedings. So, at this stage, the expert has no duty to the court; the duty is to those instructing them. Thus, there is a distinction between an expert *advisor* who prepares a pre-action *advisory* report outside CPR and an expert *witness* who prepares an *expert* report following the issue of proceedings. It is different *in Ireland*, where the Rules of the Superior Courts (RSC) Ord. 39, r 46(1), as interpreted in *Payne v Shovlin* [2006] IESC 5, requires the production of all reports of an expert intended to be called as a witness which contain in whole or in part the substance of the evidence to be given, and not just a 'will say' report. So, *in Ireland*, the distinction between an *advisory report* and an *expert report* just does not arise. All reports (good, bad, discursive, advisory or otherwise and which contain the substance of the evidence to be adduced) are disclosable if the expert is to be called as a witness. An expert report produced in response to the expert report of the other party is also disclosable. So, in Ireland, the better view is that the expert's duty to the court arises at every stage.

The *Pre-Action Protocol for Disease and Illness Claims* (Vos 2019) sets out similar processes for claims involving 'any illness physical or psychological, and any disorder, ailment, affliction, complaint, malady or derangement other than a physical or psychological injury solely caused by an accident or other similar single event' whether or not in the workplace. Under this protocol, the letter of claim may, but need not, be accompanied by a medical report. It allows for medical reports to be obtained dealing with one or more of the following: knowledge, fault, causation and apportionment; condition and prognosis; and valuation of the claim.

The Liability (Breach of Duty and Causation) Report

Most breach of duty and causation reports in clinical negligence cases are reports on papers, although some, sooner or later, may require a consultation.

The medical expert may be supplied with little more than the medical records and, perhaps, a draft witness statement from the potential claimant or family members and a sudden untoward incident report. In a fatal case, there may be reports and statements prepared for the inquest and a note of the inquest proceedings. Sometimes, the report is requested before the inquest and to assist as to questions to be asked and issues to be explored.

The first stage in preparing a breach of duty and causation report, in a clinical negligence case, is to construct, from the documents, a chronology, and particularly detailed for the period of allegedly negligent care. The amount of historical detail will depend on the nature of the allegations. If what was done, or not done, should have taken into account what happened earlier, the previous history will need to be set out in sufficient detail to demonstrate its relevance.

The next task is to go through the chronology, sometimes even minute by minute, looking for any evidence that care has fallen below the standard expected of a doctor, or other health professional, acting with ordinary care or competence (*Chin Keow v Government of Malaysia* [1967] 1 WLR 813). This criterion reflects the case law on negligence (see Box 2.4). Even the standard of usual or prudent practice may be too high

Box 2.4 The Tests for Negligence

In the realm of diagnosis and treatment there is ample scope for genuine difference of opinion and one man is clearly not negligent merely because his conclusion differs from that of other professional men . . . The true test for establishing negligence . . . on the part of a doctor is whether he has been proved guilty of such failure as no doctor of ordinary skill would be guilty or if acting with ordinary care . . . To establish liability by a doctor where deviation from normal practice is alleged, three facts require to be established. First of all, it must be proved that there is a usual and normal practice; secondly it must be proved that the defender has not adopted that practice; and thirdly (and this is of crucial importance) it must be established that the course the doctor adopted is one which no professional man of ordinary skill would have taken if he had been acting with ordinary care.

Hunter v Hanley, 1955 SC 200

The test is the standard of the ordinary skilled man exercising and professing to have that special skill. A man need not possess the highest expert skill at the risk of being found negligent. It is well-established law that it is sufficient if he exercises the ordinary skill of an ordinary competent man exercising that particular art . . . he is not guilty of negligence if he has acted in accordance with a practice accepted as proper by a responsible body of medical men skilled in that particular art . . . a doctor is not negligent if he is acting in accordance with such a practice, merely because there is a body of opinion that takes a contrary view.

Bolam v Friern Hospital Management Committee [1957] 1 WLR 582

The use of these adjectives ('responsible', 'reasonable', 'respectable') all show that the court has to be satisfied that the exponents of the body of opinion relied upon can demonstrate that such opinion has a logical basis. In particular, in cases involving, as they so often do, the weighing of risks against benefits, the judge before accepting a body of opinion as being responsible, reasonable or respectable, will need to be satisfied that, in forming their views, the experts have directed their minds to the comparative risks and benefits and have reached a defensible conclusion on the matter.

Bolitho v City and Hackney Health Authority [1998] AC 232

a standard (*United Mills Agencies v Harvey, Bray and Co.* [1951] 2 Lloyd's Rep 631). Where the expert is critical of what was done, they should address the risk/benefit ratio so as to justify subsequently, if it be so, the conclusion that there was a breach of the duty of care. Vague expressions as to 'poor' or 'inadequate' care are insufficient. The fuller and more specific the criticisms, the greater the likelihood that the defendants will appreciate the thoroughness with which the claim has been investigated. This will reduce the likelihood of delay due to a request for further details and increase the likelihood of the defendant making or agreeing an offer to settle.

In answering specific questions or responding to a general question as to breach of duty, the 'Opinion' should then set out detailed opinions as to the occasions when care fell below the expected standard, specifically what care fell below the requisite standard, what the requisite standard was, including what treatment should have been provided, how the course of the potential claimant's condition would have been different but for the failing and what effect, if any, this failing has had on the patient's condition.

These questions will assist as to causation. This is because, in personal injury cases in general, even if the claimant can establish a breach of duty, she has to show on a balance of probability that this caused injury. This is because liability means breach of duty and causation. This means: (1) that the injury would not have occurred but for the defendant's negligence (the 'but for' test); (2) that the defendant's negligence made a material contribution to the injury sustained; (3) where relevant, that the defendant's negligence materially increased the risk of future injury; and/or (4) if consent is at issue, had the claimant been adequately informed, she would not have accepted the treatment at that time.

'Material contribution' is important because there may be, as it were, a 'negligent component' and a 'non-negligent (unavoidable) component'. The courts' approach is that: 'A factor by itself may not be sufficient to cause injury but, if with other factors, it materially contributes to causing injury, it is clearly a cause of injury' (*McGhee v National Coal Board* [1973] 1 WLR 1).

In Ireland, however, 'material contribution' is not part of the law on *causation*, which applies the simple 'but for' test. Thus, if there is a negligent and non-negligent cause for an injury, it is necessary to establish that but for the negligent cause, the injury would not have happened. In reality, however, this may be circumvented by recovery for a loss of opportunity, which is not recognised in English law. For example, in a delayed cancer diagnosis or a delayed treatment case, it may not be possible to establish, as a matter of probability, that the delay resulted in a worse outcome, whether in terms of survival or otherwise. Differentiating between psychological harm attributable to the cancer diagnosis, *per se*, and the delay in treatment, may be difficult, or impossible. *In Ireland*, however, if it can be established that the claimant was deprived of an opportunity for a better outcome – even one that is not probable – that will sound recovery in damages. It is considered that opportunity which has been lost is in itself of value.

Although it is not scientifically possible to say how much of a contribution is made from a particular cause, the assessment has to be more than *de minimis*. However, medical experts should be wary of apportioning causation, for example, x per cent to the previous medical history, y per cent to the accident or breach of duty and z per cent to some unrelated life event or circumstance lest they are asked to provide the legitimate and scientific proof for the percentages. Such approaches to apportionment may not be helpful albeit that, for example *in Ireland*, the Injuries Board asks the clinician to do just that and apportion causation in 25 per cent blocks.

Where the medical expert identifies what appears to be inadequate care by other health professionals, they should indicate that expert evidence may be needed from other health professionals. This is not the expert stepping outside their expertise. It is assistance to the lawyers who might not otherwise identify the issue.

Usually, the expert will be asked to anticipate what responses the defendant may make to the allegations and set out what their responses would be. This enables the lawyers to form a preliminary view as to the likely success of the case. This will influence their response to any pre-action offer by the defendant to settle and the decision to issue proceedings.

The test for negligence is a two-stage test. First, apply the direction in *Bolam v Friern Hospital Management Committee* [1957] 1 WLR 582 (Box 2.4). Is there a body which would have done the same? If there is, second, apply the judgment in *Bolitho v City and Hackney Health Authority* [1998] AC 232 (Box 2.4). Instructing solicitors and counsel need to know how likely it is that the defendant will find, as an expert, a responsible and respectable doctor who will argue that it was reasonable or logical to have done what it is alleged should not have been done or not to have done what it is alleged should have been done. This expert may represent a minority position, but the defendant needs only one such responsible and respectable doctor.

Other than in Ireland (see 'Disclosure in Ireland' below), this report should be a 'Draft – for discussion with solicitors and counsel only (not to be disclosed)'. If proceedings are issued, a subsequent version may be disclosed, but, other than exceptionally, not the pre-action draft because it is subject to legal professional privilege that protects from disclosure confidential communications between lawyers and third parties with a view to advising clients. However, any expert's report, however it is titled or headed, may be exposed in cross-examination.

Sometimes, causation and breach of duty reports are obtained consecutively. The causation report is used to assess the viability of the claim, particularly if causation is unclear, and then, if it is likely that causation will be proved, breach of duty is assessed. However, if causation is glaringly obvious, the breach of duty report may come first.

Disclosure in Ireland

There are important differences in Ireland's disclosure rules. In personal injury cases where a plaintiff is entitled to a jury trial, for example, in claims of trespass to the person (assault, battery, false imprisonment and, probably, intentional infliction of emotional suffering, which may arise in historical abuse cases, or defamation), the expert may give evidence without the report ever having been disclosed to anyone, whether defendant or the court. Otherwise, in personal injuries and fatal injuries actions, RSC Ord. 39, r 46(1) requires that a plaintiff furnish the other parties with a schedule listing all reports from expert witnesses intended to be called and, following the reciprocal disclosure of the defendant's schedule, the parties must then exchange copies of their listed reports. This is a process of mutual, not sequential, exchange. This rule is an exception to litigation privilege.

Where a party certifies in writing that no report exists which requires to be exchanged, the other parties must then proceed to deliver their reports to all other parties to the proceedings (r 46(3)). If, having received an expert report, in such circumstances, the defendant then wishes to obtain his own report, it may not disclose the plaintiff's report to him or her in advance (*Harrington v Cork City Council* [2015] IEHC 41). There is no requirement for disclosure of reports prior to their exchange.

If any party obtains a report after delivery to the other side, they must forthwith deliver a copy of the report to the other parties (r 46(4)). Any report that has been delivered may be withdrawn by confirming in writing that the party does not now intend to call the author of the report to give evidence in the action. In such a case, the same privilege (if any) which existed in relation to the report is deemed to have always applied to it notwithstanding any exchange or delivery which may have taken place (r 46(6)).

The Rules of the Supreme Court Order 39, r 45(1) provides that 'report' means a report or reports or statements (or copy/ies thereof) from, *inter alia*, dentists, doctors, occupational therapists, psychologists and psychiatrists, and containing the substance of the evidence to be adduced and also including any drawings, photographs etc. referred to in the report.

If at any stage of the hearing of an action it appears to the court that there has been non-compliance, it may make such an order as it deems fit, including an order prohibiting the adducing of evidence in relation to which the non-compliance relates. It may also adjourn the action to permit compliance on such terms and conditions as seem appropriate and may make such order as to costs as appears just in the circumstances (r 48).

In any case, application may be made to the court for an order that in the interests of justice the disclosure provisions are not to apply in relation to any particular report in the possession of a party and which it is maintained should not be disclosed and served as required. The court may, upon such application, make such an order as to it seems just (r 50(1)).

In the event of non-compliance, a party, absent the consent of the other party, may apply to the court for an order seeking leave permitting the adducing of evidence that has not been disclosed. The court may make such order on such application as appears just in the circumstances (r 50(2)).

The Letter of Claim

If it appears to the potential claimant's solicitor, and their client agrees, instead of, or in addition to pursuing other remedies, the solicitor may send a 'letter of notification' to advise the potential defendant that it is a claim where a 'letter of claim' is likely to be sent and, in a clinical negligence case, because breach of duty and/or causation has been identified. This enables the potential defendant to consider obtaining expert evidence.

Next, a 'letter of claim' is sent setting out the grounds for the claim. The *Pre-Action Protocol for the Resolution of Clinical Disputes* cases advises that this should include a clear summary of the facts on which the claim is based, including the alleged adverse outcome; an outline of the allegations or a more detailed list in a complex case; the potential claimant's injuries and present condition and prognosis; and an outline of the causal link between allegations and the injuries. The *Pre-Action Protocol in Personal Injury Claims* states that the 'letter of claim' has to include an indication of the nature of any injuries suffered and the way in which these impact on the claimant's day-to-day functioning and prognosis. The expert should ensure that she deals with these matters.

In Ireland, under the Injuries Board scheme, the equivalent is an application for assessment by the Injuries Board notifying the proposed respondents of the claim and seeking payment of compensation, along with a report by a medical practitioner who has treated the claimant in respect of the injuries that are the subject of the claim. The same requirement for a letter of claim also arises in non-Injury Board cases.

In practice, in clinical negligence cases, it is common for the solicitors to rely on a records-based report that assists as to the main allegations of negligence and which does not deal with condition and prognosis in much more detail than is necessary to show that the potential claimant has suffered significant injury. If proceedings are issued, the medical expert will be instructed at some point to prepare a 'condition and prognosis' report (see below).

The Condition and Prognosis Report

The condition and prognosis report will require a consultation with the potential claimant who has allegedly suffered injury. In a clinical negligence case relating to a patient who has died, it will be a 'report on papers' providing expert opinion on what the patient's diagnosis was and what their prognosis would have been but for the alleged failings. For a claim in England and Wales under the Fatal Accidents Act 1976, or in Ireland under the Civil Liability Act 1961, the opinion should include when the deceased could have been expected to return to work and, if so, what it would have entailed.

Unless otherwise directed, for example, to prepare a 'draft' report, most pre-action condition and prognosis reports are prepared as if proceedings have been issued and therefore have to comply fully with the CPR. This is because the *Pre-action Protocol for Personal Injury Cases* promotes the practice of the claimant obtaining a medical report and disclosing it to the defendant, who then asks questions and/or agrees it and does not obtain their own report. However, if the case does not settle, the report may be relied on in the proceedings. Solicitors will refer to 'the claimant' (hereinafter in this section, 'the claimant' rather than 'potential claimant') even though no claim has been made. The expert may expect questions for the purpose of clarification of the report and the answers to which should be sent simultaneously to both parties. The expert's fees for answering questions are the responsibility of the questioning party. But the civil procedure rules in personal injury cases *in Ireland*, set out in the District Court Rules, Circuit Court Rules and the RSC, do not provide for questions to be put to the expert at such a stage.

In a clinical negligence case, the consultation will be used, with the assistance of the medical records, to decide whether the claimant has suffered any damage over and above their underlying disorder or whether the course of the underlying disorder has been changed for the worse. If compensation is offered or awarded, it will be for the injury sustained as a result of the alleged negligence and not for damage that would have been suffered in any event. In the case of a road or industrial accident, it is similar: identify any injury that has resulted and answer detailed questions about the claimant's condition and prognosis.

The Response to the Letter of Claim

Upon receipt of the letter of claim, the defendant has a limited period to investigate the case and respond.

In a clinical negligence case, in response to the letter of claim, NHS Resolution is likely to commission a brief overview report within a short timescale so as to respond quickly and avoid the cost of further negotiations or even civil proceedings in a case that ought to settle quickly and without dispute. An expert so instructed is asked to prepare a short report, without a detailed recitation of the facts. However, the task is the same as for the expert instructed by the potential claimant's solicitors. The main difference is that little or nothing of the chronology is set out in the report.

Upon receipt of this report, NHS Resolution may admit the claim. If the claimant's solicitors have already made an offer to settle, NHS Resolution may respond with its own offer to settle or make such an offer of its own motion. If the case is settled, no further expert opinion is likely to be needed. If the claim is admitted, but there remain issues as to condition or prognosis, the claimant's solicitors will need to provide the 'condition and prognosis' report.

In accident cases, solicitors acting for the insurers of the defendant may seek to settle the claim upon receipt of a letter of claim and without proceeding to litigation, but they may instruct their own psychiatric expert to prepare a report on the claimant. Sometimes, they provide a copy of the report prepared for the claimant's solicitors; sometimes, they prefer their expert to prepare their report 'blind'.

In Northern Ireland, claims are handled by the Directorate of Legal Services (DLS), which upon receipt of a letter of claim and/or pre-action protocol letter will investigate and obtain necessary expert reports and legal advice.

In Ireland, the Injuries Board arranges for the claimant to be assessed by a doctor or doctors from its own panel. It is rare for the Board to rely on the report from the claimant's own doctor. Occasionally, it seeks a second report from its doctor(s). Upon consideration of this medical evidence, an appointed assessor makes an award.

Serving Proceedings

If the claim cannot be settled, or the dispute otherwise resolved, or if *in Ireland* either party rejects the Injuries Board's award, or the Board declines to assess the claim, it is open to the claimant's solicitors to 'issue proceedings'. From this point onwards, *in England and Wales*, the CPR apply.

In Ireland, it is very unusual for any claim to settle prior to an application to the Injuries Board or the issuing of proceedings, other than in straightforward road traffic accident incidents. As already noted, the Injuries Board may issue an authorisation other than in circumstances where one or other party has rejected the assessment. It is invariable that proceedings issue in clinical negligence claims.

Within four months of the issue of proceedings, the 'claim form' must be served and, if the 'Particulars of Claim' are not served simultaneously, they must be served within fourteen days of the service of the 'claim form'. *In Ireland*, the Personal Injuries Summons with an extensive Indorsement of Claim must set out, *inter alia*, the acts of the defendant constituting the wrong against the plaintiff and the circumstances constituting the wrong, particulars of personal injury and particulars of negligence, breach of duty, etc. It is not necessary to append any medical report to the summons, but the plaintiff is required to verify the contents of the summons on affidavit.

In Northern Ireland, under the RCJ, within one year of the issue of proceedings, a writ must be served endorsed with the basis of the claim. A Statement of Claim must be served within six weeks of the service of the writ. It is broadly similar to a CPR Particulars of Claim.

The Particulars of Claim

The Particulars of Claim must include a concise statement of the facts on which the claimant relies and be accompanied by a medical report regarding the alleged personal injuries. Where causation issues may be complicated, a further report dealing with causation, condition and prognosis may be requested at a later stage.

Although the Particulars of Claim will be drafted in the light of the expert's opinion and closely aligned with it and can be amended at a later stage as necessary, a medical expert who has been instructed in a clinical negligence case may be sent draft Particulars of Claim for comment. There may be some urgency as the Particulars of Claim have to be served within a specified period. The draft Particulars of Claim will probably reflect closely the 'Opinion' in the draft liability report, especially if the expert has responded with sufficient clarity and precision to any questions that were put to them, but as this report is a draft, pre-action document, it will not be disclosed with the Particulars of Claim.

The expert should check the accuracy of the summarised medical history. It will not be the whole medical history and not as detailed as in the medical report. Its factual section has to be concise; the factual circumstances will generally be pleaded in a pithy, concise manner. However, when setting out the allegedly negligent acts or omissions, it will be necessary to rely on the facts and matters in this section. So, the expert must make sure that the appropriate parts of the medical history have been summarised.

The expert must point out if they cannot support all of the allegations of negligence. They should point out any criticisms of the claimant's care that are not reflected, but there may be good reason for not including them. Albeit that they relate to failings, they may not amount to a breach of duty or they may not be failings that it will be proved have been causative of damage.

Cooperation and assistance at this stage can avoid the defendant making a preliminary request for further information or clarification to which the claimant's lawyers may be unable to respond without the expert's assistance and which necessitates the expert going back not just to their report, but perhaps also the case records, for the necessary answers.

In Ireland, however, any further report generated by the expert will be disclosable. Therefore, the usual approach is for the advocate to try to speak to the expert, elicit her views in a privileged conversation and then, as needs be, have the solicitors specifically commission a supplemental report addressing the defendant's case. Frequently, being satisfied as to how the expert will address the counter-arguments, no report will be formally sought.

The Defence

If a Defence is going to be served, this has to be done so within a specified period. Where the expert is instructed by NHS Resolution in a clinical negligence claim, the Defence will probably reflect some of the points they have made in the overview report. It may be denied that a legal duty existed, that any such duty was breached, that any such breach was the cause of the injury, loss or damage or that any damage is as great as has been alleged. The Defence might be that the claimant, by their acts or omissions, was responsible to some extent for their injury ('contributory negligence') or that, by not attending for treatment, they have failed to mitigate their loss.

Where you are instructed by the claimant's solicitors, you are likely to be sent the Defence and asked to comment. It may be apparent that the defendant's solicitors have got an opinion from an expert who has taken a very different view of the case. The Defence may fairly make some points that undermine the allegations of negligence based on your opinion. If you consider that some of your opinions are going to be undermined or that your position on certain points may not after all be tenable, point this out immediately. Time and money may be wasted and justice delayed if this does not emerge until the experts' meeting. Even more may be lost, particularly your reputation, if this only emerges under cross-examination. But the points made in the Defence may not take into account information of which you are aware from the medical records or statements or they may be only the most favourable, for the defendant, of a number of interpretations of what happened. So, your role is to assist those instructing you to decide what points in the Defence may have to be conceded and what points may become trial issues.

Exchange of Lay Witness Statements

Next, and by a date fixed by the court, is the exchange of lay witness statements. In many straightforward personal injury cases, these will not be relevant. But in a complicated employment stress case and especially in a clinical negligence case, they may be critical. The Court of Appeal has repeatedly stated that experts must take into account witness statements served by the other party (e.g. *Johnson v John* [1998] MLC 0224, CA). This is when the parties appreciate the full evidential basis for each other's position. As the exchange of witness statements usually precedes by several months the exchange of expert reports on breach of duty, liability and causation, it may be necessary to amend your report in the light of this evidence.

In Northern Ireland, the RCJ do not provide for witness statements to be ordinarily produced in the preparation for litigation. This evidence is primarily obtained via examination-in-chief during the trial.

In Ireland, there is no provision for lay witness statements in personal injuries actions, other than in relation to witnesses by whose evidence special damages will be proved if they cannot be appropriately vouched.

Covert Surveillance

Such is the level of fraud in civil litigation that solicitors acting for defendants and insurance companies sometimes organise covert surveillance of claimants, although this is often unnecessary where claimants make their fraud or exaggeration obvious on social media.

The story is told of an Australian case in which a severely disabled, wheelchair-bound claimant was shown by his solicitor a film that appeared to be of him standing on top of a wagon and catching and neatly stacking sacks which were being thrown up to him. He quickly pointed out that this was his identical twin brother. He was told that if his twin brother did not provide a statement and come to court, his claim was in difficulty. His twin brother came to court and the claimant won his case. Leaving court, his barrister commented that he was very lucky that his twin brother had come to his rescue. The claimant commented that he was lucky indeed because if the camera had panned down to ground level he would have been filmed standing throwing the sacks up to his brother!

Should the expert advise covert surveillance? Probably not. This makes the expert a hostage to fortune because it might lead to a very obvious cross-examination suggesting inappropriate involvement in the litigation process. If there are reasons to doubt the credibility of the claimant and they derive from the application of the doctor's expertise, they should be set out in the report (see Chapter 8, 'Exaggeration and Malingering'). Genuinely held, reasoned opinions should be expressed in the report and can be acted upon by the solicitors. If the report has been requested by the defendant's solicitors, they may organise covert surveillance. If it has been requested by the claimant's solicitors, they may repeat their standard warning to their client about covert surveillance! Dealing with this in a 'side letter' might lead to the same cross-examination. They are usually best avoided.

Experts are commonly asked to comment on covert surveillance evidence, but seldom as interesting as in the Australian case. Usually, it is hours of supermarket shopping, enough to make anyone 'paranoid' about supermarkets, or views of a house in the dark, curtains closed and reaching the stunning climax that the subject had not been observed that day. Occasionally, it is miles of driving, but rarely as interesting as reality television programmes about 'traffic cops'. Do not expect anything like the covert surveillance in *Kavanagh QC* when his client was filmed in his wheelchair being pushed in and out of the sex shops and massage parlours of Soho.

Experts instructed by defendants' solicitors and insurance companies will usually be asked to comment on the covert surveillance after they have prepared their report even though some or all of it pre-dates their consultation with the claimant. This avoids the expert being influenced in their approach to the claimant and it avoids the expert having to conceal from the claimant the fact that they have seen this evidence, which usually will not yet have been disclosed to their solicitors. It is certainly unsatisfactory and probably unethical to see surveillance evidence, not disclose this to the claimant, not list it as evidence you have considered and try to ignore it when reaching your opinions. As it may be difficult not to be influenced by such evidence and therefore unconsciously biased, it will be misleading not to list it as evidence upon which the opinions are based. Experts instructed by claimants' solicitors are likely to see this evidence much later, as it is not usually disclosed to the claimants' solicitors until late in the proceedings. Trial by ambush may have gone (although not completely in Ireland), but defendants' solicitors will try to keep their ammunition dry for as long as possible.

Most significant covert surveillance evidence is evidence of the claimant apparently being less disabled than they have claimed to be. Its expert analysis is limited to certain experts such as orthopaedic experts. If it casts doubt on the claimant's credibility, this may have implications for reliance on the claimant's self-reported and otherwise largely, or entirely, uncorroborated history given to other experts. If so, it should be made clear that if the claimant has also been unreliable in the report of their symptoms, there must necessarily be some doubt as to the presence of the condition(s) diagnosed, its/their severity and conclusions as to its/their causation. But credibility is ultimately a matter for the trial court and it is unwise for an expert to express a view as to credibility in bald terms. In any case, it may be fair and sensible for the expert to ask for the claimant's comments on the surveillance before offering an opinion on its significance.

Exchange of Expert Reports

Expert reports may be exchanged simultaneously or sequentially. *In Ireland*, it is simultaneous exchange only on the basis that sequential exchange could be abused to enable one party to gain an advantage over the other.

If it is sequential exchange, the defendant's expert's report will usually be prepared in response to the claimant's, although *in Scotland*, it is permissible for a party to lead only oral testimony of their expert. According to the Guidance (para. 63), if it is sequential exchange, the defendant's expert report 'should then':

a. confirm whether the background set out in the claimant's expert report is agreed, or identify those parts that in the defendant's expert's view require revision, setting out the necessary revisions. The defendant's expert need not repeat information that is adequately dealt with in the claimant's expert report;
b. focus only on those material areas of difference with the claimant's expert's opinion. The defendant's report should identify those assumptions of the claimant's expert that they consider reasonable (and agree with) and those that they do not.

Exceptionally, a party may decide not to rely on its expert's report and obtain the permission of the court to instruct a different expert. However, should a party wish to rely on a new report, the first report must also be disclosed (*Edwards-Tubb v JD Wetherspoon plc* [2011] EWCA Civ 136). The author of the first report might then be called to give evidence by the opposing party. *In Ireland*, however, an expert's report may be withdrawn at any stage if it is proposed no longer to call her as a witness. The permission of the court to instruct a different expert is not required.

Written Questions to Experts

Rule 35.6 of the CPR permits a party to put questions to an expert instructed by another party for the purpose of clarification of their opinions or, if the court gives permission or the other party agrees, for other purposes (see Chapter 6, 'Answers to Questions'). This does not prevent a party putting questions to its own expert (*Stallwood v David* [2006] EWHC 2600 (QB)). If the expert does not answer the questions, the court may order that the party may not rely on their evidence and/or the party may not recover the expert's fees and expenses from another party. At this stage, the expert's instructing solicitors are responsible for payment of fees for answering the questions and not the party putting the questions.

In Ireland, the provisions are similar, although personal injury actions appear to be expressly excluded.

Discussions between Experts

Under CPR in *England and Wales* and under the RCJ in *Northern Ireland*, at any stage the court may direct, or the parties may agree to, a discussion between the experts. This may soon apply in *Scotland*. There are similar provisions in *Ireland*, but it is unclear if they apply to personal injury actions.

The purpose is not for the experts to settle the case – 'trial by expert' must not replace 'trial by judge'; it is for the parties or the court to resolve the dispute. The discussion is for identifying and discussing the expert issues in the proceedings, reaching a conscientiously agreed opinion on those issues where possible and, if not, narrowing the issues, identifying the disagreed issues, with a summary of their reasons for disagreement, and identifying what action, if any, may be taken to resolve any outstanding issues. Identifying the issues may be important in a complex case where the experts can assist by clarifying the questions before answering them. It is not in the interests of justice for experts to compromise or fudge an important issue, nor should experts strain to reach agreement. Also, an expert must not accept instructions to avoid, or defer, reaching a conclusion.

Where there has been sequential exchange of reports and the defendant's expert report has been prepared in response to the claimant's (see above), the joint statement should focus on the areas of disagreement (Guidance, para. 73).

Arrangements for discussions have to be proportionate to the value of the case. Letter, email or telephone should often suffice and, unless the court directs otherwise, it is for the experts, not the parties, to decide how the discussion takes place. Face-to-face meetings will be more likely in high value cases, where there are several experts and where the experts are going to have to look together at a significant number of records which may be sorted and paginated differently. The courts have long since decided that the attendance of the parties' lawyers is inappropriate. But if in attendance, they should not normally intervene other than to answer questions put by the experts or to advise on points of law. A large and potentially complicated experts' discussion with a number of experts or a number of parties may be chaired by an independent lawyer.

There may be an agenda. They are the exception rather than the rule, especially in simpler and lower value cases. In higher value and more complex cases with complex negligence and causation issues, they are almost always required, and the Guidance (para. 75) expects 'the parties, their lawyers and experts [to] cooperate to produce an agenda ... although primary responsibility ... should normally lie with the parties' solicitors'.

The court can give directions if the parties cannot agree the agenda promptly or if a party is unrepresented.

The statement has to be signed by both experts within seven days of the conclusion of the discussion and copies have to be provided to the parties within fourteen days of signing.

The experts' meeting is not a preliminary skirmish ahead of the main battle. In *Siegel v Pummell* [2015] EWHC 195 (QB), there was criticism of the 'mutual intransigence and disrespect' between the parties' experts and 'their mutual unwillingness to cooperate with one another'. A joint statement prepared in a spirit of mutual respect and cooperation, even resulting in continued disagreement, will be of greater assistance than one which says more about the relationship between the experts and does not advance the case beyond the positions in their respective reports.

The Single Joint Expert

The CPR encourage the use of SJEs who are instructed jointly by both the claimant and the defendant(s). Unless otherwise ordered by the court or agreed by the parties, they are jointly and severally liable for the expert's fees.

In Scotland, the Scottish Civil Courts Review 2009 approved of the idea. Theoretically, a court could order an SJE, but this would not currently be the norm. Both the Sheriff Court and Court of Session rules provide for case management, and a judge may encourage, or even ordain, joint meetings of experts. There are also rarely used powers in Scotland for the Court of Session to appoint an assessor and for a sheriff to remit to a person of skill for a report on any matter of fact, but again these powers are rarely used. *In Northern Ireland*, there are no provisions for SJEs, although there is nothing stopping the parties using one if they both agree to be bound by their evidence. *In Jersey and Ireland*, SJE provisions are similar to those in England and Wales, although so far rarely, if at all, used in Ireland.

The parties are encouraged to try to agree joint instructions; the default position is that each party can give instructions. If instructions are received from only one, the expert can give notice that unless the other instructions are received within, normally, seven days, they will begin work. If the instructions are received before the report is completed, the expert will have to decide whether it is practicable to comply with them without adversely affecting the timetable or incurring what may be further disproportionate expense. The expert should inform the parties if they are not going to comply with late instructions; the parties may seek guidance from the court. If instructions are late, or not received at all, make this clear in the report.

The SJE, like any expert, owes their first duty to the court. However, the requirements of independence, impartiality and transparency call for special measures. All correspondence should be copied to both parties simultaneously, including the claimant's letter of appointment. Telephone conversations with solicitors on either side are best avoided. If unavoidable, remind the solicitor of your joint status, advise that you will make a record, make such a record and send a brief 'minute' to both parties. SJEs should not attend any meeting or conference which is not a joint one without the written agreement of the parties or an order from the court. Also, ascertain who will be paying the fee for your attendance. The report should be sent simultaneously to both parties.

The SJE ploughs a lonely furrow. Although it is rare for an SJE to give oral evidence, it is a 'Billy No Mates' experience. The SJE cannot leave that lonely furrow to go either side for advice or support. If neither party is satisfied with the opinion or outcome of the case, the SJE may be blamed by both parties, who may feel that trial by expert has replaced trial by judge.

Asking the Court for Directions

The CPR allow an expert to file a written request for directions to assist her in carrying out her function. This will usually be a last resort after discussions with instructing solicitors have failed. It should be in the form of a letter to the district judge or deemster of the relevant court and be headed 'Expert's request for directions'. It should begin with the title of the claim, the claim number and full details of why directions are sought, and should enclose copies of any relevant documentation.

A draft should be sent to the instructing solicitors or advocates at least seven, and to all other parties at least four, days before it is filed at the court. This gives the parties a last opportunity to take steps to avoid the court having to deal with the matter.

An expert might ask the court for directions where an SJE is provided with incompatible instructions by the opposing parties, where they have identified some particular document as being critical and a party refuses to make it available or where grossly inappropriate or disproportionate questions are put by the opposing side and for which the instructing solicitors will to have to pay.

Interim Payments

An interim payment is one made on account to fund, for example, immediate care, accommodation or treatment while the overall value of the claim is still being calculated. In an application for an interim payment, it will usually be necessary to rely on expert evidence, but not *in Ireland*, where interim payments are usually made in advance of disclosure. For such a report, it is not necessary to give a long-term prognosis, but, as it is not usual for oral evidence to be given at an interim payment application, the report should otherwise be a full report and capable of withstanding scrutiny without the opportunity to test the evidence.

Family Justice Processes

Family courts make crucial decisions that affect the safety and future lives of children and their families. All jurisdictions adhere to the principle that the welfare of the child is paramount. Expert evidence in such cases is often integral to the safeguarding of children. Box 2.5 shows the family courts of all of the main jurisdictions.

England and Wales have the most highly developed rules, directions and standards relating to family court procedure and this section refers mainly to England and Wales. As these rules and directions largely replicate CPR and the Guidance, this section is mainly limited to requirements that are specific to family cases. These are set out in the FPR, Practice Direction 25B, *The Duties of an Expert, The Expert's Report and Arrangements for an Expert to Attend Court*, its annex the *Standards for Expert Witnesses in Children Proceedings in the Family Court* ('the Annex'), Practice Direction 25C, *Children Proceedings – The use of Single Joint Experts and the Process Leading to an Expert Being Instructed or Expert Evidence Being Put Before the Court* and the statutory requirements in the Children and Families Act 2014 (CFA 2014).

Northern Ireland has the Family Proceedings Rules (Northern Ireland) 1996, but it also relies on the RCJ for generic matters. *In Ireland*, the High Court Practice Direction in Family

Box 2.5 Family Courts in the Main British Isles Jurisdictions

	England and Wales	Northern Ireland	Ireland	Isle of Man	Scotland	Guernsey	Alderney	Sark	Jersey
Courts	Family Court High Court, Family Division	Magistrates' Court/Family Proceedings Court High Court, Family Division	District Family Court Circuit Family Court High Court	Magistrates' Court High Court of Justice, Civil Division, Family Business	Sheriff Court/ Family Court	Magistrate's Court Royal Court, Matrimonial Causes Division	Court of Alderney	Court of the Seneschal of Sark	Royal Court, Family Division

Law Proceedings and its Schedule deal with the preparation and exchange of a book of expert reports and other matters relating to experts and for childcare proceedings, which are mainly dealt with in the District Court, a practice direction dealing with case management, but applicable only in the Dublin Metropolitan District, deals with expert evidence.

The Nature of Family Proceedings

In England and Wales, family proceedings relating to children (hereinafter, 'family proceedings') are 'public law' care, placement and adoption proceedings and 'private law' proceedings, which are mainly concerned with disputes between separated parents about their children, such as with whom they should live or when they should see a parent with whom they do not live. Since 2014, there is now a single Family Court which hears all such proceedings save for those matters reserved to the powers of the High Court.

Family proceedings are regarded as non-adversarial, and therefore more inquisitorial. However, it may still feel adversarial because one or more parties may seek, through questions put following disclosure of the expert report or through cross-examination at the hearing, to undermine your opinion in the interests of the party they represent. If you feel that pressure is being put on you by the solicitors acting for one of the parties, either by restricting your investigations or as to your opinion, resist and make a careful note. For example, experts may be asked to assess parents who are recently separated and when the expert says that they need to interview the parents together, a solicitor may refuse.

Court Control

In England and Wales, the CFA states that in children proceedings the court's permission is required before instructing an expert (s 13(1)) and for a medical or psychiatric examination of a child by an expert (s 13(3)). Permission can only be given to instruct an expert when expert evidence is 'necessary to assist the court to resolve the proceedings justly' (s 13(6)). Thus, it is the court which must give permission for the instruction of an expert, decide what documents can be disclosed to the expert, authorise any examination of a child and, if an assessment has taken place without the court's permission, decide whether evidence arising out of such an assessment can be adduced. The court may, and usually does, order that there is only one psychiatric examination of the child.

In Ireland, such control by the court does not arise, although the court may direct the instruction of experts (see below).

The Role and Duty of the Expert

Expert evidence in family cases is often integral to the safeguarding of children and the courts rely heavily upon the objectivity, professional competence and integrity of experts. The overriding duty of an expert in family proceedings is similar to that in other legal fora, but bear in mind that under the Children Act 1989, if not in all family proceedings and in all jurisdictions, the interests of the child or children are paramount. This is why the parent cannot tell you anything 'off the record'. They need to be aware that any information that you regard as relevant to the child's interests will be shared with the other parties and may be given as evidence in court. If, in the course of the assessment, you learn something which, in your opinion, should be disclosed as a matter of urgency to the police or any child protection agency, rather than only putting it in the report, the confidentiality of the proceedings does not preclude such action, but it is advisable to discuss this with instructing or lead solicitors and, if they disagree with your course of action, seek the advice of your medical defence organisation (MDO).

In Ireland, in child care proceedings in the Dublin Metropolitan District, the letter of instruction must advise the expert of their duty to help the court on matters within their expertise and that this duty overrides any obligation to the person from whom they have received instructions or by whom they are paid.

A number of the expert's duties are similar, or identical, to their duties in other courts and proceedings. Some particular duties are laid upon experts in family cases. The FPR PD25 adds obligations to provide advice to the court that conforms to the best practice of the expert's profession (FPR 25B PD 4.1(b)) and to confine the opinion to matters material to the issues in the case (FPR 25B PD 4.1(e)), but these are of wider application. If it is recommended that a second opinion should be sought on a key issue, the expert's duty includes advising, if possible, what questions should be put to the second expert. It is the expert's duty, in expressing an opinion, to identify not only the facts upon which the opinion is based, but also any literature, research or other material upon which reliance is placed. There is a particular requirement to identify materials that have not been supplied to the expert or which are not medical or other professional records as they may raise issues as to standard of proof, admissibility of hearsay evidence or other important legal issues. Requests to third parties for information and their responses should be identified.

Eligible Experts

Opinion may be sought from perinatal psychiatrists, child and adolescent psychiatrists, forensic psychiatrists and general adult psychiatrists, along with the opinions of other related professionals such as psychologists, psychotherapists and social workers. The FPR 25B PD provides for reports to be commissioned from what the FPR call a multi-disciplinary 'expert team' rather than an individual expert (FPR 25B PD 2.2). However, the final report must give information about those persons who have taken part and their respective roles and who is responsible for the report.

Pre-Instruction Enquiry and the Expert's Response

In accordance with FPR 25C PD 3.2, '[t]he party or parties intending to instruct the expert shall approach the expert with some information about the case'. This includes the nature of the proceedings, the questions for the expert, the time when the expert's report is likely to be required, the timing of any hearing at which the expert may have to give evidence and how the expert's fees will be funded.

In response, the expert has to confirm (FPR 25B PD 8.1):

(a) that there will be no conflict of interest;

(b) that the work required is within their expertise;

(c) that they can do the relevant work within the suggested timescale;

(d) when the expert is available to give evidence, of the dates and times to avoid and, where a hearing date has not been fixed, the notice the expert will require to make arrangements to attend (or to give evidence by telephone conference or video link) without undue disruption to their normal professional routines;

(e) the cost, including hourly or other charging rates, and likely hours to be spent on the case;

Box 2.6 *Standards for Expert Witnesses in Children Proceedings in the Family Court* (Annex to FPR 25B PD)

1. The expert's area of competence is appropriate to the issue(s) upon which the court has identified that an opinion is required, and relevant experience is evidenced in their CV.
2. The expert has been active in the area of work or practice (as a practitioner or an academic who is subject to peer appraisal), has sufficient experience of the issues relevant to the instant case, and is familiar with the breadth of current practice or opinion.
3. The expert has working knowledge of the social, developmental, cultural norms and accepted legal principles applicable to the case presented at initial enquiry, and has the cultural competence skills to deal with the circumstances of the case.
4. The expert is up-to-date with Continuing Professional Development appropriate to their discipline and expertise, and is in continued engagement with accepted supervisory mechanisms relevant to their practice.
5. If the expert's current professional practice is regulated by a UK statutory body they are in possession of a current licence to practise or equivalent.
6. . . .
7. The expert is compliant with any necessary safeguarding requirements, information security expectations, and carries professional indemnity insurance.
8. . . .
9. The expert has undertaken appropriate training, updating or quality assurance activity – including actively seeking feedback from cases in which they have provided evidence – relevant to the role of experts in the family courts in England and Wales within the last year.
10. The expert has a working knowledge of, and complies with, the requirements of Practice Directions relevant to providing reports for and giving evidence to the family courts in England and Wales. This includes compliance with the requirement to identify where their opinion on the instant case lies in relation to other accepted mainstream views and the overall spectrum of opinion in the UK.

(f) any representations which the expert wishes to make to the court about being named or otherwise identified in any public judgment.

The Annex also sets out standards with which the expert is expected to apply (Box 2.6).

Instructions

In England and Wales, instructions will usually come jointly from all of the parties through the solicitor instructed by the children's guardian in a public law case or as a joint instruction from one of the parties (usually acting for the parent who is being assessed), but agreed with the other party in a private law case. If instructions are received as a party expert, the expert can invite their instructing solicitors to consider whether joint instruction would be feasible. Instructions to an SJE must be through a jointly agreed letter. A party cannot independently instruct the SJE unless the court so directs. If the parties cannot agree the instructions, they have to write to the court, which will then compile the instructions. In keeping with the less adversarial proceedings, all instructions to experts are disclosable (FPR 25.14(3)). They are not legally privileged. Where an order or direction requires an expert to do something, or otherwise affects an expert, they have to be served with a copy of the order.

In Ireland, in childcare and secure care proceedings, the court may, of its own motion or on the application of any party, give such directions as it thinks proper to procure a report from a nominated person on any question affecting the welfare of the child. The report may be received in evidence and the author may be called as a witness. The court directs who will be responsible for the report fee (Child Care Act 1991 (CCA), s 27). In addition, the court may make such order on any question affecting the welfare of the child as it thinks proper (CCA, s 47) and directions can be given as to consultation between experts (see below, 'Experts' Meetings and Discussions'). As to private law proceedings, the court, in a variety of private family law proceedings may, of its own motion or on the application by a party to the proceedings, direct a report on any question affecting the welfare of a party or any other person to whom they relate (Family Law Act 1995, s 47).

The Court's Timetable

The report should be prepared and filed in accordance with the court's timetable. This is important in any legal forum, but more so in cases involving children, as the timetable has to have regard to the speed of childhood development and the potential impact of its decisions at different stages of the child's development. This urgency is reflected in the very short period of time during which the parties can put questions to the expert.

Discussions

The letter of instruction should identify the relevant people concerned with the proceedings (e.g. the treating clinicians) and any other expert instructed in the proceedings and advise the expert of their right to talk to the other experts provided that an accurate record is made of the discussions (FPR 25C PD 4.1(f) and (g)):

> What the court is anxious to prevent is any *unrecorded* informal discussions between particular experts which are either influential in, or determinative of, their views and to which the parties ... (including perhaps other experts) do not have access. This also applies to any documentary evidence to which you have access. (Wall 2007, emphasis in the original)

If, in addition, the expert discusses the case with any of the solicitors, there should also be a record. The expert should make their own record of any discussion and decide who will produce an agreed note of the discussion. If it is with a solicitor, they will make an 'attendance note', but the expert must still make their own note. The expert should ask the solicitor to send them a copy and, if they disagree with it, write to the solicitor and keep a copy of the letter. Such notes and records have the potential to become the subject of examination or cross-examination and they must be disclosed if so requested.

The Standard of Proof

The standard of proof in family proceedings is the civil standard, but sometimes it is more appropriate to say that something is *consistent* with a particular set of facts, albeit bearing in mind that the court will decide the facts and, depending on what facts the court finds, the conclusion may be weakened. Sometimes, it is necessary to give more than one opinion depending on which set of facts is accepted by the court.

Report Content

There are some particular report requirements in family cases.

The opinion should take into consideration all of the material facts, including any relevant factors arising from ethnic, cultural, religious or linguistic contexts at the time the opinion is expressed (FPR 25B PD 9.1(f)(i)). The expert has to describe their processes of professional risk assessment and differential diagnosis, highlighting factual assumptions, deductions therefrom and any unusual, contradictory or inconsistent features of the case (FPR 25B PD 9.1(f)(ii)). They have to indicate whether any proposition is a hypothesis (in particular a controversial hypothesis), or an opinion deduced in accordance with peer-reviewed and tested technique, research and experience accepted as a consensus in the scientific community (FPR 25B PD 9.1(f)(iii)). In relation to the range of opinion, they have to identify and explain, within the range of opinions, any 'unknown cause', whether arising from the facts of the case (e.g. because there is too little information to form a scientific opinion) or from limited experience or lack of research, peer review or support in the relevant field of expertise (FPR 25B PD 9.1(g)(ii)) and give reasons for any opinion expressed, perhaps using a balance-sheet approach to the factors that support or undermine an opinion (FPR 25B PD 9.1(g)(iii)).

Some of these requirements have been formulated in response to difficulties that have arisen with expert evidence in child abuse cases, but they are worthy of more general application.

Compliance and Truth

In England and Wales, the report must comply with Practice Direction 25B. It has to include a statement at the end that the expert 'understands and has complied with the expert's duty to the court'. It should be verified by a statement of truth (see Chapter 6, 'Statement of Truth').

Compliance with the FPR is not a formality. In *Re F (A Child: Failings of Expert)* [2016] EWHC 2149 (Fam) (see Chapter 1, 'The Duties of the Expert Witness'), a very experienced psychologist, using quotation marks, included in his report extensive excerpts said to have been directly from the mother. But they were a collection of recollections and impressions, turned into phrases, adopting the mother's idiom, and attributed to her. At a finding of fact hearing solely dedicated to the expert's conduct, the judge was very critical of the psychologist and named him in the judgment.

Delivery of the Report

The expert sends the report to the instructing solicitors or, if jointly instructed, the lead solicitors. They will make copies and distribute them. This will happen irrespective of which party has commissioned the report and what the expert's opinion is. Even if the opinion is detrimental to the case of the instructing party, the report will be disclosed to the other parties and to the court.

Questions to the Expert

Questions must be put to the expert within ten days of the service of the report. The requirement that questions be put only once, be put within ten days and be just for clarification can be waived only by the court or where a Practice Direction permits.

Experts' Meetings and Discussions

In England and Wales, Practice Direction 25E covers discussions between experts in family proceedings. They are likely to occur as the result of a direction from the court for an experts' meeting. The lawyers should liaise with the experts to arrange the date and timing of the meeting and furnish the experts with an agenda and list of questions not later than two working days before the meeting. The meeting may be face to face, by telephone or by live link. These meetings differ from experts' meetings in civil and criminal cases in that they usually involve experts from different disciplines and so there may be a global discussion relating to those questions that concern most or all of the experts. This does not preclude separate discussion between or among experts of the same or related disciplines. A further difference is that the parties do not have to agree in order for the content of the discussion to be referred to at trial and there is no rule that the parties cannot be forced to accept the agreement reached by the experts.

The aim is to identify areas of agreement and disagreement and, in the case of the latter, to discuss whether any action needs to be taken to resolve the disagreement, such as the obtaining of further evidence. A nominated professional will chair the meeting, and it may be minuted or recorded for professional transcription.

A nominated lawyer will usually then draw up a statement of agreement and disagreement which will be circulated to the experts for amendment, approval and signing. This should be filed and served not later than five days after the meeting.

Jointly instructed experts should not attend experts' meetings unless all of the parties have agreed in writing or the court has ordered it, if there is an agreement or direction as to who is to pay the expert's fees and such attendance is proportionate to the case.

In Ireland, in childcare proceedings in the Dublin Metropolitan District Court, the court may direct experts to consult with one another for the purpose of identifying the issues in respect of which they intend to give evidence, where possible reaching agreement on the evidence that they intend to give in respect of those issues, and considering any matter which the court may direct them to consider, and require that they record in a memorandum for joint submission particulars of the outcome of their consultations.

In England and Wales, in public law Children Act proceedings the court can direct a meeting between the local authority and any relevant experts in order to assist the local authority in the formulation of plans and proposals for the child. The court directs the arrangements, nominates the chair and the minuting. However, the expert should make their own detailed notes of the meeting.

If the parties' solicitors are present at the meeting, they will be partisan and their questions will seek to advance their client's position. Restrict your answers to the questions on the agenda. This is not a mini-trial. Your answers to their questions will be 'on the record', whether the meeting is in person or by telephone, and subsequently you may be cross-examined on them. This even more so makes it essential that there should be a proper record of the meeting.

In Ireland, there is no provision for such discussions.

Getting on the Learning Curve

Some medical experts will have started, as this chapter has done, in the criminal court, probably in a less serious case, and eventually found their expertise called upon in civil and family courts. For some like me, it will have been largely a process of learning by experience and, I freely admit, from my mistakes. In the next chapter, we set out suggestions for education and training which offer today's and tomorrow's medical experts a steeper and hopefully smoother learning curve.

Further Reading

Buchan, A. (gen. ed) (2019) *Lewis and Buchan: Clinical Negligence. A Practical Guide*, 8th edn (Bloomsbury Professional).

Powers, M. and Barton, A. (eds) (2015) *Clinical Negligence*, 5th edn (Bloomsbury Professional).

Training, Development and the Maintenance of Expertise

Keith Rix

Clear professional standards, appropriate training, credentialing and quality control for expert witnesses have the potential to address more directly the sorts of problems that arise from the evidence of unqualified, careless, overworked or even unscrupulous experts.

The Honourable Thomas A. Cromwell in Macfadyen Lecture 2011

Training as an Expert Witness

In AWLP, the GMC states: 'You should consider undertaking training for the role (of expert witness)'. This does not go far enough. You must be trained:

> It is the expert's responsibility . . . to undertake training on the role of the expert and how to perform properly. The courts do not require it, but in the interests of raising standards and of reducing the risk of failed justice, expert witnesses will be advised to engage in training and education about the expert witness system. (Cooper 2006)

Such training can begin during general professional training and it should form part of higher training. It requires appropriate supervision. The doctor who takes up expert witness work in retirement may find it difficult to obtain appropriate supervision and training and can anticipate judicial criticism, except in cases where the events occurred when they were still in practice.

Necessary Competencies

The Royal College of Psychiatrists (2010) identifies as competencies to be acquired in higher training in forensic psychiatry the abilities to:

- Prepare reports for . . . Courts of Law . . . [and] criminal justice agencies,
- Interpret legislation and explain the implications in jargon free language at a level for the specific situation,
- Receive and negotiate instructions to prepare reports,
- Develop a formulation of a case and write a report to a high standard,
- Testify as an expert witness within limits of own expertise.

Consultants who are experienced expert witnesses are well-placed to supervise trainees in the acquisition of these abilities. This is similar to how psychiatric trainees in England and Wales learn to prepare reports for the First-tier Tribunal (Health, Education and Social Care) Mental Health (Rutherford *et al.* 2015). Higher trainees in all medical specialties should be able to obtain similar training and supervision by secondment or attachment to appropriately experienced trainers.

Box 3.1 Approaches to Training as an Expert Medical Witness: Preparing Medicolegal Reports

- Prepare an expert 'opinion' based on one of a library of reports covering the range of commonly encountered issues in their speciality and from which the opinion section has been removed. This can be carried out as a group exercise; prior to the group discussion, trainees can exchange and assess each other's opinions.
- Attend a medicolegal consultation with supervisor and draft a report based on the consultation and consideration of all documents and materials available to the supervisor.
- Conduct a medicolegal consultation under the direct observation of the supervisor and draft the consultant's report ('ghost report') incorporating any additional information elicited, or signs identified, by the supervisor.
- Conduct a medicolegal assessment 'solo' and present history and examination findings to the supervisor, who should verify them; then draft the supervisor's report ('ghost report') incorporating any information elicited, or signs identified, by the supervisor.
- Conduct a medicolegal assessment 'solo' and prepare a report in own name and counter-signed by the supervisor who can, if necessary, arrange to clarify or confirm the trainee's findings.

Adapted from Rix, Eastman and Haycroft 2017

Training in Report Preparation

Trainees can begin by writing expert opinions based on the facts in specimen reports and preparing 'ghost reports'. Higher trainees can progress to reports prepared in their own name and countersigned by their supervisor (Rix 2011a) (see Box 3.1).

Particularly where reports are prepared in accordance with the Rules, there are similar requirements 'where the expert has based an opinion or inference on a representation of fact or opinion made by another person' to '(i) identify the person … (ii) give the qualifications, relevant experience and any accreditation of that person, and (iii) certify that that person had personal knowledge of the matters stated in that representation' (CrPR 19.4(e)). This applies where the supervisor relies on a trainee's examination of the subject. It must also apply where the supervisor relies on the history taken by the trainee. Therefore, the supervisor should include a paragraph along the lines set out in Box 3.2 and the trainee's curriculum vitae (CV). The supervisor must distinguish their own examination findings from those of the trainee so as to 'make clear which of the facts stated in the report are within the expert's own knowledge' (in accordance with CrPR 19.4(d)) or to comply with the obligatory statement of truth required by CPR.

Reports prepared by sufficiently experienced trainees must be countersigned by their supervisor and should include as an appendix the consultant's own page CV (see Box 3.3) own one page.

Training to Give Live Testimony

One of the best ways for trainees to familiarise themselves with court procedure and the giving of evidence, and get some judicial tuition, is to sit on the bench as a judge's marshal. So, training scheme organisers should establish a relationship with the resident judge at their local combined court hearing centre. Trainees should shadow consultants who act as expert witnesses, including attending conferences with counsel and listening to their testimony.

Box 3.2 **Suggested Format for Consultant's Statement as to Their Reliance on Trainee's Assistance in Preparing an Expert Report**

In preparing this report I have relied on an assessment of the [defendant*] carried out by Dr William Battie, Specialty Registrar in Forensic Psychiatry, who is attached to me for the purposes of his higher training in forensic psychiatry. Dr Battie's qualifications and relevant experience are set out in Appendix 2. The assessment was/was not carried out under my direct supervision, i.e. I was/was not present when Dr Battie carried out the assessment. I did/did not supplement Dr Battie's assessment with my own assessment in the form of my own enquiry and examination of the [defendant*]. In the section 'Psychiatric examination' I have set out Dr Battie's findings (and distinguished these from my own mental state findings, these being the only facts within my own knowledge) [if applicable]. I certify that Dr Battie had personal knowledge of the matters upon which I have relied insofar as they are matters ascertained by him through history taking and examination.

* Or 'complainant', 'claimant', 'applicant', 'plaintiff', 'pursuer' or 'defender', etc.

Rix, Eastman and Haycroft 2017

Box 3.3 **Countersignature Statement by a Consultant Who Has Supervised a Trainee's Report**

I confirm that I am the consultant psychiatrist to whom Dr Henrietta Maudsley* is attached for the higher training, which she is undertaking as the final stage of preparation for her appointment as a consultant psychiatrist. Hence, I am responsible for supervising her training and performance; and I have acted in that capacity in her preparation of this report. However, the opinion expressed in the report is her own, albeit I have supervised her in coming to that opinion. Only in the event that a new question were to be raised within the case that is not addressed in the report, and which Dr Maudsley considers herself not competent to answer, would I expect to be required to give expert evidence to the court in my own stead; albeit of course a different competent expert could be called to deal with such a question. At all times we would both be guided by any relevant court direction. My own CV is to be found as Appendix 2.

* Note that name has been changed from the original.

Rix, Eastman and Haycroft 2017

For psychiatrists, experience of giving evidence at a tribunal hearing is invaluable, but must be gained in accordance with the Tribunals Judiciary guidance (Rutherford *et al.* 2015). However, this is insufficient on its own.

Trainees should only exceptionally give oral evidence without the supervision of their trainer, who should be present to provide feedback. However, this can only take place after they have completed the entirety of their evidence, as a witness is not allowed to discuss their evidence during the course of their testimony.

A number of bodies provide training in courtroom skills. Such an induction is essential.

Trainer Vigilance

The trainer must keep the trainee's competence under frequent review. At every stage, they must be satisfied that what is expected of the trainee is consistent with their level of experience and competence and matches the complexity of the case. This determines the nature and amount of supervision.

Maintaining and Developing Expertise

It is necessary to keep up to date, not just up to date and fit to practise in your medical speciality, but also as a doctor. Court users in Bradford, and not least a particular judge, will remember the late Dr Ray Travers, not for his expert psychiatric evidence, but for his speed of response and clinical skill when he rushed forward and immediately rendered assistance as the judge collapsed to the floor.

Maintaining Clinical Practice

It is important to maintain clinical practice and 'be familiar with guidelines and developments that affect your work' (GMP). Heed the judgment in *R v Henderson* [2010] EWCA Crim 1269:

> The fact that an expert is in clinical practice at the time he makes his report is of significance. Clinical practice affords experts the opportunity to maintain and develop their experience. Such experts acquire experience which continues and develops. Their continuing observation, the experience of both the foreseen and unforeseen, the recognised and the unrecognised, form a powerful basis for their opinion. Clinicians learn from each case in which they are engaged. Each case makes them think and as their experience develops so does their understanding. Continuing experience gives them the opportunity to adjust previously held opinions, to alter their views. They are best placed to recognise that that which is unknown one day may be acknowledged the next. Such clinical experience . . . may provide a far more reliable source of evidence than that provided by those who have ceased to practise their expertise in a continuing clinical setting and have retired from such practice . . . They have lost the opportunity, day by day to learn and develop from continuing experience.

Registration and Licensing

Maintain your registration with the GMC or the MC. Except in family cases, a licence to practise is not required in order to give expert evidence, but you should have one, especially if it is a condition for indemnity insurance. It is not necessary if your only role is to come out of retirement to give evidence as to normal practice at the time when you were in practice or when giving evidence on scientific causation when currency in clinical practice is not relevant. *In Ireland*, the issue of licensing does not arise.

Indemnity and Insurance

You should have indemnity or insurance cover from an MDO or insurer for your medico-legal work. The Supreme Court in *Jones v Kaney* [2011] UKSC 13 abolished immunity from suit for expert witnesses at least in respect of claims by a litigant to whom the expert owes a duty. *In Ireland*, it has long been the case that an expert may be liable in negligence to the subject of their report (*McGrath v Kiely* [1965] IR 497), although in the case of a court-appointed expert, immunity from suit may be conferred on a negligent expert provided they have not attempted to abuse their position as an expert witness (*O'Keefe v Kilcullen* [2001] IESC 84). But getting something wrong is not the same as negligence. It may not even incur judicial criticism. *AW v Greater Glasgow Health Board* [2015] CSOH 99 illustrates how the courts may regard experts' errors understandable 'having regard to the volume of material the experts are required to consider and the complexity of the subject matter'.

Approved Medical Practitioner Status

It is advisable to maintain approved medical practitioner (AMP) status where applicable. *In England and Wales*, this means 'special experience in the diagnosis or treatment of mental disorder' (Mental Health Act (MHA) 1983, s 12) (often rendered in reports with 'and' instead of 'or' and sometimes even less accurate variations, which can open up embarrassing, but easily avoidable, cross-examination). The more rigorous requirement *in Scotland* is for 'special experience in the diagnosis and treatment of mental disorder' (Mental Health (Care and Treatment) Scotland Act 2003, s 22). In some circumstances, medical evidence is not admissible from a registered and licensed medical practitioner unless they are an AMP. There is no equivalent status *in Ireland*, where not all psychiatrists employed as consultants are necessarily on the Register of Medical Specialists or possess a certificate of completion of specialist training.

I was in court for a fitness to plead and stand trial enquiry when my opposite number, called by the defence, admitted that his s 12 approval had expired six weeks previously. As evidence had to be given by a s 12 approved doctor, the defence was unable to rely on his evidence.

Peer Groups and Personal Development Plans

In your peer group, you need at least one other member who is also a medical expert witness. You can help each other formulate personal development plans (PDPs) that cover your medicolegal work. If not, join or form an informal peer group of medical expert witnesses.

Courses, Training and Conferences

Your PDP should include regularly updated training in report writing and witness skills, teaching on developments in statute and case law and court procedure, and updates on areas of medicolegal practice related to your speciality. The record for your annual appraisal (but there is no formal annual appraisal *in Ireland*) will also be the evidence you may be required to provide that you are engaged in continuing professional development (CPD) geared to maintaining competence as an expert. You may be asked to 'demonstrate training in and/or knowledge of [your] duties to the court as an expert' (Inns of Court College of Advocacy 2019).

At *The Grange*, we developed a monthly meeting at which we presented cases and updated ourselves on areas of the law. We still organise an annual conference with mainly invited speakers from medicine and the law. The programme is generated by our peer group and others who attend the Conference. Thus, there is a close correspondence between our PDPs and the conference programme. It usually means that, if we identify a need for education or training on a particular subject, we meet that need at the next Grange conference.

Books, Journals, Law Reports and Libraries

Law reports illustrate better than any textbook what happens in court when a particular medical issue is in dispute and the judge or judges have to resolve the dispute. But law reports are limited to what the judge considers important for the public record and as a record of their decision-making. Furthermore, cases in the lower courts and cases that do not go to appeal are only occasionally reported.

Build up a library of books and law reports relevant to your expert witness practice. Look up the relevant law reports quoted in this book. You can often supplement these when you go to court as the parties often produce a bundle of 'authorities' that are usually thrown away at the end of the case.

Membership of a law library ensures access to the largest range of law reports and also law journals. Many law reports are accessible on the websites of the British and Irish Legal Information Institute (BAILII) at www.bailii.org, Her Majesty's Courts Service at http://search.hmcourts-service.gov.uk, Mental Health Law Online at www.mentalhealthlaw.co.uk and Family Law Week at www.familylawweek.co.uk.

Medicolegal Societies and Expert Witness Organisations

Join your local medicolegal society or the Medico-Legal Society of London. If you have a law degree, join the Society of Doctors in Law and appreciate the combination of fine dining in the Inns of Court and topical after-dinner medicolegal discourse.

Join the Academy of Experts or the Expert Witness Institute. They provide training for experts, publish journals or newsletters and organise annual conferences at which judges, lawyers and experts talk about the latest developments affecting experts. This will enable you to 'keep up to date with, and follow, the law . . . and other regulations relevant to your work' (GMP) as an expert witness.

Further Education

A number of universities now offer post-graduate degrees relevant to experts. There are Master of Laws degrees in Medical Law, Medical Law and Ethics and Mental Health Law. Consider obtaining Membership of the Faculty of Forensic and Legal Medicine of the Royal College of Physicians.

Audit and Case-Based Discussion

The most powerful audit tool is a few days in court where three or more of the most incisive legal brains, assisted by a small army of experts, analyse your report and test your opinions.

For day-to-day practice, case-based discussions of expert reports are needed. In an assessment of your credibility as an expert, you may be asked about your participation in such peer review. Box 3.4 provides a framework for assessing a medicolegal report in a case-based discussion.

Some items are rated on a three-point scale: Requires attention/improvement – Adequate – An example to others. For others, it is a two-point scale. It is or it is not within their expertise. It is a formative experience with emphasis on improvement and the pursuit of excellence. It is not a pass/fail test.

The free text section of the form begins with 'Good practice'; it starts with the most positive and affirming outcome. It then moves on to: 'Suggestions for improved practice'. When these sessions are incorporated into a conference, they can be followed by a plenary session at which examples of good practice are collated. However, the discussions themselves are confidential.

Box 3.4 A Framework for Assessing a Medicolegal Report in a Case-Based Discussion

- within the doctor's expertise;
- evidence of consent where appropriate;
- acceptable structure and properly presented;
- 'user-friendly';
- compliance with relevant rules;
- methodology explained and includes such information as the court may need to decide whether the opinion is sufficiently reliable to be admissible;
- knowledge, understanding and correct application of legal tests;
- facts and opinions clearly separated;
- issues addressed;
- evaluation of quality of evidence/clinical veracity;
- opinions supported by reasons and withstand logical analysis;
- includes range of reasonable opinion;
- summary of opinion/conclusions;
- glossary (if applicable)/terms explained;
- evidence of independence and impartiality;
- expedition at all stages, particularly achieving all deadlines;
- probity (terms and conditions, record of time spent, detailed, itemised billing).

Feedback and Appraisal

Eyre and Alexander (2015) observe that '[m]edical expert reports are written in a communication void in which it can be readily – but wrongly – assumed that lack of comment from the lawyers arises from their satisfaction with the report', but '[a]s with any process that exists without feedback, mistakes will be repeated and dysfunctional aspects of professional practice soon become "the way it is done".'

Annexed to FPR 25B PD are *Standards for Expert Witnesses in Children Proceedings in the Family Court*. They include the requirement for the expert to have undertaken appropriate training, updating or quality assurance activity – including actively seeking feedback from cases in which they have provided evidence – relevant to the role of expert in the family courts in England and Wales within the previous year. Obtaining such feedback should overcome the problem identified by Eyre and Alexander.

As recognised by the Royal College of Psychiatrists (Rix *et al.* 2015): 'Appraisal directed towards revalidation requires that all aspects of a doctor's work be assessed . . . Hence, there is a duty on psychiatrists who give expert testimony to ensure that such work is included in their appraisal and revalidation.'

Make use of the online feedback system, the *Multi-source Assessment Tool for Expert Psychiatric Witnesses* (MAEP) (www.rcpsych.ac.uk/improving-care/ccqi/multi-source-feedback/maep). Box 3.5 shows the domains in which the expert is rated.

Rating is on a six-point scale:

- excels at standards;
- exceeds expected standards;
- satisfactory;

Box 3.5 Feedback Domains for the *Multi-Source Assessment Tool for Expert Psychiatric Witnesses*

- professionalism/professional demeanour;
- ethics;
- skills;
- reliability of opinion;
- presentation of opinion/report;
- understanding of law, procedure and rules of evidence;
- oral testimony;
- business manners and affairs.

- unsatisfactory;
- very unsatisfactory;
- extremely unsatisfactory.

Feedback also includes a comparison with the performance of other psychiatrists.

Compliments, complaints and criticisms should be included in any appraisal file and form the basis of reflective practice.

Knowing When to Stop

Always be willing to learn from other experts. If you find that you have nothing more to learn, it is probably time to give up being a medical expert and read no further or just 'be willing to share your knowledge with colleagues who might be called to give evidence in court, to help build their confidence and willingness to give evidence in the future' (AWLP). Otherwise, read on – about the business of being an expert.

Business Matters

Danny Allen and Keith Rix

Experts should be spared piles of documents which [are] of little relevance. The cost of expert involvement [is] unnecessarily inflated by over-burdening them with insignificant papers.

Thorpe and Hughes LJJ in *Re S (Care Proceedings: Assessment of Risk)* (2008) Times, 7 April 2008, CA

Job Planning

It is from the UK's National Health Service (NHS) or Ireland's Health Service Executive or public voluntary hospitals that you are likely to start your expert witness career. Be mindful of your contractual obligations. You cannot get on with your medicolegal work and say nothing or your probity will be in question. However, many employers, in agreeing a job plan, are happy for consultants to do some medicolegal work in 'work' time. If you want to do it on your employer's premises, you need permission. Your employer may want payment, but this will be a deductible business expense.

Setting Up Your Business

In terms of good business practice and tax efficiency, consider setting yourself up as a business. In the UK, Her Majesty's Revenue & Customs (HMRC) will tax you at your highest rate without the possibility of claiming expenses against your earnings until you register as self-employed. There is some leeway to register retrospectively in the first year. You will need a name – something simple like Dr Andrea Duncan Forensic Practice.

Decide on your accounting year. If it finishes on 30 April, you then have over a year to collect the money from your debtors before tax is due. This is particularly important in the UK where you pay tax on what you invoice, whether or not you have been paid, whereas in Ireland generally income tax arises on receipts, not invoicing.

Document and keep evidence of your expenses to set off against income. Employ an accountant whose fees should be offset with the money you can save! Open a business account, to keep business earnings separate, with a deposit account to save for tax. If you take money from clients directly, best practice is to keep this in a 'no. 2 account' until 'spent'.

If you need to raise money from your bank or just as good discipline, you will need a business plan. If you adopt a mission statement, do not fall foul of GMC or MC rules, which require you not to make exaggerated claims.

But a business is not synonymous with a company. If you want to form a company, consult an accountant. But be careful how you show the company name in reports. If the report is from Dr Andrea Duncan Forensic Psychiatric Reports Company, cross-examination may begin with 'Whose report is this? Is it the company's report?', bearing in mind that a company has a different and separate legal status.

Indemnity or Insurance Cover

Obtain indemnity or insurance cover from an MDO or insurer for your medicolegal work (see Chapter 3, 'Indemnity and Insurance Cover'). It should extend to claims brought after your death. In *McHugh v Gray* [2006] EWHC 1968 (QB), there was an issue as to whether the deceased psychiatrist's inaccurate and falsely optimistic prognosis for the post-traumatic stress disorder (PTSD) of a Hillsborough Stadium disaster spectator had, through his negligence, resulted in an undervaluing of his claim.

Working and Being Contactable

You need somewhere to conduct your assessments (see Chapter 5, 'The Venue'). It could be your daytime place of work, an independent hospital, your own premises or a set of 'doctors' chambers', with the advantage of sharing an established infrastructure and having a peer group.

Consider how people will contact you and what sort of address you will use. You must separate your expert witness work from any NHS work. Using your home address should be ruled out. Consider a PO (Post Office) Box. This can be literally a place where you collect mail, or it can redirect to a geographic address. However, the underlying 'real' address is not secret.

Link your business to an available internet domain name and purchase this in as many iterations as possible. You will use one to promote your business; the others will 'point' there. Create a professional email address, such as enquiries@drandreaduncan.co.uk.

Consider getting a computerised telephone number. You can get a local or a non-geographic number which initially can simply be routed to your telephone. Later you can direct it to other numbers (e.g. your assistant) or a computerised switchboard. Another advantage is that its operation can be restricted to working hours. A second number can be used as a 'fax to email'. Solicitors still seem to expect it. Your telephone can automatically be directed to voicemail if you are not available. A DX (Document Exchange) address is tremendously useful as solicitors use this as an alternative postal system because they are not charged by weight.

Staff

The expert who tries to run their practice alone is a fool! They are expending energy on things at which they are probably not very good and probably wasting important time when fees could be earned or time off enjoyed. Medicolegal work is reasonably lucrative, so employing staff should be possible and desirable. For detail of how to employ people, see *Business for Medics* (Allen 2014). Consult an accountant; most have payroll departments to assist small businesses. They will deal with tax, national insurance, pensions, contracts and grievance procedures and advise you on other matters, such as employers' or public liability insurance.

Responding to the Letter of Enquiry

To Accept or Decline

Upon receipt of an enquiry, ask yourself a number of questions (Box 4.1). You should decline instructions from friends so as to avoid a conflict of interest. You must have

Box 4.1 Questions to Be Answered in the Affirmative before Accepting Instructions to Prepare an Expert Medical Report

- Am I in good standing with the College?
- Have I been appraised in the last year (if applicable)?
- Am I up to date with CPD?
- Does my personal development plan address the issue of my competence as an expert witness?
- Have I had an introduction to expert witness work?
- Have I received or refreshed training in the role of an expert witness in the last five years?
- Am I available to attend the trial (if the trial date has been fixed)?
- Do I have the time to devote to this case?
- Can I deliver the report by the required deadline?
- Can I declare that I have no actual or potential conflict of interest or personal interest?
- Am I sure that I have no prior knowledge of this case?
- Do I understand exactly what questions I am being asked or what the issues are?
- Do I have relevant knowledge or direct experience of, and expertise in, this area of psychiatry?
- Does the question or issue fall within my own expertise?
- Am I able to give an honest, trustworthy, objective and impartial opinion without it being prejudiced by any views I may have as to the subject's age, colour, culture, disability, ethnic or national origin, lifestyle, marital or parental status, race, religion or beliefs, gender, gender orientation or social or economic status?
- Can I provide sufficiently detailed information as to my proposed fees to those instructing me in order for them to decide if they are proportionate to the matters in issue and ensure value for money?
- Do I understand the specific framework of law and procedure within which this case is taking place?
- Am I familiar with the general duties of an expert?
- Do I understand my duty to the court?

sufficient time. The party which instructed the expert neurologist in *Williams v Jervis* [2009] EWHC 1837 (QB) was financially penalised because of his 'failure to spend adequate time in properly analysing the case'. Be clear about timescales. *In the Isle of Man*, you are expected to see the subject and report within eight weeks of receiving confirmation that your fees are agreed. Failure to comply with court deadlines risks an adverse costs order. If the proposed timetable would cause a problem or if your other commitments would prevent you giving sufficient time to the case, the onus is on you to identify this problem at the outset (*Re X and Y (Delay: Professional Conduct of Expert)* [2019] EWFC B9 HH).

If these questions can be answered in the affirmative, you may decide to accept instructions. In any event, the Guidance (para. 22) requires experts to confirm without delay whether they accept their instructions. *In the Isle of Man*, you are expected to respond within twenty-one days of the date of the letter of enquiry.

But make sure you have clear instructions as to the type of expertise required, the purpose of the report, the nature of the matter to be investigated, the questions to be answered and the history of the matter, including any factual matters that may be in dispute. In AWLP, the GMC says: 'You must make sure you understand exactly what questions you are being asked to answer. If your instructions are unclear, you should ask those instructing you to explain. If the instructions are still not clear, you should not provide expert advice or opinion.' There is no equivalent guidance from the MC, but this guidance is of general application.

Acceptance may be conditional on the questions the solicitor wants to ask but which may not yet have been formulated. Be proactive in ensuring that you can answer the questions eventually agreed. You may need to suggest questions or modifications. There may be a subtle difference between the question being asked by a solicitor who has no medical training and what you as a medical expert think it is. Assist by using your medical expertise to identify hitherto unrecognised issues that may be material to the case.

Notwithstanding the clear obligation on an instructing solicitor and counsel to ensure that the expert is appropriate for the case and aware of their duties (*Kennedy v Cordia (Services) LLP* [2016] UKSC 6), they can only do so if they have sufficient, accurate information as to your qualifications, training and experience so as to match the expertise with the needs of the court. This creates a complementary obligation on you to ensure you are satisfied that you have sufficient expertise and to be honest about it. The expert's 'lack of current experience' in *R (Duffy) v HM Deputy Coroner for Worcestershire* [2013] EWHC 1654 resulted in the quashing of the coroner's verdict. In *Rhodes v West Surrey and North East Hampshire Health Authority* [1998] 6 Lloyd's Rep Med 24, an obstetrician was found not to have told the truth about his surgical or expert witness experience. The GMC has an interest in these matters: 'You must always be honest about your experience, qualifications and current role' (GMP). So do the criminal courts. A forensic computer expert was convicted of perjury after misrepresenting his qualifications (*R v O'Shea* [2010] EWCA Crim 2879). Only finally agree if you are happy that the questions are within your expertise.

If you consider that you might fall short of providing sufficient expertise, be honest about it; conceal it at your peril. If in doubt, discuss this with a colleague or your MDO. If still in doubt, decline. Do not fear that you will not be instructed again. Knowing that you can be trusted will enhance your reputation. If the case calls for highly specialised expertise and you know someone better qualified, recommend their instruction or you may find them on the other side.

In a criminal case in England and Wales (CrPR 19.3(3)(c)), you must, and in any case or jurisdiction it is advisable to, mention anything which might reasonably be thought capable of undermining the reliability of your opinion or detracting from your credibility or impartiality as an expert. This includes any potential conflict of interest, anything to suggest that you are biased, any criminal convictions and any previous judicial criticism. GMC, MC or medical practitioners tribunal (MPT) proceedings that have resulted in a finding of impairment should be disclosed. Arguably, complaints that have not been upheld do not have to be disclosed because they may not be thought capable of detracting from your credibility. Most medical experts will at some time be in receipt of a complaint, subsequently not upheld, from a dissatisfied litigant.

The enquiry may come from a litigant in person (LIP). Often, they lack the sophistication of professionals and may not understand your duty to the court or tribunal. If they do not like your report, they may be disinclined to pay and likely to complain. The Civil Justice Council (CJC) (2011) makes the point that in England and Wales experts can ask for payment in advance. But, this is only part of the problem. Contracting with an LIP requires understanding of, and compliance with, the complexities of consumer law; if they have a right to cancel, avoid commencing any work during the cancellation period. Also, since 1 April 2019, people who *give advice* or *make representations* on behalf of others come under a new Financial Conduct Authority regulatory regime. Whilst this does not apply to 'pure' expert evidence, it would seem prudent to avoid giving pre-action advice to LIPs.

Many experts do not accept instructions from LIPs. However, the CJC discourages experts from declining instructions from LIPs, unless there is good reason, as this can limit access to justice for a disadvantaged group. For psychiatrists, who may find their evidence being challenged by the person about whose mental health they are reporting and who has instructed them so to report, with the risk of consequent harm to them, there may be good reason to decline.

The Positive Letter of Response or Engagement Letter

Send your positive letter of response to an enquiry or engagement letter with your terms and conditions. Box 4.2 sets out what should be included in the letter generally. A sample letter is in online Appendix 1. It can be adapted to take into account guidance or requirements specific to the jurisdiction.

the Guidance (para. 17) advises that terms of appointment should be agreed and it sets out what they should normally include (Box 4.3). It is of general applicability except that the last two points do not apply *in Ireland.*

If you are asked to attend a preliminary hearing to determine the admissibility of your evidence, expect a searching enquiry, but do not see it as a challenge to your expertise or a criticism and go on the defensive. This is the court or tribunal satisfying itself that you are the appropriate expert.

Box 4.2 Matters to Be Covered in Positive Letter of Response to an Enquiry

- Confirm that there is no conflict of interest, or draw attention to any that, it has been agreed, does not disqualify you.
- State that the work is within your expertise.
- State that you can comply with the timetable.
- If the trial has been fixed, indicate dates and times to avoid if possible. If it has not been fixed, indicate how to obtain an up-to-date commitments list.
- If evidence is to be by telephone conference or video link, indicate how much notice will be needed to make arrangements.
- If, for example in a family case, you do not want to be named, or otherwise identified, in any public judgment, say so.

Box 4.3 Terms of Appointment to Be Agreed at the Outset in a Civil Case

- the capacity in which the expert is to be appointed (e.g. party-appointed expert, single joint expert or expert advisor);
- the services required of the expert (e.g. provision of expert's report, answering questions in writing, attendance at meetings and attendance at court);
- time for delivery of the report;
- the basis of the expert's charges (either daily or hourly rates and an estimate of the time likely to be required, or a total fee for the services);
- travelling expenses and disbursements;
- cancellation charges;
- any fees for attending court;
- time for making the payment;
- whether fees are to be paid by a third party;
- if a party is publicly funded, whether or not the expert's charges will be subject to assessment by a costs officer.

Fees

Experts usually charge by the hour. Fees may be fixed or negotiable. If the latter, their level will depend on how you value your time, your experience and reputation, the scarcity of the relevant expertise, the source of funding, the value and importance of the case and what the market will withstand. The court may place a limit on your fees. If you consider it unreasonable, your instructing solicitors, with supporting evidence from you, may be able to have it increased.

You may seek to agree that you will be paid what you have reasonably estimated the cost of the report to be irrespective of any limit set by the court, but this may necessitate your instructing solicitors, or their client, making up the shortfall. So, solicitors will often state up front that fees should be subject to costs assessment or limited; they may not agree to becoming responsible for the shortfall.

You have a duty to record the time you spend and the Legal Aid Agency (LAA) has the right to audit your records. So, keep readily accessible, detailed and accurate records. Online Appendix 2 is an example of a time sheet for the initial report. It can be adapted for addenda/amendments, experts' meetings and joint statements, attendance at conferences and court, etc.

You may be asked to accept deferral of payment to the conclusion of the case. If you have to pay income tax on those fees before they are paid, consider a percentage increase to reflect the fact that effectively you are providing a loan which, if obtained from a bank, would attract interest.

Aim to provide an estimate based on preparation, the length of the consultation and drafting the report. *In England and Wales*, in a civil case, a party applying for permission to rely on expert evidence has to provide an estimate of the cost. In high value cases, the court makes a 'costs management order' at the first procedural hearing. This sets a costs budget for the whole case. For solicitors' 'cost estimates', they need estimates for each defined step in the litigation process: the initial report; additional work pre-trial, including supplementary reports, answers to questions, reviewing surveillance and other evidence such as expert reports; conferences with counsel; experts' meetings; and trial attendance. Use your detailed records to work out averages and likely maxima; use these to estimate fees for different types of case. Beware estimating on the basis of the average case; half the time you will be out of pocket. You can provide a copy of your analysis if you are asked to provide the information for cost estimates (see online Appendix 3). As the court decides the *maximum* amount of expert costs, you can negotiate on the basis of your *maximum* fee and then charge for the *actual* time spent. Far better to overestimate and charge less. Do not underestimate. Solicitors will find it difficult and annoying going back to the court to ask for an increased fee; in itself this will add to the costs. However, in fixed fee cases you may want to agree a fee based on average time and absorb the differences for the sake of clarity and expediency.

Terms and Conditions

The United Kingdom Register of Expert Witnesses, the Academy of Experts and the Expert Witness Institute all produce model terms and conditions. These can be adapted to cover all matters in Box 4.3. Best practice is to obtain independent legal advice in the drafting of such a document.

If you take instructions from LIPs, consumer legislation requires a formal contract. For clients seen in your rooms, this is usually in the form of an 'on-premises contract' within the meaning of the Consumer Contracts Regulations 2013 and the Consumer Rights Act 2015. A sample contract is shown in online Appendix 4.

Whilst the overall aim of anyone in business is to make a profit, the ethical expert will want to balance the obligation to assist in the administration of justice against pecuniary gain and to ensure that expertise is available to people of limited financial means. Be willing to undertake some cases *pro bono* and others at uneconomic rates, but it must be pure *pro bono* and not work on a 'no win, no fee' basis, in which case your impartiality (as in a contingency fee arrangement) might be in issue.

Curriculum Vitae

Prepare tailored *curricula vitae* (CVs), perhaps a page or two long, focused on the training and experience relevant to a particular type of case. They can also be used to create Appendix 1 in your report (see Chapter 6, 'The Writer' and Appendix 1 in Appendices A and B). Offer a list of relevant publications with the option of sending copies. It can make the difference between you or a less erudite expert being chosen.

Your CV must be accurate and up-to-date. Check carefully the wording of qualifications and memberships. Beware claiming membership of a body of which you have ceased to be a member. Some judges have been highly critical of such errors. A simple error can lead to a complaint to the GMC of dishonesty. Carefully distinguish between memberships by subscription and memberships by examination. The GMC will not wish to see any untruths, exaggerations or material omissions. Your honesty should not be an issue. 'A poorly drafted CV can provide substantial ammunition to an attorney set on discrediting an expert' (Babitsky *et al.* 2000, p. 77). If you have exaggerated your CV, it can be argued that you have exaggerated your opinion.

Balance of Claimant and Defendant Work

In civil (mostly personal injury) work, you may be asked about your balance of claimant, defendant and SJE instructions. You may be asked about the balance of defendant and prosecution reports in criminal cases. Lawyers see this as a mark of impartiality or otherwise. But getting a balance is not always that simple, especially at the beginning. The Crown Prosecution Service (CPS) requests relatively few reports as these are generally reactive to defence reports; many defence reports are not disclosed as they do not support the client's case. You are more likely to be instructed by the prosecution in England and Wales if you are on the National Crime Agency's list of expert advisors. In personal injury cases, insurers and their solicitors will judge you by the reports disclosed by claimants' solicitors, unaware of your reports which have not been disclosed. So, you must be honest when asked and be open to taking cases from both sides.

In order to avoid an imbalance of claimant and defendant instructions in personal injury cases, run two waiting lists, as Dr Donald Johnson taught one of us (K. R.), so that the number of claimant and defendant reports is approximately equal.

Qualified Acceptance of Instructions

If your answers to some questions in Box 4.1 are in the negative, it may be for want of further information, which may be forthcoming on request. Trials can be moved and evidence can be given by video link or even by telephone on occasion. Do not ignore deadlines, but do not be shy of asking for more time at the outset. Usually, all it takes is for the solicitors to apply to the court once they know they have an otherwise willing expert.

Have a low threshold for declaring potential conflicts of interest and before accepting instructions. Your evidence will not automatically be rendered inadmissible; it is the nature and the extent of the interest that matters (*Armchair Passenger Transport Ltd v Helical Bar plc* [2003] EWHC 367). Clearly, if there is a genuine conflict of interest – for example, their client is a relation – you must refuse, but less obvious ones, such as being acquainted with an expert, should be declared. Always try and view it from the perspective of the ordinary person. In *EXP v Barker* [2015] EWHC 1289 (QB), the defendant and his neuroradiology expert had doctored their CVs to conceal any prior relationship. The expert had trained the defendant, written at least one paper with him and assisted him in securing posts. Although the trial judge considered that this went to the weight of the expert's evidence, the Court of Appeal would not have disagreed if he had found it inadmissible. However, in the urogynaecology clinical negligence case of *Haughey v Newry and Mourne Health and Social Care Trust* [2013] NICA 78, the Northern Ireland Court of Appeal refused to deprecate the practice of calling local expert witnesses where there were only six specialists in the jurisdiction, all known to each other and all members of the Ulster Gynae Urology Society of which the defendant had been chairman and whose successor had been his expert witness. But where possible this should be avoided. If you already know something of the case, or have knowledge of related proceedings, it may be advisable to decline instructions. If you consider accepting, you must fully inform those instructing you. They need to be aware of the fact that, if you know of other relevant evidence, you may well have a duty to give the court a full account of it and indicate how, if it has, it has influenced your opinion.

In Scotland, experts must disclose to their instructing solicitors whether they have worked with the expert instructed by the opposing party (if known).

Sooner rather than later you should have administrative help. Your assistant will soon learn which templates to use and which questions to ask, but you must always check the final letter to make sure it is correctly tailored to the case; this can make the difference between being accepted or rejected.

Getting Ready for Starter's Orders

If your terms and conditions are accepted, it is time to prepare.

First, reconsider the issues to be addressed. They may relate to a particular statutory or common law legal test. You may need it explaining: 'it is a good thing for the expert to have before him the legal test' (*Routestone Ltd v Minories Finance Ltd* [1996] 5 WLUK 237). This is particularly important if your report is for an unfamiliar jurisdiction. Experts *in Scotland* are required to 'ensure that they are up-to-date with the current legal criteria before they give an opinion as to insanity or diminished responsibility, although it is the responsibility of the commissioning agent to ensure that the medical practitioner is provided with the relevant information' (Scottish Executive 2005, ch. 3, para. 13). This is just good practice.

Second, make sure that you have all the relevant documents. The Guidance (para. 30) requires experts to try to ensure that they have access to all relevant information held by the parties, and that the same information has been disclosed to each expert in the same discipline. Experts should seek to confirm this expeditiously, notifying instructing solicitors of any omissions. Do not be bullied into starting without all necessary materials. You may realise that there are likely to be in existence relevant documents of which your instructing solicitors are unaware and if so they should obtain them sooner rather than later. Almost always it will be necessary to see the subject's general practice records or some other medical records, otherwise the history will be uncorroborated and thereby vulnerable to attack by either party.

If something becomes obvious after you have seen the subject, inform your instructing solicitors what you need to see before you complete the report. Be prepared to see the subject again or even speak to an informant (with appropriate permission), if subsequent disclosures raise issues which need resolving.

Records

Your records should be stored safely and securely, readily retrievable and in compliance with the General Data Protection Regulation (GDPR) and the Data Protection Act 2018 (DPA). This can be in digital form. Keep records for at least seven to ten years depending on your attitude to risk. This is because there is a six-year limitation period for bringing a professional negligence claim or making a complaint to the GMC (but no limitation period for the making of a complaint to the MC). Furthermore, the limitation period begins to run from the date of accrual of the cause of action, which may be considerably later than the date of the assessment or report.

Following the introduction of the GDPR, it may be sensible to keep only those records that relate to your own examination. The evidence bundles, including the medical records, can be either returned to the instructing solicitors or, with agreement, confidentially destroyed. Retention requirements for records in criminal cases are shown in Box 4.4. Any subsequent communications and replies should be carefully filed, including any notification that a report has been disclosed to the other side. Have an index/contents page on which you can record the progress of the case and the location of subsidiary material such as DVDs or files (see online Appendix 5).

Deadlines and Timetables

Ensure that your report is delivered by the agreed time or otherwise to your own standards. Solicitors in criminal cases may need your report to discuss with their client on a prison visit

Box 4.4 Retention Requirements for Records in Criminal Cases in England and Wales

- Cases involving homicide, riot, Official Secrets Acts, treason and other offences against the state, terrorist offences, offences listed in Sch 1 of the Children and Young Persons Act 1933, kidnapping and all cases in which a sentence of life imprisonment has been imposed: twenty years.
- Other criminal cases tried on indictment: ten years.
- All cases tried summarily: one year.
- All other criminal cases: one year.

These times are from the date on which the court or tribunal finally disposed of the case.

pre trial. Solicitors in civil cases may need to confer with insurance companies. Solicitors in family cases are likely to be under the thumb of a judge trying to impose strict time limits. Judges may need your report as part of the 'bundle' which they study a day or so before the case. If there are likely to be problems in meeting deadlines, hopefully due to understandable problems rather than your own laziness, inform your instructing solicitor as soon as possible so they can ask for an extension if appropriate. If you miss a deadline, there may be a costs penalty for you or your instructing solicitors, your report may not be admitted and, even worse, the case may collapse. Any serious lack of engagement can lead to a complaint to the GMC, which expects you to 'cooperate with case management, making sure you meet the timescales for producing reports and going to conferences, meetings or court hearings' (AWLP) or the MC.

Information Technology

The practice in the Commercial and High Court of providing electronic copies of reports is spreading. It is not unusual, because of the speed with which reports are required, for electronic reports to be sent to solicitors ahead of the paper copy. Have appropriate security in place, with documents in non-editable form and some form of encryption. Passwords should be sent by another mode of communication.

Commitments and Holidays

Solicitors should enquire about your availability for trial when seeking to instruct you. Often, this is impossible because the trial date has yet to be set. Occasionally, solicitors are frankly too ill-organised, even when they find out the dates of trials, to mention it to you. Then they panic at the last minute! Even then, the commitments of a busy medicolegal expert are continually changing and it is not unheard of for there to be clashes between two cases. In those circumstances, the solicitor who has served a witness summons always wins. In the absence of such, the solicitors may have to argue it out between themselves and their respective courts. If a witness summons requires you to attend for a longer period than required for you to give evidence, you can appeal against it. Even if there is no summons, you can have discussions about which day in a trial you can attend.

There is no substitute, though, for having a very clearly organised diary and no better person for organising this than a very efficient personal assistant. An important part of this diary will be your holiday and conference dates. In *Matthews v Tarmac Bricks & Tiles Ltd* [1999] EWHC Civ 1574, Lord Woolf MR declared that:

> It was important that in cases where doctors were involved as much notice as possible was given for the date of the hearing. However, it was essential that it was appreciated that, whereas the courts would take account of the important commitments of medical men [sic], they could not always meet those commitments in a way which would be satisfactory from the doctor's point of view ... Doctors who held themselves out as practicing [sic] in the medicolegal field had to be prepared to arrange their affairs to meet the commitments of the courts where that was practical.

So, other than in Ireland, where the judiciary is still quite indulgent of the needs of 'medical men' and will seek to accommodate their availability, medical experts may sometimes have to interrupt their holidays either physically to appear in court or to give evidence by live link or telephone. However, this arrangement is certainly not reciprocal. Judges' holidays are apparently sacrosanct as HHJ Robert Taylor wrote in *The Times* (7 July 1999): 'A holiday is for recreation, being deprived of which is not going to make people better judges. As an American Supreme Court Justice once said: "I can do a year's work in 10 or 11 months – but not in 12!".'

Getting Paid

The best way to get paid is to be an expert in Ireland. The legal costs landscape there is very different from that in England and Wales and such that you should not release your report until payment has been received. Next best is to be an expert in the Isle of Man, where the instructing advocates will obtain a cheque from their client payable to the expert before authorising the expert to start work and then release it by return upon receipt of 'a satisfactory report' and fee note.

Remember that if you are taxed on what you charge rather than what you have been paid, you will need some money in the bank for the tax bill.

Have a clear invoicing system with numbered sequential invoices and remember that the more detailed a breakdown you are able to give, the less likely your fees are to be queried or challenged.

Mainly, you have to trust that solicitors will live up to their obligations. But it is as well to accept their disregard of your contracted timescale. Occasionally, they, and more frequently medicolegal reporting agencies, go bankrupt. Faced with a non-paying solicitor, you need to distinguish your desire to be paid from your duty to the court. You may even need to ask the court for guidance – for example, when the solicitor asks you to re-examine the subject despite not having paid for a report. Rather than 'chasing' solicitors yourself, have a low threshold for delegating it. Where possible, try and build the cost of this into your pricing structure.

There will be a minority of cases where you have no real choice but to threaten, or even take, legal action to recover your debt. You may well lose the relationship, but if the solicitor is on the verge of bankruptcy, being an official creditor will put you at the front of the queue for later payment. Or, if you have been served a witness summons, point out that, other than very exceptionally, the court will set aside a witness summons served on the expert by a solicitor who has not paid their fees (*Brown v Bennett*, Times, 2 November 2000 (QBD)).

Marketing

The best way to market your services as an expert witness is to prepare reports and give testimony of such high quality that solicitors and barristers recommend you to their colleagues. In the meantime, there are several things you can do to get yourself known.

Consider advertising, but bear in mind the GMC and MC guidance on advertising. It must be factually accurate and evidence-based; do not make claims which are false, misleading or unsubstantiated, or which suggest that you are better than colleagues or have the potential to raise false expectations. Include your GMC/MC registration number. *In Ireland*, your letter head should not include membership of associations or societies other than those recognised or accredited by appropriate training bodies.

Get your name into one of the better-known expert witness registers and have a website. If you are really keen, write a blog, but all forms of writing, articles for 'trade journals', peer-reviewed papers and articles in the press raise your profile, as do talks to learned societies, groups of solicitors or conferences. Social media can be used for business purposes (you must create business pages or sites, not use your personal status). Announcements can be made on multiple platforms and social media can also be used to 'drive' traffic towards your website or to contact your practice by other means such as email or phone. Old-fashioned business cards can be useful. Produce promotional material about your practice for physical or electronic delivery to solicitors.

Probity and Compliance

Expert witness work brings with it responsibilities beyond those of being a good doctor. You have a duty to comply with the legal rules surrounding the work that you do. Be as careful in your business dealings as you are in your medical practice; this means careful compliance with all appropriate laws and regulations. Your business dealings may not escape the notice of the GMC or MC. A retired professor of microbiology indicated an intention to mislead the Legal Services Commission in order to obtain financial advantage and expressed a willingness to provide a false estimate of the number of hours likely to be worked in order to obtain an enhanced fee. He was suspended from the Medical Register for three months.

Register with the appropriate information or data protection commissioner's office. You must comply with the GDPR and the DPA. At the least, you will need a data protection policy, a privacy notice and advisedly a separate consent form for data processing.

Keep your insurer abreast of your earnings, as the fee you pay may depend on this to some extent.

Take out appropriate insurance, including employers' liability and public liability insurance, and almost certainly insurance against a costly tax investigation. You must keep accurate and clear financial records and, in case of a revenue audit, for at least six years. If or when you approach the threshold, you must register for and charge value added tax (VAT).

A well-known psychiatrist was asked, at the opening of his cross-examination in a murder trial, how long he had spent with the prisoner. After he had replied, the QC reached down and lifted up a huge and heavy tome, with much huffing and puffing, and through the pages of which he slowly leafed, building up a sense of suspense, until he came to the date of the psychiatrist's visit to the prison. This was the prison's 'gate book', which recorded the time of the psychiatrist's arrival at, and the time of his departure from, the prison!

With your business affairs in order, you are ready to look at the medicolegal consultation.

Further Reading

Allen, D. (2014) *Business for Medics: How to Set Up and Run a Medical Practice* (Kindle Direct Publishing).

The Medicolegal Consultation

Keith Rix

I must say that, as a litigant, I should dread a lawsuit beyond almost anything else, short of sickness or death.

Judge Learned Hand, quoted by Shapiro (1993, p. 304)

In cases involving medical issues, the medicolegal consultation, comprising history-taking and examination, supplemented sometimes by tests or investigations and, wherever possible, information from an informant, lies at the heart of the process of assisting the court. It provides the psychiatric expert with the opportunity to use training, skill and experience to explore by effective questioning the subject's symptoms, in the context of their family, personal and medical history and personality, and, through careful observation of the physical and mental state, to assess their current condition. The consultation requires the highest standards and should be conducted with an awareness and understanding of the potential effects of the proceedings on the subject. Without a personal consultation with the subject, you are reliant on the records made by others as to the subject's history and condition.

The consultation is an important and potentially stressful experience for the subject. The litigation may have dominated their life for years. Their liberty, reputation, career or financial security may be at stake. They may have been waiting for the appointment for some time, have had to travel a long distance and suffered other inconvenience to get to it. If you are seeing a prisoner, they may not be expecting you or they may have been wrongly informed as to who you are and the purpose of the visit. If you are instructed by 'the other side', they may be expecting a hostile consultation. It may be the first time that they have seen a psychiatrist. They may have some of the popular misapprehensions of psychiatry. They may resent the psychiatric label or be angry that their solicitors have sent them.

Arrangements for the Consultation

Fix a date for the consultation and send an 'appointment letter' (online Appendix 6). The subject needs due notice, although sometimes it is necessary to arrange appointments at short notice. Allow for how far away they live and, where appropriate, their capacity for complicated journeys using different forms of public transport.

The appointment letter should include or enclose:

- the nature and purpose of the consultation;
- the likely length of the consultation;
- who has requested the consultation;
- where, when and at what time the consultation will take place;

- a request for details of any special requirements (such as a downstairs consulting room, an interpreter);
- any requirements as to proof of identity and advising as to whether it is intended to take a photograph for identification or other purposes;
- contact details sufficient to enable the appointment to be changed, a warning to be given of late arrival or for directions to be sought en route;
- how to complain;
- travel directions, details of car-parking arrangements and, if appropriate, information as to how and where refreshments may be obtained.

Online Appendix 7 sets out the information that you could consider providing on your website.

The Essential Ingredients

Courtesy

It is surprising how often subjects report that experts they have seen 'for the other side' have treated them unpleasantly, abruptly or condescendingly.

Respect

However distasteful or objectionable the subject's actual or alleged behaviour, whatever your views about the merits of the litigation, or however appalled you feel about a parent's alleged behaviour towards their child, the subject is a fellow human. It is not for you to judge them; treat them with respect.

Sympathetic Objectivity

A sympathetic approach helps you to build rapport and elicit a reliable history. The subject wants to know that someone is prepared to listen, to believe them, if they are telling the truth, and to try and understand what it feels like for them. But sympathy must be combined with objectivity. It is not necessary to believe everything they say. It is a forensic investigation; the doctor's usual therapeutic objectives must almost always take second place to the requirement for evidence that assists in achieving the overriding objectives of justice and fairness.

Patience

Some people find it difficult enough giving their history to any specialist, even more so a psychiatrist and particularly if it is for the first time. A hurried and inaccurate history is not in the subject's interests, in the interests of justice or in the interests of the expert who may have this failing exposed in the witness box. They need time, patience and often encouragement to tell their story.

The Venue

Your safety is paramount. Aim for a reasonable balance between the safety measures in a hospital emergency consultation room and an environment in which the subject feels as comfortable as possible. Have an agreed method of summoning assistance. If you are consulting outside usual clinic hours, consider whether it is safe to do so or what special precautions are needed.

If the subject is in a prison or a psychiatric facility, ask whether you should see them on their own. You may need to be accompanied or have a personal safety alarm. In prison, ascertain the arrangements for summoning help.

You may decide to hire a room in a hotel or a meeting room in a business centre. Where someone is housebound or unable to travel, a home assessment may be necessary, but ask if the solicitor would see the subject in their home. Consider taking someone with you. Ensure that someone knows the time and location of your consultation. Solicitors are often willing for you to see their client at their offices.

You are advised not to see the subject in your own home. A retired consultant psychiatrist was killed in his home by a former patient. His name was on a gate-post. The patient had been looking for another of his former consultants; fortunately, he had moved.

A formal consulting room allows you to get used to how people respond in that setting. Make it welcoming. Carpet, curtains and fresh flowers help. Have a chair identical to that of the subject or at least sit at the same level. If it is also an office, organise it so that the subject feels that they are your priority, that you were expecting them and you were prepared. Paper tissues are essential. If the subject cannot bring in a hot beverage, there should at least be water available.

If you conduct the assessment by video link, draw attention to how this can limit the assessment of appearance and behaviour and prevent the utilisation of the senses of touch and smell.

Be Prepared

Medical Records

Only exceptionally, conduct the consultation without seeing the subject's medical records. As Boyle (2016, p. 129) says:

> The import of the medical records is huge:
>
> - Did the claimant actually seek treatment when he said he did?
> - What did he tell the doctors about his accident?
> - Did he mention the sites of pain which he latterly complains were injured?
> - Did he attend the doctor with other complaints whilst not mentioning his current problems?
> - Does he, in fact, have a long history of similar, or related, complaints which cast doubt on his assertions about causation of his current injuries?
> - Have there been subsequent accidents?

Inconsistencies between what is in the records and the subject's history and questions about unexpected entries are best addressed at the initial consultation rather than by having to recall the subject.

The subject may consider as inadequately prepared an expert who has not considered their medical records and this can compromise the consultation.

If there are redactions, consider asking for an unredacted version.

Chaperones and Interpreters

Consider, and if necessary make, arrangements for a professional interpreter or chaperone. It is inadvisable to use family or friends as interpreters. Chaperoning may be necessary for physical examination, where there is a history of abuse, where gender issues arise or in order to respect cultural conventions.

Security Clearance and Related Requirements

If the subject is in prison custody, allow time for security clearance. Heed what you are not allowed to take into a prison. If you have to return several times to leave behind yet more items, do not be surprised if it is 'dinner time' shortly after, or even before, you get to the prisoner.

Timetabling

Have sufficient time available. Consider the need for more than one consultation. Be able to contact the subject if the consultation is going to be delayed or postponed. Allow time to read the documentation either a day or so ahead or just before the consultation. The appointment should take place when you are unlikely to be interrupted; if an interruption is expected, explain this. Start on time; a delay may make the subject more anxious, give the impression that they are not important or cause them to rush.

Opening the Consultation

Your Professional Demeanour

Remind yourself that their solicitor may ask their client how you treated them. Cultivate, or display, an appropriate professional demeanour. Introduce yourself and find out how they wish to be addressed.

Should Anyone Else Be Present?

Usually, it is best to see the subject on their own. Sometimes, a chaperone may be advisable. Occasionally, the subject may be too nervous to be seen on their own. In *Whitehead v Avon County Council (No. 1)* [1995] 4 WLUK 267, the Court of Appeal refused an application by a nervous subject to have a friend present, although in *Hall v Avon Health Authority* [1980] 1 WLR 481, it was held that the attendance of a third party would be particularly appropriate if the claimant 'were in a nervous state or confused by a serious head injury, or if the defendant's nominated doctor had a reputation for a fierce examining manner'. What matters is that the subject should be sufficiently at ease to form a rapport and give a reliable history. The presence of a partner or friend may inhibit them from giving a full and frank history. Experts who have allowed a family member to be present have sometimes been criticised in court because the history may have come not from the subject, but the accompanying person, or may have been influenced by their presence or non-verbal communication. Sometimes, it is advisable to see the subject and accompanying person for the introduction to the consultation and then, if the subject is willing, for the accompanying person to leave. There are exceptions. With severely brain-injured claimants, it is commonly regarded as essential to have a family member or another familiar person present. When assessing capacity, it may be necessary to establish what the claimant can achieve with the assistance of a relative, friend or professional who works with them.

If a third party is present, arrange the seating so that you can observe and control communication.

Introducing Yourself, Explaining and Obtaining Consent

Explain who you are, who has instructed you, the nature of the consultation, its purpose and the limits of confidentiality.

Before you can engage as an expert in a consultation for the purpose of producing a report and disclosing information about the subject to a third party, informed consent must be obtained from them or a person with the legal right to consent on their behalf. Consent is required for (1) assessment and obtaining any collateral history, other records, etc., (2) compiling a report based on (1), and (3) furnishing that report to the commissioner. Ensure that they are not attending under duress, which renders any consent invalid. Consent should not be assumed simply because you have been instructed to prepare a report on the subject.

Make it clear that the subject may refuse at the outset. They must be aware that upon its disclosure the report may advance or damage their interests and that by consenting to the report being prepared, they are consenting to it being used for the purpose for which it is requested, which will usually be to advise the instructing party, and, unless it is the report of an occupational health physician (OHP) to an employer following a management referral, or an independent report for an OHP (see Chapter 13, 'Consent and Confidentiality'), their consent to a medical assessment/report on behalf of a third party may mean that they have no right to see the report or have any control over its content or disclosure to that third party. They should be made aware that refusing a reasonable request of a defendant/respondent for a medical assessment and report, or making consent conditional in some way, may result in their claim being stayed until such time as consent is given (CPR 3.1(2)(f)). Although the staying of proceedings, until they do so, effectively requires that the requested assessment and report be carried out if the proceedings are to be progressed (and otherwise making the claimant a *spoliator* in their own cause), such is the price of litigation. In short, a claimant who puts their medical condition in issue would be obliged to consent to examination and would have no control over the contents of the resulting report or any right to see it. A report commissioned by a defendant/respondent is covered by legal professional privilege. Its purpose would be destroyed were there to be an obligation to the subject to obtain their consent before its disclosure to the defendant/respondent. It is where consent to the assessment, the compilation of the report and the furnishing of it to the commissioner is insufficiently specific and not fully informed that difficulties may arise.

If the subject wishes to make furnishing of the report to the commissioner conditional on (1) prior review and/or (2) prior approval, there is no consent to doing otherwise, irrespective of views as to the impropriety of doing so in any situation. This is best addressed, however, by the commissioner in advance. Thus, if it is a condition of the commissioning of the report that it be furnished without prior review and/or approval, and the subject refuses, there is no consent to the process and seeking to prepare a report is a futile exercise. If the commissioner is agnostic on the point, or is satisfied that a report be furnished subject to prior review and/or approval by the subject, there can be no complaint if it is not furnished. But, at the outset, the expert should clarify with the commissioner, in agreeing their terms and conditions, that even if the subject does not consent to the report's release, they expect to be paid for work undertaken.

Consent does not have to be in writing, but it is always preferable for reasons of proof and it assists if the subject complains, for example, that something was not explained or that they did not know the purpose of the consultation. Create or adapt a written consent form (online Appendix 8). It is a useful framework for explaining the nature and purpose of the consultation. It may be advisable to have a separate consent form for GDPR purposes (online Appendix 9).

Make clear that the subject does not have to answer any questions, although this may severely limit the usefulness of the report. If they choose not to answer *some* questions, this may limit its usefulness, but perhaps not significantly. They may disclose sensitive information. Agree to identify this in the report, but they need to know that the solicitors and court may not be able to restrict its circulation. They need to know that nothing is 'off the record'; any relevant information must be disclosed; the expert 'cannot receive information "in confidence" from anybody . . . The watchwords should be openness and sound preparation' (*County Council v SB*). If they make an 'off the record disclosure', this is a withdrawal of consent and the instructing solicitor should be advised accordingly, although the disclosure still attracts a quality of confidence and cannot be articulated to the solicitor without further consent.

In the case of an LIP, it is particularly important to be satisfied that the LIP is able properly to consent and that you have clearly set out your role and the applicable court rules. Everything must be properly recorded, and extra care taken to confirm the instructions they have given and ensure that consent is fully informed.

Occasionally, a subject may not be able to consent and lack the capacity to do so. In a criminal case, this may be someone who is unfit to plead and stand trial. In a civil case, it may be a brain-injured claimant who lacks the capacity to litigate.

In such a case, it may be a breach of confidence but in the subject's best interests to prepare a report without their consent. The GMC states: 'You may disclose personal information if it is of overall benefit to a patient who lacks the capacity to consent' (GMC 2017b). Justify this in the report. Consider consulting with others, such as carers or relatives, before deciding whether to proceed in an incapacitated person's best interests.

In Ireland, best interests may also be applicable (Assisted Decision-Making (Capacity) Act 2015 (ADM(C)A), s 8), but in the context of, for example, criminal or catastrophic injury proceedings, there is also a public interest in disclosure of relevant matters; it facilitates the proper administration of justice, be it the acquittal of a person who was incapable of forming the *mens rea* for an offence, addressing fitness to plead or facilitating the proper compensation of a tortiously injured claimant. When balanced, public interests tend to outweigh private interest that may incline in the opposite direction.

History Taking and Examination

Usually, avoid discussing the alleged offence or the cause of the action (i.e. an accident or allegedly negligent treatment) at the beginning. In a criminal case, take the whole history prior to the alleged offence and then ask, if appropriate, about the alleged offence. In a personal injury case, take a background history prior to the accident or allegedly negligent treatment and then ask about the incident or circumstances giving rise to the claim.

In a criminal case, the subject's history between the alleged offence and the consultation must be distinguished from the history prior to the alleged offence. In a personal injury case, the subject's history subsequent to the accident or allegedly negligent treatment will be of critical significance, but it will need to be considered against the background of their history up to the potentially injurious event or events and compared to what their personal and medical history might have been but for the accident or allegedly negligent treatment.

Sometimes, subjects attempt to dismiss any enquiry as to their lives prior to the alleged offence or the accident. Explain that you need to understand them as a person: in a civil action, their unique reaction to a traumatic event may be more, or only, understandable in the light of their previous history; in a criminal case, their life up to the alleged offence may assist in understanding why they acted as they did. Also, in many civil cases, explain that, to give an opinion as to the effects of the accident on how they cope with life, relationships, employment and social functioning, you need to understand what their life was like before the accident. Perhaps explain also that such a detailed history is essential for choosing between treatment options, predicting their likely response to treatment and giving an overall prognosis.

The medical expert is best placed to obtain a detailed and accurate history of physical, psychological or psychiatric symptomatology, including a painstakingly detailed account of an event, or series of events, such as a criminal offence or a road traffic accident, their effects on activities of daily living and any limitations attributable to injuries. Only the medical expert has the skill to establish this factual evidence as to injuries, symptoms, effects and consequences. Record it carefully in the subject's own words. This part of your report is likely to be analysed in depth by the lawyers and compared with the account given to the other side's expert, perhaps accounts given to other experts, the contents of the medical records or police interviews, the subject's proof of evidence or witness statement and perhaps even a covert recording of the consultation.

A full mental state examination is mandatory and extended cognitive testing may be needed. The examination starts when you meet the subject in the waiting room and it finishes when you return them to the waiting room. The nature and extent of the physical examination will depend on the nature of the case.

Certain investigations may be indicated. It may be appropriate to use rating scales and questionnaires, although their interpretation and validity may be questioned because they are unlikely to have been validated in a medicolegal setting and where they are even more prone to bias than in clinical practice. They provide fertile ground for cross-examination. Many screen for psychiatric disorder, but, if a full psychiatric assessment is carried out, screening is unnecessary.

Limit investigations to those of a medical nature. A psychiatrist appeared before the GMC when a complaint was made that he had organised the covert surveillance of a police officer in a police pension case. In *Charnock v Rowan* [2012] EWCA Civ 2, the court disagreed with the suggestion that 'the doctor's role is routinely that of a sleuth' and observed that forensic medical practice had been disfigured by the practitioners who took such a role. It may be permissible to record the subject's gait as they walk to the gate, but do not follow them down the road. The private investigator will probably already be there.

A History from an Informant

It is often helpful and sometimes advisable, even essential, to obtain a history from an informant. In family cases, it is assumed that collateral information will be sought, and that in reports for sentencing in criminal cases a history and information will be obtained from the defendant's family. Albeit not usually an uninterested party, it is helpful to hear about the impact of the person's condition from the person who may know them best. It provides a check on the accuracy of what they say. This is not just about being alive to exaggeration. Especially in the case of the brain-injured, people with dementia and the intellectually disabled, memory problems, lack of insight, confabulation, slow information processing, etc. can lead to an under-estimate or misunderstanding of their disability.

Records

Record the consultation on paper or a PC. Records should be structured, clear, legible and comprehensive so they can be studied by another expert to see why and how opinions have been reached. They should be accurate. A neurologist was criticised in *Williams v Jervis* [2009] EWHC 1837 (QB) for mis-recording some of what the claimant had told him as was demonstrated by the claimant's transcript of a covert tape-recording of the consultation. In consequence the party calling him was penalised with an order for indemnity costs. Record the times of the start and finish of the consultation.

Further Enquiries

Do not hesitate to recommend a further consultation, obtaining further records or obtaining further evidence without which you will have to express only a provisional or qualified opinion. Occasionally it may be necessary to recommend the instruction of another expert.

You are now ready to draft your report.

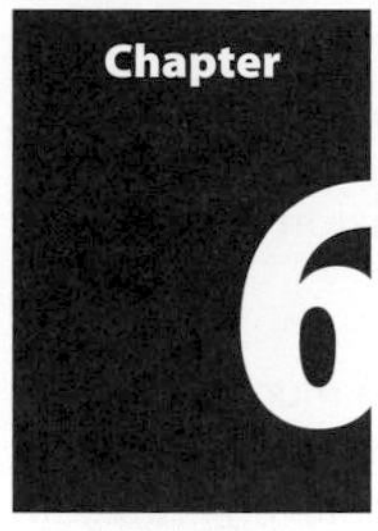

Chapter 6 The Report, Amendments, Answers to Questions, Experts' Meetings and Conferences

Keith Rix

[T]he purpose of an expert report and the giving of expert opinion evidence is to assist the court; it is not to advocate on behalf of the patient.

Barton J in *Flanagan v Minister for Public Expenditure and Reform* [2018] IEHC 208

The Report

The purpose of the report is to communicate your opinion so as to assist the court as to the matters in issue and enable it to do justice. Consider the likely readership, which will usually be the intelligent lay person with no medical knowledge, but if in doubt aim for the lowest common denominator. Write in plain English. Make it comprehensible to the first-time reader and easy to follow. 'People who do not have a medical background may rely on your advice and evidence to help them make decisions. Where it is possible to do so without misleading anyone, you should use language and terminology that people who are not medically qualified will understand' (GMP). Especially for a jury, it has to tell a story they can follow and hold their interest. As the jury rarely sees the report, you will be able to précis it in suitable language when you give your evidence.

Use one of the model forms. Those of the Academy of Experts and the Expert Witness Institute have been drawn up by judges. If cases go to trial, the 'judge-friendly' format may be critical. But in any event, readers are assisted by easily navigable reports which are easily compared because of their similar format. In reports for the criminal jurisdiction in England and Wales, there are a number of 'necessary inclusions' (*R v B* [2006] EWCA Crim 417). All are reflected in this chapter.

Sometimes, depending on the nature of the case or the instructions, or for a particular jurisdiction, you can depart from the model format.

See the appendices for specimen reports, one on Daniel McNaughtan (Appendix A) and one on Charles Dickens (Appendix B), laid out according to the model form.

Length of the Report

It was once said that a report should be no more than two pages of foolscap. Today's reports are much longer, but this is changing. Judges prefer short reports and may reduce experts' fees for excessively long reports. His Honour John Cockroft said, quoting a Spanish saying: 'Something good, if it is short, is twice as good.' Judges say that they have little time to read reports. They look for findings and conclusions. Some suggest that the facts, or assumed facts, which justify the conclusions, but which counsel need for examination and cross-examination, can be confined to appendices. Arguably, any facts that are not linked to an opinion can be removed.

What Sir James Munby (2013) said when President of the Family Division of the High Court of England and Wales is more widely applicable:

> [T]oo many reports . . . are simply too long, largely because they contain too much history and too much factual narrative . . . I want to send out a clear message: expert reports can in many cases be much shorter [and] be more focused on analysis and opinion than on history and narrative. In short, expert reports must be succinct, focused and analytical [as well as being] evidence based.

In *Re IA (A Child) (Fact finding; Welfare; Single hearing; Experts' reports)* [2013] EWHC 2499 (Fam), where the judge had stipulated a report of ten to twelve pages and it ran to thirty-five pages, he criticised the expert for devoting a considerable number of pages to issues he had not been asked to address, concluding:

> His report contained an abundance of tedious, even mind numbing detail . . . as well as senseless questions . . . I could scarcely believe what I was reading . . . The modern way exemplified by Dr X's over-inclusive and doubtless expensive report is no longer acceptable. Experts must conform to the specifics of what is asked of them [. . .] I struggle to recall a single instance when such expansive and all inclusive analysis has been of real utility in a case of this kind.

The judge contrasted this expert with 'Professor Christine Hall at Great Ormond Street Hospitals [who] was masterly in her ability to distil essential information and opinion within an impressively succinct report'. In the Family Court, reports are now limited to forty pages (FPR 27A PD 5.2A1).

Solicitors also need shorter reports, otherwise 'the parties and the Court [spend] a disproportionate time reading the reports which results in an increase in costs. Furthermore, the likelihood that important points are lost in the vastness of the context is unhelpfully increased' (*Harman (A Child) v East Kent Hospitals NHS Foundation Trust* [2015] EWHC 1662 (QB)).

Constrained by costs budgets, solicitors will increasingly instruct experts who provide concise reports allowing them to assess their opinions in the minimum of time and judges are likely to 'specify the maximum length of . . . an expert's report' (*Re L (A Child) (Procedure: Bundles: Translations)* [2015] EWFC 15).

Structure

It matters how well-organised the report is. In *Tsui Ning Jacky v Wong Yat Sun* [2006] HKCU 133, where the judge had to choose between the opinions of two experts, he relied not only on the fact that one expert's reasoning was more cogent and rejected the opinion of the other expert as really no more than speculation, but he also took into account how the first expert's report was far better organised and professional. 'The body of the report should be categorised, classified and sub-divided, preferably in numbered points or paragraphs to as great a degree as possible within the confines of the subject matter' (Hodgkinson and James 2015, p. 248).

Box 6.1 Presentation, Content and Style of the Report

- typed;
- first person;
- active voice;
- short sentences and paragraphs;
- headings and sub-headings;
- fact distinguished and separated from opinion;
- clear, concise, succinct, focused, analytical, logical, objective, reliable, evidence-based and of high quality;
- straightforward and not biased, intentionally misleading or false;
- not promoting the view of the instructing party or advocacy;
- transparent and not omitting material or information that does not support the opinion expressed or conclusions reached;
- it should be, and should be seen to be, the product of an independent investigator, regardless of the pressures of the litigation;
- showing the weaknesses as well as the strengths of the case;
- properly and fully researched;
- a 'stand-alone' document;
- good quality paper;
- margins wide enough for written comments – at least 5 cm;
- font size 11 at least (12 obligatory for family proceedings – FPR 27A PD 5.2A1);
- 'Arial' typeface;
- line spacing 1.5 (saves paper) or 2;
- numbered paragraphs (obligatory for family proceedings – FPR 27A PD 5.2A1);
- paper hole-punched for use in a standard lever arch file or ring binder;
- a slide binder because it allows the report to be removed for copying – avoid comb binders, staples and paper clips;
- plastic covers;
- front cover clear so that the title page can be read without opening the folder;
- printed on one side of the page only (obligatory for family proceedings – FPR 27A PD 5.2A1); and
- use of 'headers' and 'footers'.

The points of presentation, content and style of the report that are preferred, if not mandated, are set out in Box 6.1.

The header zone (on all pages except the front page) should set out at the right in bold:

Report of: Dr. J. Hunter
Specialism: Morbid anatomy
On the instructions of: Messrs. Inge and Webb, Solicitors
Prepared for: The Assizes, Warwick

Because most people flick through the bottoms of pages when looking for a document, or a page in a document, in the trial bundle, the footer zone (on all pages except the front page), also in bold, is set out as here on page 2 of the report:

Report of Dr. J. Hunter concerning Sir Theodosius Boughton, Bart **25 February 1781**
R v CAPTAIN JOHN DONNELLAN **2**

If it is not the first report, it should state: 'Second report of . . .'.

Box 6.2 shows a suggested structure.

Box 6.2 The Structure of the Report

Front Page
Contents Page

1. Introduction
   - 1.1 The Writer
   - 1.2 Synopsis
   - 1.3 Instructions
   - 1.4 Summary of Conclusions/Executive Summary (obligatory for family proceedings and a maximum of four pages – FPR 27A PD 5.2A1)
   - 1.5 Disclosure of Interests
2. The Background to the Case and Issues
   - 2.1 The Relevant People
   - 2.2 The Assumed Facts and Substance of All Material Instructions
   - 2.3 The Issues (Questions) to Be Addressed
   - 2.4 The Assumptions Adopted
3. Investigation of the Facts and Assumed Facts
   - 3.1 Methodology
   - 3.2 Interview and Examination/Basis of Report
   - 3.3 Investigations
   - 3.4 Documents and Materials
   - 3.5 Medical Terms and Explanations
4. The Facts and Assumed Facts/Factual Analysis
5. Opinion
6. Summary of Conclusions
7. Declaration
8. Statement of Truth

Signature Block
Appendix 1: Qualifications, Training and Experience of the Writer
Appendix 2: The Process of Psychiatric Assessment
Appendix 3: History and Examination
Appendix 4: Documents and Materials Studied
Appendix 5: Glossary of Medical and Other Terms
Appendix 6: References
Appendix 7: Chronology

Front Page

The top section shows the title of the action:

- the name of the court top left (e.g. 'In the Central Criminal Court');
- the case number top right; and
- the party or parties below and central (e.g. R v Daniel McNaughtan).

The second section identifies the author of the report (e.g. 'Report of Dr. E. T. Monro, Consultant Psychiatrist'). It can be omitted and incorporated in the fourth section, but it must stand out. I once saw a report which was signed illegibly and nowhere in the report was the name of its author.

The third section should include:

- 'On the instructions of' – name and address of those instructing the expert;
- 'Who act on behalf of' – person or party, such as 'The defendant';
- 'Their reference';
- 'Specialist field' (e.g. 'Child and adolescent psychiatry');
- 'Subject matter' (e.g. 'Psychiatric assessment of the Defendant');
- 'Date(s) of instruction(s)';
- 'Date of report';
- 'Report reference';
- 'Date of consultation';
- 'Place of consultation';
- Mode of consultation – 'Face-to-face' or 'Live link';
- 'Consent' – 'Written', 'Verbal' or 'Not applicable'.

The fourth section should include:

- Name of expert;
- Post-nominal qualifications;
- Status/appointment;
- GMC/MC number;
- Contact details, including:
    - full professional/correspondence address;
    - telephone number(s);
    - email address;
    - perhaps also name of secretary/personal assistant,
        - their email address; and
        - telephone number if different.

Contents Page

Help the reader to navigate their way round the report. How detailed it is will depend on the report's length and complexity. Only in very short reports is this unnecessary.

Introduction

'The Writer'

Briefly introduce yourself sufficiently to orientate the reader and explain why you may be regarded as having relevant expertise by reference to 'the range and extent of the expertise

Box 6.3 Information to Be Provided in a Report for Criminal Proceedings in Scotland

- Name
- Current post
- Current employer
- Qualifications
- Fully registered with the General Medical Council
- Approved under section 22 of the 2003 Act and with which health board
- A statement that the report is given on soul and conscience
- A statement as to whether the expert is related to the person
- A statement as to whether the expert has any pecuniary interest in the person's admission to hospital or placement on any community-based order

Mental Health (Care and Treatment) (Scotland) Act 2003, Code of Practice, Vol. 3: *Compulsory Powers in Relation to Mentally Disordered Offenders* (Scottish Executive 2005), ch. 6, para. 102

and any limitations upon the expertise' (*B v Nugent Care Society* [2009] EWCA Civ 827). In a report complying with CrPR 19.2(3)(a), you have to define your area or areas of expertise. Your full details are in your report's Appendix 1. Identify any relevant area of which you have a working knowledge. You must also 'make clear the limits of your competence and knowledge when giving evidence or acting as a witness' (AWLP).

In Scotland, there is a requirement under the *Mental Health (Care and Treatment) (Scotland) Act 2003, Code of Practice*, Vol. 3: *Compulsory Powers in Relation to Mentally Disordered Offenders* (Scottish Executive 2005) ('the Scottish Code of Practice') that reports in criminal cases should include specific information (Box 6.3).

'Synopsis'

Set out concisely the general nature of the case in a sentence or two.

'Instructions'

This makes it clear at whose request the report has been prepared and for what purpose. It can be very brief. If you have received supplementary instructions, add: 'I received further instructions on [date].'

'Disclosure of Interests'

Either state any actual or potential conflict of interest or personal interest which might be considered as influencing your opinions (see Chapter 4, 'Qualified Acceptance of Instructions') or state that there are none (see also the Declaration, below). Make it clear if you have treated, or are currently treating, the subject of the report (see Chapter 1, 'Impartiality').

'The Background to the Case and Issues'

'The Relevant People'

This is often limited to the names of the defendant in a criminal case or the claimant and defendant(s) in a civil case. Often, it probably adds nothing and can be omitted. It is of use in a more complex case where it is a list of those who feature in your narrative account, for example: 'Dr. Alexandra Morison – on call senior house officer', 'Mary Ferrers – estranged wife of the Defendant'.

'The Assumed Facts and Substance of All Material Instructions'

This is a background narrative of the facts provided by the instructing party. Recite them as received, even if they may not be accurate, so that the basis of your opinion is explained. Responsibility for any inaccuracy rests with those instructing you. Include any information given orally, for example, by telephone. Omission of 'off-the-record' oral instructions is not permitted. Usually, this section is based on the letter of instruction. Although some experts attach a copy, it is legally privileged, and this needs the approval of the instructing party. Usually, it is not disclosed, but if there is reason to believe that your statement of the substance of the instructions is inaccurate or incomplete, or that you have misled the court as to your material instructions, the court can order disclosure and allow cross-examination on the matter. As this section can considerably lengthen the body of the report, consider setting out here only a very brief statement and then set out the full instructions in an appendix (illustrated in the specimen report at Appendix B).

'The Issues to Be Addressed'

This is a list taken from the letter of instruction. So, the opinion is confined to the matters material to the disputes between the parties or the issues before the court. It reminds you not to waste time and money and incur criticism for dealing with other matters. If you think that another matter should be addressed, ask those instructing you. In order to avoid questions or criticism about matters on which you have not expressed an opinion, consider a footnote: 'Unless I have indicated otherwise, these are the only matters I have been asked to address. The absence of an opinion on a particular issue does not mean that I have no opinion on the issue. It means only that I have not been asked to address the issue.'

It may be useful to include here a statement of the relevant law as you understand it. You are not proclaiming expertise in the law, just indicating that you know the relevant legal tests. If you get it wrong, the instructing solicitor can put you right and ask you to adjust the opinion accordingly.

If any issue falls outside your expertise, make it clear, although your instructing party should already know.

'The Assumptions Adopted'

This may be the assumptions that what the subject has said is true and that the contents of the medical records are accurate unless otherwise indicated. If you have made such assumptions or any other assumptions as to facts or made any deductions from factual assumptions, make this clear. Occasionally, you are asked to adopt an assumption. Set this out fully. If it is unreasonable or unlikely, make this clear. Beware, because in cross-examination 'probably the most useful grounds that [counsel] can focus on are the validity and merits of any assumptions applied by the expert' (Smethurst 2006). 'An expert report is only as good as the assumptions on which it is based' (Bell 2010).

Investigation (of Facts and Assumed Facts)

The purpose of this part of the report is to explain how the expert opinion has been reached. Some readers may not know, or may misunderstand, how a psychiatrist works. Furthermore, the expert has a duty to 'furnish the Judge or jury with the necessary scientific criteria for testing the accuracy of their conclusions, so as to enable the Judge or jury to form his own independent judgment by the application of these criteria to the facts proved in evidence' (*Davie v Edinburgh Corp. (No. 2)*, 1953 SC 34).

The first section is about 'Methodology'. In criminal cases, even though the Law Commission's proposals on the determination of evidentiary reliability (Law Commission 2011) have not become law, they are now embodied in the CrPR (see Chapter 1, 'Reliability'). They may affect practice in other jurisdictions. It may therefore be wise, if not necessary, to indicate that clinical practice depends partly on knowledge for which there is a sound scientific evidence base and partly on experience-based knowledge which has stood the test of time, but lacks a robust foundation in the rigorous research that forms the basis of 'evidence-based medicine'. Indicate that, in relying on both categories, you have done so in accordance with a responsible body of psychiatric practice.

Thus, explain how the diagnosis has been reached, explain how, for example in a personal injury case, the opinion on causation has been reached, explain how the particular prognosis has been reached and explain why you recommend particular treatment or have commented, as you might, on the treatment already given.

Particularly in relation to treatment, in family cases, it is now usual to ask that recommendations for treatment comply with National Institute of Health and Clinical Excellence (NICE) guidelines. This is not always going to be possible. Thus, it may be necessary to point out that you have relied on approaches that have wide acceptance by doctors and, where possible, given weight to treatments for which there is the strongest evidence base with regard to effectiveness and safety. However, there are many treatments that are accepted as effective, but for which there have not been trials that satisfy the most stringent criteria of evidence-based medicine or have been endorsed by NICE.

In family cases, you must describe your professional risk assessment process, but indicate its limitations (Royal College of Psychiatrists 2008), and the process of differential diagnosis. Other courts may soon expect this. The key is transparency.

All of this can be moved to your report's Appendix 2, 'The Process of Psychiatric Assessment'.

Under 'Interview and examination', set out the details of the consultation. Say whether anyone else was present and, if so, what part, if any, they took *during* the consultation. State that, unless otherwise indicated, the history is that obtained from the subject *at the consultation*. It is hearsay, which will either be admitted or may have to be proved (see Chapter 1, 'The Role of the Medical Expert Witness'). If the consultation was by live link make this clear and refer to any technical or other difficulties or limitations.

Refer to any particular circumstances such as the place, time or any constraints, such as inadequate time due to prison routine or the potentially inhibiting presence of someone such as a police or prison officer, partner or care worker.

If a trainee has assisted, name her and cross-refer to an extra appendix giving details of her qualifications, training and experience (see Chapter 3, 'Training in Report Preparation'). If you have obtained the views of colleagues, identify them. You must disclose the fact and nature of any discussion of 'the content of a proposed report in detail with another expert under a peer review arrangement' (*Pinkus v Direct Line Group* (EWHC QB, unreported, 2 January 2018). This only applies where the peer provides 'constructive input'; it does not apply to proof reading.

Make clear that, apart from your knowledge of the practice of psychiatry, unless otherwise indicated, the only facts within your own knowledge are your findings on examination of the subject.

If an informant has been interviewed, identify them and explain this.

Occasionally, reports are prepared without consulting with the subject, because the subject is dead, the court has ordered it or the subject has consented.

If so, head this section 'Basis of Report'. Make it clear that the report is based on a study of records only, why this is so and indicate any potential limitations. Justify the decision to proceed on such a basis. Indicate a willingness to reconsider your opinion following a consultation. In AWLP, the GMC states: 'If you are asked to give an opinion about a person without the opportunity to consult with or examine them, you should explain any limits this may place on your opinion. You should be able to justify the decision to provide your opinion.' A report which is prepared without consulting with the subject of the report may be ruled inadmissible or little weight attached to the opinion therein. In *R v Ibrahim* [2014] EWCA Crim 121, the decision of the trial judge not to admit expert psychiatric evidence as to the appellant's attention deficit hyperactivity disorder (ADHD), in part because it would be 'very unsatisfactory to admit expert evidence from a medical expert who had not interviewed or met the defendant', was upheld and the Court of Appeal added that the expert's 'speculation about what the appellant was thinking and why he acted as he did was of no great assistance. He had never met the appellant.'

If someone has carried out testing, she should be identified here with a cross-reference to the extra appendix which sets out her qualifications, relevant experience and any accreditation (CrPR 19.4(1)(e)). State whether or not you supervised the testing (CPR 35 PD 3.2(5)). *In Scotland* (Crown Office and Procurator Fiscal Service), whether or not you supervised the work, you have to notify the prosecutor as the court will accept such evidence as hearsay evidence.

Under 'Documents and Materials', refer to your report's Appendix 4 in which are listed at least the 'documents, statements, evidence, information . . . which are material to the opinions expressed or upon which those opinions are based' (*B v Nugent Care Society*) and which may also include audiotapes, DVDs, photographic exhibits, etc. It must be accurate. In *Williams v Jervis* [2009] EWHC 1837 (QB), the judge imposed a financial penalty on the defendant whose orthopaedic expert was unclear in his evidence as to what medical records, reports and witness statements he had seen prior to writing his report.

Some counsel and solicitors hold that all documents and materials should be listed. Others hold that if you list everything, the other side is entitled to see everything and so you should not refer to documents that your instructing solicitors do not intend to disclose for the time being, such as draft witness statements or a report on liability and causation in a medical negligence case because, if they are listed, the other side will be entitled to see them. Boyle (2016, p. 57) says that 'any document referred to by the expert on the face of the report is, in effect, disclosed', but the actual test is whether the other side needs the document to understand your opinion or if you have used that document as a significant part of the process of forming your opinion. In *Anglia Water Services Ltd v HMRC* [2017] UKFTT 0386 (TC), an expert was criticised for listing in his report only the documents which he considered relevant, but the court observed that CPR 35 PD 3.2(2) 'requires details only of material *relied upon*' (emphasis in the original).

In Ireland, the listed documents may or may not be disclosable. In *Doherty (A Minor) v North Western Health Board* [2005] IEHC 404, it was held that there was no obligation to disclose some of the documents referred to by the experts as they did not come within the definition of a report and could not be considered as a like matter to a map, drawing, photograph, graph, chart or calculation.

You must not fail to list a document containing information that is relevant to your opinion. If you do not, there is the danger that you will include in your report information which could only have come from an undisclosed document which would make you vulnerable in cross-examination. In an application for disclosure of a document or report, other than in Ireland (see above), the other side will probably succeed if you have seen it and relied on it, but not if you have seen it, read it and definitely not relied on it. If you make clear that a particular document is not material to your opinion, it ought to remain privileged. An application for disclosure may succeed if there is some reason to believe that there is something inaccurate or misleading about your statement of the instructions you have received.

If you are sent 'background material' and asked not to refer to it in your report, return it to the solicitors unread. It may contain information relevant to your opinion, in which case you will have to refer to it.

In a criminal case *in England and Wales*, the expert cannot rely on the contents of a witness statement if a notice has been given under the Criminal Justice Act (CJA) 2003, s 127 that it is not in the interests of justice for the expert to base an opinion or inference on the statement.

As 'instructions' include all materials sent to the expert, reports in civil cases prepared in compliance with the Guidance (para. 55) should include the dates on which the materials were received.

If documents are missing, illegible or incomplete, point this out. Identify materials that have not been produced with the report, such as original medical or other professional records. This may include any questionnaires completed by the subject of the report, but good practice is to attach them as an appendix. Be prepared to reveal everything.

If important documents have not been supplied or obtained, say so, explain why they have not been obtained and indicate why they are important, how information from them may make a material difference to your opinion.

A reference to 'Medical Terms and Explanations' can be included here or go at the end of the Introduction. Explain that any medical or technical terms will be highlighted, for example **emboldened**, and included in a glossary that appears as your report's Appendix 5 or give the definition or explanation as a footnote when it is first used. It should satisfy the GMC's AWLP: 'You should explain any abbreviations and medical or other technical terminology you use. Diagrams with explanatory labels can be useful.' It may include acronyms, symptoms, signs, diagnoses, drug names, forms of treatment and definitions of grades such as 'speciality registrar', etc.

If you rely on published or unpublished research or other authoritative material, state this under 'Research' or 'Authorities' and cross-refer to your Appendix 6, a list of references. These are references to cited work which supports your opinion or the underlying reasoning. It is not a generalised list, but you can list here any '[r]elevant extracts of literature or any other material which might assist the court' (*B v Nugent Care Society*). In a clinical negligence case in England and Wales, if you rely on unpublished work, you must provide a copy of it with the report. This is good practice in general. Supply copies or extracts, with sufficient pages from before and after the extract for it to be seen in context.

The Facts and Assumed Facts/Factual Analysis

So far, you should not have expressed any opinion. Similarly, here, there should be no opinion – not even a snippet. You may comment, but do so in brackets and follow the comment with your initials.

This section sets out facts and assumed facts, the grounds upon which your opinion will be based. Your opinion is only as strong as the facts upon which it is based and it is your responsibility to set out the grounds for your opinion because 'unless a witness states in his or her evidence . . . the grounds and reasoning that have led to the opinion, the opinion is valueless' (*Cadbury Schweppes v Durrell Lea* [2007] FCAFC 70). Unless the court can prove the facts underlying an opinion, it is deprived of 'an important opportunity of testing the process by which the opinion was formed, and [this] substantially reduces the value and cogency of the opinion evidence' (*Bell v F.S. & U. Industrial Benefit Society Ltd* (Supreme Court of New South Wales, unreported, 9 September 1987)).

Separate headings are advisable to distinguish the history (assumed facts) and the mental state/psychiatric examination (facts).

Some facts will be agreed by both or all parties. They are 'agreed facts'. Disputed facts will have to be proved to the required standard of proof. They are 'asserted' or 'alleged facts'. You may not know which facts are agreed, so by using the term 'assumed facts' you are acknowledging that some of the facts on which you rely may be agreed and others may not be agreed by the parties or found by the court. What the subject of the report or any informant tells you, and what the witnesses say, are assumed facts which may be agreed facts or asserted or alleged facts that have to be proved in evidence. The judge or the jury decides the disputed facts: 'Where an expert relies on the existence or non-existence of some fact which is basic to the question on which he is asked to express his opinion that fact must be proved by admissible evidence' (*R v Abadom* [1983] 1 WLR 126). And as Bell (2010) has observed, 'Whether or not the expert believes in that sub-stratum of facts or knows them to be true or is satisfied that they are true, is completely beside the point.' The corollary is that: 'If the doctor's evidence is based entirely on hearsay and is not supported by direct evidence, the judge will be justified in telling the jury that the defendant's case . . . is based on a flimsy or non-existent foundation' (*R v Bradshaw* (1986) 82 Cr App R 79) and '[i]f the expert has been misinformed about the facts or has taken irrelevant facts into consideration or has omitted to consider relevant ones, the opinion is likely to be valueless' (*R v Turner* [1975] QB 834).

Hearsay, or 'second-hand' evidence, is evidence by one person of the evidence of another and statements in documents that are offered to prove the truth of what is written. The general rule is against the admission of hearsay. This is because it has not been given under oath and its reliability cannot be tested by examination, cross-examination and re-examination of the person who made the statement or created the document. However, there are statutory and common law exceptions to the exclusion of hearsay evidence known as 'admissible hearsay assertions'. In civil cases, most hearsay statements are admissible, other than in Ireland, and medical records are admissible as evidence of the facts stated in them. *In Ireland* (see Chapter 1, 'The Role of the Medical Expert Witness'), the records must be admitted or proved in the usual way (*McGregor*). In criminal cases, under the CJA 2003, s 114, hearsay is admissible if there is a statutory provision for its admission, if there is a common law exception to its inadmissibility, if all the parties agree or if its admission is in the interests of justice. Where a medical expert gives evidence as to the condition of a person, she can report the symptoms she has elicited and rely on these to explain her diagnosis, but if their existence is in issue, they must be proved by admissible evidence. Likewise, although medical records are admissible in evidence, they are only evidence that the patient reported the symptom or that a doctor observed the sign. If there is an issue as to whether the patient had that symptom or sign, the symptom or sign will have to be proved by admissible evidence.

Where you rely on assumed facts, identify your source.

In this section, you may set out assumed facts which are not otherwise within the knowledge of the court, specifically the contents of medical records and, at least to some extent, the history you have obtained from the subject.

Usually, the only 'facts' to which you can testify are facts within your own knowledge, such as your examination findings and your experience of the practice of psychiatry, and facts taken from the work of other experts and from specialist literature or research within your field of expertise or of which you have a working knowledge.

Views differ as to how much of the subject's history goes in this section.

Some hold that this should be a full and detailed account of medical history, family history, personal history and personality, so as to bring the person alive and to show that all potentially relevant aspects of the history have been considered. But this results in the excessively long reports of which judges are critical. This format is illustrated by the specimen Daniel McNaughtan report in the first edition of this book (Rix 2011b).

Others hold that this section should be relatively brief and limited to the information which is necessary to demonstrate, and allow reference to, the evidence base for the opinions reached. The body of the report at least is much shorter. The full history and mental state go in an appendix. This is illustrated in this edition's specimen report on Daniel McNaughtan (Appendix A). The specimen report on Charles Dickens (Appendix B) goes further and excludes the full history and examination (online Appendix 11) from the report, but the record is retained for reference and, if required, disclosure.

Usually, relevant information from the medical records should be set out under the heading, or in an appendix, 'Medical history as taken from medical records' and not combined with 'Medical history as given by the defendant/claimant'. If much depends on the comparison of the subject's account with the documented history or if it would otherwise be difficult to convey the relevant chronology, they can be integrated, but only so long as the different sources of information can be distinguished. The guiding principle is that different types of fact must be identified and distinguished. This can be achieved either by using different headings and, in particular, by separating what the subject has told you from what others have said or is in other documentary sources, or by using a number of separate appendices. It can be confusing if the reader cannot distinguish between what, for example, the defendant told you about his state of mind, what he told the police when interviewed and what he told another expert. If these are different accounts, the court may have to decide how much weight to attach to each one.

However, if, for example, in a clinical negligence case, where a detailed chronology needs to integrate what staff recorded at the time and what they subsequently say they did at the time, different type can be used, such as ordinary type for information from the contemporaneous records and italic for information taken from their witness statements or their evidence at the inquest. If this is set out in a table, the right-hand column can be used to identify the source of the information.

Computers and word-processing have now made it unnecessary for the psychiatric expert to use a roll of ceiling paper, as Dr Neville Gittleson did in the benzodiazepine litigation, with one end at the front door and the other end at the back door, upon which he set out, by hand, the chronology of the case, usually finding that, at one or more points, he still could not squeeze all of the relevant information into the space he had allowed. So, set out information from medical records chronologically with information from general practitioner and specialist records integrated. With computerised word-processing, there is no excuse for setting it out in the same haphazard way in which documents have been filed or entries made on the general practice or hospital computer.

Where information comes from multiple sources, it is important that the source of each piece of information or quotation can be found in the records, so such a paragraph is likely to include a number of page references in brackets. If you do not include them in the first draft, you will spend hours trying to track a single elusive reference at a later stage. If the medical records are not paginated, ask your instructing solicitors to provide paginated records. This is because the model practice direction for clinical negligence cases requires that all references to medical notes in any report should be made by reference to the pages in the paginated bundle of records prepared by the claimant's solicitors.

Take care in checking the facts and address the facts at issue. The GMC's AWLP states: '[Y]ou must take reasonable steps to check the accuracy of any information you give, and to make sure that you include all relevant information.' In *Harris v Johnston* [2016] EWHC 3193 (QB), there was an issue as to injury caused by a *Cobb* dissector, but the claimant's expert referred throughout his report to the entirely different *Cobb* retractor, a mistake which he ought not to have made if he had read the defence and the witness evidence or sought clarification. The judge found that the expert had failed in his duty under CPR Part 35 and this was made worse because he had previously been criticised for factual inaccuracy. His evidence was disallowed in its entirety. In *Williams*, an orthopaedic expert was criticised, and his instructing party financially penalised, for a number of inaccuracies in the report which were due to not having read the source material, including the claimant's statement.

Summarise here the findings of any investigations you have carried out or caused to be carried out; the details go in an appendix.

In this part of the report, where you rely on the opinions of other experts, such as a neurologist, make this clear so that their opinion is one of your assumed facts.

This section should usually end with the examination findings.

This section is the launch-pad for the 'Opinion'. The reader will need to see how each and every opinion can be properly deduced from the facts in this section (or an appropriate appendix) supplemented, perhaps, by facts in the material instructions.

Include all material facts. 'You must not deliberately leave out relevant information' (GMP) – for example, material that is inconsistent with, or does not support, your opinion. In *Frazer v Haukioja* [2008] CanLII 42207 (ON SC), the court observed that cherry-picking facts which supported a diagnosis that just happened to support the cause of the client who retained the expert and failing to include the facts that hurt the cause, whether or not those latter facts were capable of explanation and elimination in the course of the development of the expert's analysis and opinion, smacked of partiality. So, do not mislead by omission. 'What the court expects from you is an objective, independent, well-researched, thorough opinion, which takes account of all relevant information and which represents your genuine professional view on the issues submitted to you' (Wall 2007).

Opinion

Addressing Evidential Reliability

The framework for the opinion is 'Issues to be addressed'. But first assess the quality of the evidence on which you rely and 'take reasonable steps to check the information' (GMP).

Your opinion is only as good as the information on which is based. Experts *in Scotland* are told (Crown Office and Procurator Fiscal Service):

> An expert witness should not provide the court with a statement of unqualified conclusions about the question of fact on which his/her opinion relies. If an expert witness does so, the effect of his/her testimony may well be diminished. It is therefore of the utmost importance that any expert witness carefully describes the source and assesses the worth of all material on which his/her opinion is based.

Under the CrPR, the report must 'include such information as the court may need to decide whether the expert's opinion is sufficiently reliable to be admitted as evidence' (CrPR 19.4(1)(h)).

This section might therefore have as its first subheading 'Evaluation of evidence'. Although it is ultimately a matter for the court to evaluate the evidence and the subject's credibility, the court may be assisted in doing so by understanding upon what evidence you have relied and what weight, according to your clinical experience, you have attached to it. You are not usurping the role of the court, but fulfilling the expectation of the judge in *Turner v Jordan* [2010] EWHC 1508 (QB) that when as '[a] consequence of the fact that diagnosis in a psychiatric case depends on assessment of what is reported by the patient [it is necessary] for the psychiatrist confronted by a patient to consider whether or not to accept at face value what the patient reports'.

This section includes but is not limited to: the completeness and legibility of records, drawing attention to any redactions and their likely significance; the clinical plausibility of the subject's history with reference, if appropriate, to inconsistencies with other accounts and inconsistencies with or between other sources such as witness statements and Department for Work and Pensions (DWP) or similar records. But bear in mind that the Citizens Advice Bureau tells claimants to describe how they are on their very worst day and this may be reflected in documents.

Assess the worth of all of the material on which your opinion is based. The court needs to know to what extent, having regard to your medical expertise, you consider that you can rely on these assumed facts, albeit that the court will make its own findings as to fact. Your level of confidence in the evidence may influence the court as to the extent to which it needs to make such findings of fact. '[T]he basis for the asserted opinion must be sufficiently clear for its reliability to be properly assessed' (*Richmond LBC v B* [2010] EWHC 2903 (Fam)). But incorporate an acknowledgement that the evaluation of evidence and the credibility of the subject is ultimately for the court and any opinion as to clinical plausibility refers only to your clinical judgement as to whether the subject's presentation rings true by reference to your clinical experience; it is not an opinion as to the subject's credibility or veracity in general.

Addressing the Issues

Each issue, or question, becomes a heading so that you address the questions asked. Under each, state your conclusion and show with clarity, logic and succinctness how this properly derives from the facts; but try to avoid their repetition and refer to them only so far as is necessary for your reasoning to be understood. You want the reader to accept your conclusion, so the important word, explicit or implied, will be 'because'; the conclusion or opinion has to be reasoned:

> [A] well constructed expert's report containing opinion evidence sets out the expert's opinion and the reasons for it. If the reasons stand up, the opinion does. If not, not.' (Jacob J in *Pearce v Ove Arup Partnership Ltd (Copying)* (2002) 25(2) IPD 25011)

> What really matters in most cases is the reasons given for the opinion. (*Routestone Ltd v Minories Finance Ltd* [1996] 5 WLUK 237)

> It is simply wrong in principle for an expert to fail to set out the way in which he has reached the conclusions in his report. (*R v T* [2010] EWCA Crim 2439)

The opinion has to be diligently researched, objectively sound, genuinely and honestly held and impartially presented.

Set out the opinion on the issue, or the answer to the question, as a short, stand-alone sentence (Canadian psychologist Stephen Hart, personal communication). Follow this by one or more sentences of argument and clear and informed reasoning. Try to have just one such paragraph for each question or issue. When you produce your 'Summary of Conclusions', this will then comprise the opening sentence from each paragraph in the 'Opinion'.

Achieving Balance

Highlight the strengths of your arguments, but also set out any material facts or matters that might undermine, or detract from, your opinion and any points that should fairly be made against it. The latter are a 'necessary inclusion' (*B v Nugent Care Society*). As already noted, GMP says that 'you must not deliberately leave out relevant information'. Do not simply ignore what you consider unimportant or irrelevant. Do not simply reject relevant material. Explain why it does not affect your opinion. Identify any unusual, contradictory or inconsistent features of the case. Take into consideration any relevant factors arising from ethnic, cultural, social, religious or linguistic contexts.

It must be a balanced opinion. The use of a balance sheet listing factors that support or undermine the opinion has been advocated in family cases, but it could be problematic and invite a degree of cross-examination that might not otherwise arise.

Avoid being over-dogmatic or using extreme forms of expression. Avoid wording that might be regarded as pejorative, prejudicial or pre-judgemental. 'A combative tone is inappropriate and only serves to undermine the likelihood of [the] conclusions being accepted' (Hodgkinson and James 2015, p. 247).

The Range of Reasonable Opinion

Where there is, and usually there is, a range of reasonable opinion, summarise it. Give reasons for your own opinion and for not adopting the other possible opinions. By identifying the weaknesses in the alternative opinions, you strengthen your own position, you assist the court by providing the means of testing the validity of your opinion (and the other alternative opinions) and you rehearse arguments that may arise in cross-examination.

Imagine the subject being presented at a case conference and imagine the most extreme views of your reasonable colleagues. Also, consider the perhaps ridiculous views of unreasonable colleagues; occasionally, they may be instructed as experts. If you have seen the other expert's report, comment briefly on their opinion and explain why, if it be so, you do not accept it. If you have not seen it, try to anticipate what it might be. This is not being adversarial; it is about providing the court with as much information as possible to allow the court to choose between competing opinions.

Boyle (2016, p. 65) uses the analogy of a tripod. The range of opinion in a personal injury case must have three extreme points:

- that the claimant has all of the symptoms of which he complains and that they are all caused by the accident;
- that the claimant has all of the symptoms of which he complains, but none of them is caused by the accident;
- that the claimant has none of the symptoms of which he complains.

A pendulum suspended from a tripod with its feet positioned at the extremes would, like the expert's opinion, come to rest somewhere in the triangle created. As Boyle says (2016, p. 66): 'The Pendulum allows, indeed insists on, a contemplation and assessment of the alternatives.'

Where there is a conflict of factual evidence, set out alternative opinions based on the different factual scenarios. Only express a preference for one if it depends on the application of your expertise. For example, there may be an inconsistency between the subject's reported symptoms and evidence from other sources which would not be obvious other than to a psychiatrist.

Addressing Unidentified Issues

Do not answer questions that have not been asked unless you have been invited to mention any other matters you consider relevant. If you waste time and money on matters that are not in issue, and you have not already been paid, you may not be paid, or at least not in full. However, it may be that a separate condition has intervened or occurred, which those instructing you may not know about or understand, that potentially changes the course of the case.

One significant exception is where the set of questions does not call for an actual diagnosis. It may be a case in which it is helpful to set out the diagnosis first as the basis for some of the other opinions. However, avoid 'straining the symptoms to fit a possible diagnosis when they [do] not fit naturally' (*Van Wees v Karkour* [2007] EWHC 165 (QB)). It may not matter. In *Noble v Owens* [2008] EWHC 359 (QB), it was held that 'the precise characterisation of Mr. Noble's ... disorder does not signify. What matters are the symptoms of Mr. Noble's condition and the prognosis.'

Another significant exception is where the subject needs treatment. An action for negligence was brought against a psychiatrist who reported on a victim of the Hillsborough football disaster diagnosing reactive depression (*Hall v Egdell* (unreported, 2004)). The claimant's experts' evidence was that he had failed to diagnose PTSD. The judge found that the expert had been negligent in gathering the data to found his conclusion and that, as the expert was the first doctor consulted by the claimant since the disaster, he had an obligation to the claimant as a patient to inform the claimant's general practitioner of his recommendation as to treatment. So, whether or not asked to do so, make a recommendation for treatment that accords with the best practice of medicine, ask that it is passed to the subject's ordinary medical attendant and ask to be informed that this has been done. If the instructing party does not pass on the recommendation, seek legal advice as to whether you should communicate the recommendation directly. Beneficence may override your duty of confidentiality to those instructing you. Beware of writing to the subject's general practitioner. If you do so, and if time permits, discuss this with your instructing solicitor, but be careful not to include any privileged information and send a copy of any letter to your instructing solicitors. Take note of *Cornelius v de Taranto* [2000] 6 WLUK 833, where a claimant was awarded £3,000 for breach of contract. The action was against a psychiatrist who had prepared a medical report on the claimant in connection with an allegation of constructive dismissal. In order to arrange treatment for the claimant, the psychiatrist sent the report, which contained material defamatory of the claimant, to her general practitioner and another psychiatrist. She was found liable and on appeal the finding was upheld. However, the judge at first instance had ordered the psychiatrist to pay £45,000 towards the claimant's costs. Due to the fact that the claimant had lost a substantial part of her claim, this order was quashed, no doubt much to the relief of the psychiatrist and her MDO.

Hypotheses

If advancing a proposition, make clear if it is a hypothesis, especially if it is controversial, or an opinion deduced in accordance with peer-reviewed and peer-tested technique, research and experience accepted as a consensus in the professional psychiatric community.

Treading on the Judge's Toes

Do not to usurp the role of the judge, jury or coroner. An expert's assistance does, and generally should, stop short of supplanting the court as decision-maker on matters that are central to the case and deciding the ultimate issue which it is for the court and not for the expert to decide – the so-called 'ultimate issue' rule.

The judge decides if the defendant hospital was negligent. The jury decides the defendant's guilt. This does not mean that you cannot give an opinion on the ultimate issue. Indeed, in a civil case the judge will want your opinion on whether the doctor exercised the ordinary skill of an ordinary competent doctor exercising her art. Under the Civil Evidence Act 1972, s 3(1), 'where a person is called as a witness in any civil proceedings his opinion on any relevant matter on which he is qualified to give expert evidence shall be admissible in evidence'.

The underlying rationale for the ultimate issue rule is, as stated in *The Ikarian Reefer*, that it is a matter for the judge's or jury's own view. But this rule has weakened. As indicated, expert opinion on the ultimate issue is admissible in civil cases and in criminal cases, the abolition of the rule has been recommended, but never put into effect. Given the ever-increasing complexity of areas of expert evidence, there has been a blurring of the line between acceptable expert opinion *per se* and upon the ultimate issue. For example, it is common for expert accountants to state that there can be no rational and honest explanation for particular transactions such that fraud is inferred. Indeed, in *R v Stockwell* [1993] 3 WLUK 119, Lord Taylor LCJ stated, as an aside, that:

> . . . the rationale behind the supposed prohibition is that the expert should not usurp the functions of the jury. But since counsel can bring the witness so close to opining on the ultimate issue that the inference as to his view is obvious, the rule can only be . . . a matter of form rather than substance.

One leading text on criminal law, *Blackstone's* (Ormerod and Perry 2019, para. F11.35), states: '[A]n expert *is* allowed to express an opinion on an ultimate issue, provided that the actual words he employs are not noticeably the same as those which will be used when the issue falls to be considered by the court' (emphasis in the original).

Where the ultimate issue may be avoided, the court will endeavour to ensure this occurs. In *Pora v The Queen* [2015] UKPC 9, the Judicial Committee of the Privy Council ruled inadmissible a forensic psychologist's evidence on the basis that in trenchantly asserting that the appellant's confessions were unreliable, he was supplanting the court's role. The expert 'could have expressed an opinion as to how the difficulties that Pora faced might have led him to make false confessions. This would have allowed the fact finder to make its own determination to whether the admissions could be relied upon ... unencumbered by a forthright assertion from the expert that the confessions were unreliable.'

By contrast, another forensic psychologist's evidence about 'a possible explanation for his having admitted to something that he did not do' was accepted as evidence which was relevant and, at least potentially, extremely helpful in determining whether Pora's confessions could be relied on.

So, there is no need to 'simply creep up to the opinion without giving it' (*Routestone Ltd*). What matters is how the opinion is expressed.

Provisional or Final?

Make it clear if this is not a final opinion, but provisional or qualified. Perhaps critical records remain to be obtained. Perhaps account needs to be taken of the opinion of another expert. If appropriate, suggest the instruction of another expert. Rarely, be prepared to recommend a second opinion on a key issue.

Summary of Conclusions

Finally, set out a summary of the conclusions.

Declaration

In England and Wales, reports in criminal, civil and family proceedings require a declaration that the expert understands and has complied with their duty to the court. So far, only the CrPR not only require the report to contain 'a statement that the expert understands an expert's duty to the court, and has complied and will continue to comply with that duty' (CrPR 19.4(1)(j)), but also set out the terms of the declaration in thirteen paragraphs (CrPR 19B CP D). Such declarations have been taught, recommended and adopted for some years and that in the CrPR is based on them. They are illustrated in the specimen reports (Appendices A and B). *In Northern Ireland*, an expert's declaration is set out in generally identical terms. *In Scotland*, such a declaration has no place, but 'the standards which it encompasses are those standards which will be expected for any expert giving evidence to a court in Scotland' (Crichton 2014). Furthermore, expert reports have to be signed under the words 'on soul and conscience'. Failure to do so risks a fine of 'one hundred merks Scots' (about £400 today). *In Ireland*, RSC Ord. 39, r 57(2) provides that every expert report delivered pursuant to the Rules or to any Order or Direction of the court, is to: (1) contain a statement acknowledging the expert's duty to assist the court as to matters within their field of expertise and which duty overrides any obligation to any party paying their fee; and (2) disclose any financial or economic interest of the expert. In addition, experts are advised to adopt a declaration as set out in *O'Leary v Mercy University Hospital Cork Ltd* [2019] IESC 48 (online Appendix 12).

In England and Wales, to comply with the CPIA, as amended, if instructed by the prosecution you also have to include a declaration confirming that you have read and followed *Guidance for Experts on Disclosure, Unused Material and Case Management* (CPS, 2019) and recognise the continuing nature of your disclosure responsibilities (see Chapter 2,

'Disclosure Obligations'). This additional declaration (online Appendix 13) should be inserted in the CrPR declaration as para. 14. It should be accompanied by a certificate setting out the answers to six questions designed to elicit matters that may affect your credibility (online Appendix 14) and an index of unused material in which you list your case notes, time sheets, case costings and records of conversations and emails with the officer in the case, police personnel, prosecutor and other CPS personnel.

The equivalent declaration in Scotland is: 'I confirm that I have read the guidance contained in the ACPOS Disclosure Manual which details my duties as an expert witness in assisting the Crown to discharge its disclosure obligations. I have followed the guidance and recognise the continuing nature of my responsibilities.'

One of the functions of the Declaration is to avoid experts acting in disregard of their duties to the court. This led to the psychiatrist in *Phillips v Symes (A Bankrupt) (Expert Witnesses: Costs)* [2004] EWHC 2330 (Ch) being threatened with the financial penalty of a wasted costs order which makes the person against whom it is made pay costs wasted by their misconduct, default or serious negligence. The application was made on the basis that he 'was in serious breach of his duties to the court by acting recklessly, irresponsibly and wholly outside the bounds of how any reasonable psychiatrist preparing an opinion for the court could have properly acted with regard to his duties'. In these Chancery proceedings relating to the capacity of Mr Symes, a bankrupt, one of the criticisms of the expert was that he had failed to act in conformity with his expert's declaration (1) to mention all matters which he regarded as relevant to his opinion, (2) to draw attention to matters of which he was aware that might adversely affect his opinion and (3) to comply with his duty to correct or qualify his report when necessary.

Statement of Truth

Reports *in England and Wales and in the Isle of Man* in criminal, civil and family proceedings and for some tribunals also require a statement of truth, without which a report may not be admitted in evidence (*Al Nehayan v Kent* [2016] EWHC 623 (QB)). The CrPR require that a report must contain the same declaration of truth as a witness statement (CrPR 19.4(1)(k)). Some of these are set out in Box 6.4.

Bear in mind the GMC's AWLP: 'You must make sure that any report you write, or evidence you give, is accurate and not misleading' and the MC's guidance: 'Reports must be relevant, factual, accurate and not misleading. Their content must not be influenced by financial or other inducements or pressures' (MC 2019, para. 40.2).

Signature Block

After the body of the report comes the signature block. The date of the report can be added.

Appendices

Appendix 1 sets out as an abbreviated CV, in no more than a page, your qualifications, relevant experience and, if any, accreditation, in three sections:

- academic and professional qualifications in full;
- your expert witness training and your clinical training and experience in your speciality, ending with your current post or appointment(s), current employer and any current positions of responsibility in, or related to, the profession; and
- details of research and publications.

Box 6.4 Statements of Truth

Civil Procedure Rules and Family Procedure Rules:

> I confirm that I have made clear which facts and matters referred to in this report are within my own knowledge and which are not. Those that are within my own knowledge I confirm to be true. The opinions I have expressed represent my true and complete professional opinions on the matters to which they refer.
>
> *And additionally in children proceedings:*
>
> I also confirm that I have complied with the *Standards for Expert Witnesses in Children Proceedings in the Family Court* which are set out in the Annex to Practice Direction 25B – *The Duties of an Expert, the Expert's Report and Arrangements for an Expert to Attend Court.*

Criminal Procedure Rules:

> I confirm that the contents of this report (consisting of ~ pages) are true to the best of my knowledge and belief and that I make this report knowing that, if it is tendered in evidence, I would be liable to prosecution if I have wilfully stated anything which I know to be false or that I do not believe to be true.

Isle of Man:

> I confirm that insofar as the facts stated in my report are within my own knowledge, I have made clear which they are and I believe them to be true and that the opinions I have expressed represent my true and complete professional opinion.

Tailor this to the case so that it is clear why it is appropriate for you to give expert evidence. At trial, it will facilitate comparison of your expertise with that of the other side's expert.

In some cases, such as a clinical negligence claim where the High Court's standard direction requires the expert to produce, at the same time as their report, a CV giving details of any employment or activity which raises a possible conflict of interest, you may also need to provide a full CV.

Even where your opinion is unopposed but forms the basis of oral testimony, your counsel will use this to seek to persuade the judge or jury to accept your evidence.

Appendix 2 describes the process of psychiatric assessment.

Appendix 3 sets out the history taken from the subject and your mental state examination findings.

Appendix 4 lists the documents and other materials provided.

Appendix 5 is your glossary.

You may have additional appendices, such as a chronology of the case, a chronology of entries in the medical records or an appendix of references.

In Scotland, in criminal cases (Crown Office and Procurator Fiscal Service):

> Passages from a published work may be adopted by an expert witness and made part of his/her evidence or they may be put to a witness in cross examination for comment. Where it will be necessary for you to refer to published work when you give evidence let the Procurator Fiscal know this so that the items can be added to the indictment as productions and disclosed to the defence. If the Procurator Fiscal is unaware that you wish to refer to published work during your oral evidence, it will not be available as a production in court.

Finally, we are all human and make mistakes, so a good proof-reader is worth their weight in gold and can correct careless errors and bring inconsistencies to your notice.

When you have checked and signed your report, have it posted with a suitable covering letter (online Appendix 15).

After-Thoughts

If you change your opinion on any material matter, you should, without delay, notify those instructing you and advise the reason. In a criminal case, if the report has been disclosed, inform all parties and the court. If the instructing party fails to disclose the change of an opinion already disclosed, inform the court, but seek legal advice as well.

Amendments

You may be asked to consider amending your report. But remember that your opinion has to be independent and uninfluenced by the exigencies of the litigation. Be prepared to remind those instructing you that the opinion is yours and not theirs. However, provided that you are not asked to devise facts or opinions which may advance the subject's case, or give an opinion which is no longer your own, independent and uninfluenced by the exigencies of the litigation, it is quite proper to make amendments at the suggestion of the solicitors or counsel and Box 6.5 lists permissible amendments.

It is also proper for counsel to seek to discuss, or annotate on a draft report, observations and questions to be considered in any revisions. Indeed, there is often much to be learned from the suggested amendments, especially when, as in a foreign language class, a better form of words is suggested. If there are factual errors or new facts to be considered, consider carefully whether they affect your opinion. As John Maynard Keynes said: 'When the facts change, my opinion changes.' But be sure that any amended opinions follow from the now different factual background. Do not hurry; you must be fully refreshed as to the totality of the facts lest any amendment, especially to your opinion, introduces inconsistency. You can charge for amendments, but not for any which result from your faulty drafting.

Experts should, however, be especially cautious about amendments in the Irish disclosure regime, where all reports are disclosable (if the evidence of the witness is to be relied on) and uncomfortable questions might arise on cross-examination in relation to amendments.

Box 6.5 Permissible Amendments to a Report at the Suggestion of Solicitor or Counsel

- correction of material errors of fact;
- address legally relevant issues;
- remove references to issues outside expertise or on which evidence is not legally admissible (e.g. the ultimate issue);
- comment on new facts;
- ensure compliance with the appropriate procedural rules;
- presentational changes;
- annexation of relevant materials (e.g. publications);
- a form of words.

Hodgkinson and James 2015, p. 250

What must have been the discomfort of the expert in *Loughlin v Singh* [2013] EWHC 1641 (QB) can be deduced from the annex to the judgment. It deals solely with the expert's evidence. The issue was the claimant's capacity to manage his own affairs. Before the court were two reports by the expert. In the first, he stated his agreement with two other experts that the claimant had capacity, although they actually said that he did not. In his revised report, prepared following a telephone conversation with instructing solicitors, his conclusion was lack of capacity, but he did not refer to his previous report or explain his change of opinion. In his oral evidence, he implied that he changed his opinion as a result of another consultation with the claimant; but there was no evidence of such a consultation, only his intention to conduct one. The judge concluded the expert lacked independence and rejected his evidence in full.

Refusal to reconsider your opinion may get you into trouble. This happened to the psychiatrist in *Phillips*. He was criticised because when he was sent further material, he refused to reconsider his opinion that Mr Symes lacked capacity. Indeed, he refused to look at it until directed by the judge to do so at the trial. After doing so, he was forced to admit that Mr Symes was capable of managing his affairs.

The real difficulty is where instructing lawyers want you to change your opinion, or how it is expressed, or exclude material, in order better to support their case. In *Marsden v Amalgamated Television Services Pty Ltd* [2001] NSWSC 510, a psychiatrist admitted under cross-examination that at the request of his instructing solicitor he had removed significant material from his report. This only came to light when an earlier version of his report was accidentally passed to cross-examining counsel. In *Liverpool Victoria Insurance Co. v Zafar* [2019] EWCA 392 (Civ), a general practitioner expert, who allowed changes to be made to a report in a whiplash case not caring if they were true or false, and who deliberately and repeatedly lied, including blaming someone else for the amendment, had his suspended prison sentence for ten offences of contempt of court upheld. The court held that 'this form of contempt undermines the administration of justice' and observed that 'breach of the trust placed in an expert witness by the court must be expected to result in a severe sanction', quoting with approval *South Wales Fire and Rescue Service v Smith* [2011] EWHC 1749 (Admin): 'expert witnesses who act dishonestly in the evidence they give to the court . . . must expect [to go to prison]'.

Lawyers' reasons may be persuasive, but be careful. You must not include anything in your report which has been suggested to you by anyone, including the lawyers instructing you, without forming your own independent view. If ever there is good reason to sleep on a report, this is it. If, after thorough and careful reflection, and after reminding yourself where your duty lies, you accept the suggestion, make the amendment and put the reasoning into your own words, then sleep on it. Look at it afresh the following day. Sometimes, on reflection, it appears that the valid and best supported conclusion is the original one. If you go ahead with the amendment, you need to be as confident about the reasoning behind it as you are about the rest of your reasoning. If not, express the amended opinion with whatever qualification is necessary to reflect your independence, impartiality and objectivity.

If you change your opinion, the reason should be crystal clear. If it is not and if the earlier version of your report has already been disclosed, or is disclosed inadvertently, or otherwise falls into the hands of another party, any change of opinion, especially if it suggests partiality, will go under the microscope and you risk being accused of being biased, partisan or even a 'hired gun'.

If you change your opinion for no other reason than to please your paymaster, the solicitor and barrister will not forget. Your next contact with the same barrister may be when she is instructed by the other side. Do not be surprised if she gives you a hard time or does not recommend you for other cases. If you acquire a reputation as a 'hired gun', you may have some short-term gains, but when the barristers are sitting as recorders or have been elevated to the bench, do not be surprised if your opinions carry little weight. If, for good reason, you refuse to budge, this will enhance your reputation and judges who have known you when they were barristers will be more likely to respect your opinions.

Answers to Questions

Experts are not expected to answer questions that are not properly directed to clarification of the report, unless the court gives permission or the other party agrees, if they are disproportionate or are asked out of time. For these reasons and because the instructing solicitor may not have been sent the questions or may consider that they call for more than clarification and they have not agreed to this, consult immediately with your instructing solicitor before answering the questions and advise as to the likely cost of doing so, as this informs any discussion as to the proportionality of the questions.

If the questions have been ordered by the court, the court order should specify the date by which the answers should be provided. If it is unrealistic, seek to negotiate an alternative date. If negotiation fails, you can apply to the court for additional time. If no deadline is indicated, plan to provide the answers within two to four weeks and if this is not practical inform the party asking the questions and the instructing solicitor.

As the court can give permission for any questions that 'assist the just disposal of the dispute' (*Mutch v Allen* [2001] EWCA Civ 76), the questions may deal with issues that you have not addressed in your report, but to which you will only answer if they fall within your area of expertise.

The questions should have been framed carefully and you should match that care in the way you provide the answers, even though this may involve a considerable amount of time reading the file. So, only when properly and sufficiently refreshed, set about answering the questions that have been asked and not the questions that you think might have been asked. Pay careful attention to the clarity of your answer and the way in which you apply any legal tests drawn to your attention.

The form in which the answers are sent should be a stand-alone document in which the following are set out:

- title of the action;
- 'answers to questions put by Messrs XXXX pursuant to CPR 35.6';
- their reference;
- expert's name;
- date;
- each question followed by the answer;
- signature block.

Do not infuriate your readers by setting out a series of numbered answers which only make sense when they locate the list of questions.

Some solicitors request their expert to send them the answers in draft form and it may be appropriate and helpful to do so. The reasons are these. Sometimes, the form or content of a question may be influenced by a particular point of law or legal test which it is important for you to understand before answering the question, and without assistance you may misunderstand the question. The instructing solicitor may also advise as to factual inaccuracies. However, you must be mindful of your duty to the court and avoid being manipulated into providing a partisan opinion.

Answers should be set out in neutral language and must not convey any annoyance you feel about being asked questions the answers to which you consider are contained in your report or which you feel could have been answered in your report if you had been asked them.

Experts' answers to questions automatically become part of their reports. So, they are covered by the statement of truth and form part of their expert evidence. Some solicitors expect that answers will conclude with the statement of truth; others consider this unnecessary.

Send answers simultaneously to the party that has asked the questions and to the instructing solicitors.

Experts' Meetings

Preparation for a discussion between experts must include comparing the materials, usually reports, records, DVDs and statements, that each expert has seen. Instructing solicitors should have advised which of the expert's reports, addenda, letters, etc. have been disclosed. Good practice is to exchange lists in advance.

It is very important that the experts should have had access to the same materials. Significant differences of opinion may disappear or change in their significance once both experts have seen the same materials. If one expert has not seen documents that the other expert has seen, it is best to adjourn. The Guidance (para. 25) requires an expert who identifies that the basis of his instruction differs from that of another expert to inform those instructing him.

Usual practice is for one expert to prepare a draft and send it to the other expert. Some solicitors are critical of this and may threaten to ask the court to order disclosure of the first draft. However, judges approve. Nevertheless, this must not inhibit meaningful discussion and some cases will call for such before any drafting. The expert who prepares the draft usually finds that its preparation powerfully concentrates the mind on the issues. Often, it will be clear that there is close agreement on a number of issues. Areas of disagreement may also be clear, but there may be difficulty identifying the reasons for disagreement. Identifying your reasons for disagreement with the other expert is often easier than identifying their reasons for disagreement with you. If an expert significantly alters his opinion, the joint statement has to include a note or addendum by that expert explaining the change of opinion and the reasons.

Box 6.6 suggests a structure for an experts' joint statement in a case where no agenda has been prepared. This is not the place to recite the details of the case. The court will be aware of the facts of the case. Where there is disagreement, the reasons for disagreement must be clear and succinct. The courts are not assisted by copying sections from a report, especially if they do not include reasons, or writing 'Please see my report for reasons' and the more so if the reasons are not there. Where there is an agenda, the body of the statement will be the experts' answers to each question and, if appropriate, reasons for disagreement.

Box 6.6 Structure of an Experts' Joint Statement

- title of the action;
- heading that identifies the document as an experts' joint statement and the speciality and names of the experts;
- brief paragraph identifying the experts and their instructing solicitors (with their file references), listing experts' reports by date and with confirmation that the experts have seen each other's reports;
- a paragraph confirming that the experts have seen the same documents and identifying any which have been seen by one but not the other expert;
- areas of agreement (with reasons if applicable – see Chapter 2, 'Pre-Hearing Discussion of Expert Evidence');
- areas of disagreement with reasons;
- any steps to be taken to resolve disagreement;
- a paragraph in these or similar terms:

We each DECLARE THAT: (1) We individually here re-state the Expert's Declaration contained in our respective reports that we understand our overriding duties to the court, have complied with them and will continue to do so. (2) We have neither jointly nor individually been instructed to, nor has it been suggested that we should, avoid reaching agreement, or defer reaching agreement, on any matter within our competence.

Conferences

If you are asked to attend a conference with counsel, prepare for it as if it is the trial. Have your file properly organised and complete. 'Nothing is more annoying than the witness who fiddles about with all sorts of tatty bits of paper, in the apparently forlorn hope of finding something relevant' (Braithwaite and Waldron 2010). Practise your recital of the reasons for disagreeing with the other side's expert. Be ready to learn from the way in which the barrister tests your opinion. She should challenge you about your work. She wants to know what you are going to say when cross-examined and your opinion is put under attack. It is in her interests to explore any potential area of uncertainty or weakness. See it as a 'dummy run'. She wants to see that you are '[c]onfident, personable, able to explain technical issues clearly and prepared to entertain alternative points of view . . . Or are [you] flustered, unsure, dogmatic and possibly just outraged at the tone of your questioning?' (Smethurst 2006).

If it is the pre-trial conference, find out the questions you will be asked. Ask how you will be expected to give your evidence, where to sit and whether you will have to hear other evidence. Usually, experts sit beside the solicitor and behind the barrister, but *in Ireland*, where the solicitor usually sits with their back to the judge, facing counsel, expert witnesses usually sit behind junior counsel. Be clear about the time at which you are expected to attend. If you are going to have to base your opinion on facts proved by the evidence of other witnesses, it is usual to be allowed to be present for their evidence, but for this the judge will have to give permission (other than in Ireland where there is no restriction on the attendance of expert witnesses during the course of any part of the evidence).

The following chapters deal with some of the circumstances in, and the issues about, which your expert opinion may be sought.

Reports for Criminal Proceedings and in Prison Cases

Keith Rix and Rajan Nathan

Medical science and the law have moved a long way since 1982. We hope that the safeguards now in place will prevent others becoming victims of similar miscarriages of justice. The courts must ensure that lessons learnt are translated into more effective protections. Vigilance must be the watchword of the criminal justice system if public confidence is to be maintained.

Henry LJ in *R v Roberts* (CA, unreported, 19 March 1998)

In a criminal case, the defence, the prosecution or the court may instruct you. You may be asked to assess an accused, a complainant or another witness or a convicted prisoner in contemplation of parole or release on licence.

Documents and Materials to Be Considered

It is usual to have access to the indictment, or in the Isle of Man the information, or charge sheet, a prosecution summary, prosecution witness statements, the record of police interview, the custody record and a list of previous cautions and convictions. *In Ireland*, the witness statements are included in a 'Book of Evidence'. There may be body-worn video of the arrest or crime scene, photographic exhibits or CCTV recording of the accused in the custody suite. It may be necessary to listen to, or watch, recordings of the interview. An extended version of the list of previous convictions may give limited detail of the offences. 'Unused material', on which the prosecution does not intend relying, may be relevant, so enquire about its availability and potential relevance. For an accused remanded in custody, ask for the prison healthcare records. Requesting the general practitioner records is essential. Educational, social services and probation records may assist. There may be a pre-sentence probation or social work report.

Consent Issues

It may be a condition of bail that the accused cooperates with the preparation of a medical report, but informed consent should be sought.

If the accused is pleading not guilty, be careful asking about the alleged offence. Explain that they are entitled not to answer questions about, or give an account of, the alleged offence. Their account may be compared with those given to the police and their solicitors. If you are instructed by the prosecution, the accused is particularly likely to exercise their right to silence, but this may make assessment difficult, for example in relation to fitness to plead and stand trial (FTP) and mental condition defences (see below). Particularly where risk to others is an issue, and potentially a conflict with the doctor's ethical duty of beneficence, the accused needs to understand the implications of such an assessment (see below).

Consent can include the report being made available to the probation service or equivalent (see online Appendix 8) and to obtaining medical and other relevant records.

Report Requirements

Box 7.1 sets out the matters to be addressed in a report. Reports for sentencing in England and Wales should comply with *Good Practice Guidance: Commissioning, Administering and Producing Psychiatric Reports for Sentencing* (Her Majesty's Court Service 2010) ('*Good Practice Guidance*').

Box 7.1 Matters to Be Addressed in a Report in a Criminal Case in Scotland

Preliminary information

- At whose request the assessment was undertaken, circumstances of assessment (place, time, any constraints on assessment such as inadequate time to complete assessment due to prison routine)
- Sources of information used (interview with the person, interviews with others, documents examined)
- The person's capacity to take part or refuse to take part and understanding of the limits of confidentiality
- If any important sources of information could not be used, there should be a statement as to why this was the case

Background history

- Family history
- Personal history
- Medical history
- Psychiatric history
- Recent social circumstances
- Personality
- Forensic history

Circumstances of offence or alleged offence

Progress since offence or alleged offence

Current mental state

Opinion: would cover some or all of the following matters:

- Fitness to plead
- Presence of mental disorder currently and whether the criteria for the relevant order are met
- Presence of mental disorder at the time of the offence
    - o The relationship between any mental disorder and the offence (this is still relevant even if the person has been convicted as it may affect choice of disposal)
    - o Whether the person was insane at the time of the offence
    - o In murder cases, whether there are grounds for diminished responsibility

- Assessment of risk in the presence of mental disorder
  - The risk of harm to self or others
  - The risk that the person might pose of re-offending
  - The relationship between this risk and any mental disorder present
  - Does the person require to be managed in a secure setting, and if so should this be at a state (high secure) hospital?
- What assessment or treatment does the person require?
  - Does the person need further assessment?
  - Where should this take place, does the person need a period of in-patient assessment and what level of security would be required?
  - Why, which issues remain to be clarified?
- Does the person require treatment for a mental disorder or condition?
  - What treatment does he/she need and where should this be given?
- State any matters that are currently uncertain and the reasons they remain uncertain

Mental Health (Care and Treatment) (Scotland) Act 2003, Code of Practice, Vol. 3: *Compulsory Powers in Relation to Mentally Disordered Offenders* (Scottish Executive 2005), ch. 6, para. 102

Specific Issues in Criminal Proceedings

Pre-Trial and Preliminary Issues

Assessments in Police Custody and for Bail

Once charged with an offence, an accused must either be released on police bail or held in police custody for a court to decide if they should be released on bail or further remanded in custody. If bail is not granted by the court, they are remanded to prison. Psychiatric reports may be requested in relation to applications for, or the granting of, bail or ordered as a requirement of bail. Residence at a psychiatric hospital may be made a bail condition. The main issues to be addressed in bail reports are set out in Box 7.2.

For such a report, it is necessary to consider and address some of the exceptions to a person's right to bail (Box 7.3). *In Ireland*, the fundamental consideration is the likelihood of the accused attempting to evade justice (*The People (Attorney General) v O'Callaghan* [1966] IR 501), although considerably modified by the Bail Act 1997.

At the accused's first appearance before the magistrates or equivalent court, the court needs an accurate diagnosis, a detailed description of the accused's condition and a prognosis so that the court is sufficiently confident, in appropriate cases, to grant bail.

Where an alleged offence involves a particular person or class of person and it appears to have arisen as a consequence of some specific psychiatric condition, the psychiatrist has to consider whether the accused is likely to commit further offences, particularly involving the original complainant or others with whom they are perceived, perhaps as a result of delusions, to have something in common, or interfere with witnesses, particularly the complainant.

Box 7.2 Issues to Be Addressed in a Report on a Person in Police Custody

- does the person *appear* to be suffering from mental disorder?
- does he/she currently pose a risk to him/herself or other people?
- does he/she require assessment or treatment in hospital?
- if so, how urgently is this required?
- is the person fit to be interviewed and if so, does he/she require an appropriate adult?
- is the person fit to plead were he/she to appear in court?
- may the person require community care mental health services?

Mental Health (Care and Treatment) (Scotland) Act 2003, Code of Practice, Vol. 3: *Compulsory Powers in Relation to Mentally Disordered Offenders* (Scottish Executive 2005), ch. 2, para. 7 (emphasis added)

Box 7.3 Some Exceptions to a Person's Right to Bail

- having been arrested for absconding or breaching bail conditions;
- for the person's own protection;
- there being substantial grounds for believing that the accused would fail to attend court/surrender to custody;
- there being substantial grounds to believe that the accused would commit an offence;
- there being substantial grounds for believing that the accused would interfere with witnesses or otherwise obstruct the course of justice.

There may be a case for offering psychiatric admission and, in the case of someone who can give informed consent to admission and comply with bail conditions, the court may be willing to grant bail because hospital treatment will make it less likely that they will commit further offences or interfere with witnesses.

For a person at court, have regard to their mental health needs and consider how they ought to be met, whether on bail or in custody. If there is a need for out-patient or community treatment, arrangements can be made to facilitate this in the event of bail being granted, but for a remand in custody, identify the need for treatment as a matter to be addressed by the prison healthcare service. So, designate one copy of the report for either the general practitioner or the prison medical officer. Consider sending it by email. Similar considerations apply to notifying the prison where there is an urgent need for hospital admission. Perhaps a bed is not available or the magistrates are not willing to allow the person to go to a bed of the level of security considered appropriate.

If bail is granted, conditions may be attached and in particular to facilitate an enquiry into the person's mental condition. There may be a requirement to attend for this purpose as an out-patient, or to reside as an in-patient, at a particular place and to comply with any directions which may be given.

If it is a bail condition to be admitted to a psychiatric hospital, pay careful regard to the wording of the bail conditions. They should incorporate requirements to obey the directions of the doctor or nurse in charge and comply with hospital rules. This is a statutory requirement in Scotland. Draw up a list of rules, including, for example, compliance with hospital policies concerning personal searches, alcohol and drug screening and following the advice of the clinical team. Obtain written agreement in the form of a contract. A patient who breaches this contract or insists on leaving when refused permission to do so may be in breach of their bail conditions. Appropriate wording and written consent should overcome any objections to notifying the police that the person is about to be discharged for failure to comply with the hospital rules. If the police cannot be informed, they will not be able to consider an arrest for breach of bail and there will be a risk of further offences on bail or interference with witnesses. Local arrangements should ensure police cooperation when a patient is being discharged under such circumstances. If there is no urgency, identify a discharge date, preferably at least three working days away, and notify the court and the patient's solicitor so that a date can be set for a hearing to consider the breach of bail.

For someone who might not comply with bail conditions, courts in most jurisdictions (Ireland excluded) have the power to remand a person to hospital for assessment. It is not an alternative to a remand on bail with a condition of residence in a psychiatric hospital, but an alternative to a remand to prison, so essentially a provision for obtaining a psychiatric report which could not be obtained by a remand on bail.

In England and Wales, for a remand for assessment (MHA 1983, s 35) an AMP must have reason to suspect that the person is suffering from mental disorder within the meaning of the MHA 1983, s 1. Only reasonable suspicion is needed. Its purpose is to inform the court as to issues such as FTP and disposal; its purpose is not to compel assessment for evidential purposes at the behest of the prosecution (*R (M) v Kingston Crown Court* [2014] EWHC 2702 (Admin)). It cannot be used to impose treatment, but response to treatment may be part of the assessment. A person remanded under s 35 can be prevented from leaving the hospital, but, if admitted to an unlocked ward, it needs to be fairly certain that they will comply with the requirement to stay in the hospital. If such cooperation can be expected, then arguably the criteria for s 35 are not met; it would not be impracticable to obtain the report if they were remanded to the hospital as a condition of bail. Thus, remands under this section are more likely to be to locked hospital facilities, as physical security may be necessary.

In Scotland, a similar provision exists under the Criminal Procedure (Scotland) Act 1995 (CP(S)A)), s 52D for an assessment order. Box 7.4 sets out the issues to be addressed in a report recommending such an order. The significant differences are that the doctor providing the evidence for making the order does not have to be an 'approved' registered medical practitioner (RMP) (under the Mental Health (Care and Treatment) (Scotland) Act 2003, s 22) and the purpose of the order is to determine if the criteria for a treatment order are met.

Northern Ireland has a similar provision in the Mental Capacity Act (Northern Ireland) 2016 (MCA(NI)), s 164(1). An order for a medical report where the accused has, or is reasonably suspected of having, a mental disorder (defined in s 305 as 'any disorder or disability of the mind') requires evidence from an AMP (i.e. a medical practitioner approved by the Regulation and Quality Improvement Authority (s 253)).

Discontinuance of Proceedings

Once a person has been summonsed, arrested on warrant or charged by the police, a prosecuting authority takes over. The *Code for Crown Prosecutors* (CPS 2013) in England and Wales identifies some common public interest factors tending for and against

Box 7.4 Issues to Be Addressed in a Report Recommending an Assessment Order under the Criminal Procedure (Scotland) Act 1995, s 52D

- Does it appear that the person has a mental disorder? The category need not be specified.
- Is it likely that detention in hospital is necessary to assess whether the following conditions are met?
  - the person in respect of whom the application is made has a mental disorder;
  - medical treatment is available which would be likely to prevent the mental disorder worsening or alleviate any of the symptoms, or effects, of the disorder ('the treatment considerations');
  - if the person were not provided with such medical treatment there would be a significant risk to the health, safety or welfare of the person, or to the safety of others ('the risk considerations').
- Is it likely that there would be a significant risk to the person's health, safety or welfare or to the safety of any other person if the assessment order were not made?
- Is a suitable hospital placement available which will be able to admit the person within seven days of the order being made?
- Is there a reasonable alternative to enable the assessment to be undertaken without making an assessment order?

prosecution. One relates to the mental health of the accused (Box 7.5) as is also the case *in the Isle of Man*. Such evidence may make a prosecution less likely, subject to the victim's views. In general, it will be in the public interest to prosecute even if an accused is mentally disordered. A similar consideration applies to victims. Proceedings can be discontinued under the Prosecution of Offences Act 1985, s 23 by withdrawal of the case or simply offering no evidence.

In Ireland, discontinuance is brought about by the Director of Public Prosecutions entering a *nolle prosequi* (see below). There is also provision under the Probation of Offenders Act 1907 to dismiss the charge or order a conditional discharge in certain summary cases where 'having regard to the character, antecedents ... health or mental condition of the person charged ... it is inexpedient' to punish the person or it is expedient to release the offender on probation without recording a conviction.

In the Isle of Man, the Attorney General would usually offer no evidence should it elect to discontinue proceedings and in the Court of General Gaol Delivery it is also possible for the prosecution to offer a *nolle prosequi* (see below).

Box 7.6 sets out matters to be considered in a report on discontinuance. But many people will be unhappy about being charged with a criminal offence and anxious about going to court. This is not the same as 'significant mental ... ill-health'. Likewise, threats to commit suicide, if the prosecution goes ahead, have to be evaluated with the utmost caution lest the prosecution is manipulated into discontinuance where there is no real suicide risk.

Nolle Prosequi

In a number of jurisdictions, but not Scotland, the prosecution has a power to stop or 'stay' a prosecution by the entry of a *nolle prosequi*. It is a power with which the courts may not

Box 7.5 A Public Interest Factor against Prosecution Relating to the Mental Condition of the Accused

Prosecutors should also have regard when considering culpability as to whether the suspect is, or was at the time of the offence, suffering from any significant mental or physical ill health as in some circumstances this may mean that it is less likely that a prosecution is required. However, prosecutors will also need to consider how serious the offence was, whether it is likely to be repeated and the need to safeguard the public or those providing care to such persons.

From the Code for Crown Prosecutors (CPS 2013), para. 4.12

Box 7.6 Matters to Be Considered in a Report on an Accused Where Discontinuance of Proceedings Is the Issue

- previous offences which may indicate an ongoing or recurrent mental disorder;
- the likelihood of mental disorder leading to further offending;
- alternatives to prosecution:
  - voluntary treatment as an in-patient, out-patient or in the community;
  - rehabilitation under a conditional caution;
- the accused's insight into their need for treatment;
- the accused's likely compliance with a conditional caution or voluntary treatment;
- the likely effect on the accused's mental state of the continuation of the prosecution.

interfere. It brings the criminal process to an end, but it does not prevent subsequent indictment for the same offence. In reality, however, it usually heralds the end of the prosecution.

A *nolle prosequi* is now usually directed to be entered where the accused cannot be produced to plead or stand trial owing to physical or mental incapacity which is expected to be permanent. Pay particular regard to severity and prognosis. Relatively severe forms of intellectual disability and some forms of dementia might be grounds.

Abuse of Process

Courts can also stay proceedings to protect the legal process from the abuse into which it might fall without such powers; it is a limited discretionary power to prevent a prosecution proceeding. It applies where it will be impossible to give the accused a fair trial, or in the particular circumstances it offends the court's sense of justice and propriety to be asked to try the accused, or a trial will undermine public confidence in the criminal justice system and bring it into disrepute (*Warren v Attorney-General for Jersey* [2011] UKPC 10). In cases of potential unfairness, the accused needs to be seriously prejudiced; there has to be a real risk that a fair trial could not be had. *In Ireland*, it is less a case of abuse of process than a requirement of constitutional justice.

This power may be exercised where the fairness of the trial would be compromised because the proceedings were going to be 'oppressive and vexatious' for the accused, such as where the accused is too ill to be tried or for their trial to continue. This could risk bringing the justice system into disrepute. Fairness might be compromised where an accused, as a result of memory impairment, cannot give an account of events because they can no longer relate to the events at the relevant time (Jackson and Johnstone 2005). In *R v L* [2013] EWCA Crim 991, where three adolescents had been trafficked to work in cannabis farms and one adult for the purpose of sexual exploitation, the court indicated that an abuse of process application would be likely to succeed where the trafficked person 'was under levels of compulsion which means that in reality culpability was extinguished'.

There is no clear distinction between what nature or degree of mental disorder should lead to an application for a stay and what should lead to an enquiry as to FTP. Inevitably, preparing a report for a stay requires consideration of matters that touch on FTP. If the application is unsuccessful, the defence may then raise the issue of FTP.

A stay is only that, so the court may order the accused to be reassessed later to ascertain whether they have recovered sufficiently to stand trial. It is not unknown for accused persons to fabricate or exaggerate mental disorder in order to postpone, indefinitely, they hope, a criminal trial. Their investigation requires the most careful examination of all the medical records of their treatment after the stay has been granted since, as time goes by, it becomes increasingly difficult to avoid saying or doing something that 'gives the game away'.

Fitness to Be Interviewed and Reliability of Police Interviews

In England and Wales, the Isle of Man and *Northern Ireland*, in order to avoid obtaining interview evidence that is subsequently excluded because the prosecution cannot prove beyond reasonable doubt that it was not obtained by oppression or in consequence of anything said or done which was likely to have made it unreliable (Police and Criminal Evidence Act 1984 (PACE), s 76, Criminal Justice Act 1991 (CJA 1991), s 11(2) and Police and Criminal Evidence (Northern Ireland) Order 1989 (PCE(NI)O), art 74, respectively) or because it would have such an adverse effect upon the fairness of the proceedings that, according to the judgment and discretion of the court (*R (Saifi) v Governor of Brixton Prison* [2001] 1 WLR 1134) it should be excluded (PACE, s 78, CJA 1991, s 13, PCE(NI)O, art 76, respectively), the police apply a number of safeguards set out in Code C of the Codes of Practice of the PACE, the PCE(NI)O and the Police Powers and Procedures Codes Order 2014 (the Manx Codes). *In Scotland*, the equivalent requirement as to the fairness of the interview is determined according to Lord Hodge's ruling in *HM Advocate v Duncan* [2006] HCJ 06:

> . . . the test is one of fairness in all the circumstances, having regard not only to the means by which the interview was conducted but also other circumstances which might place the accused in a position of such disadvantage that he could understand neither the situation he was in nor his right not to answer the questions which were put to him.

In England and Wales, it is recognised that although 'vulnerable persons are often capable of providing reliable evidence, they may, without knowing it or wishing to do so, be particularly prone in certain circumstances to providing information that may be unreliable, misleading or self-incriminating' (PACE Code C, Note for Guidance 11C; PCE(NI)O Code C, Note for Guidance 11C; similar provision at 11C in the Manx Codes). The

England and Wales Code C includes particular provisions relating to persons who 'may be vulnerable as a result of having a mental health condition or mental disorder' and the Northern Ireland Code C also makes provision for detainees who have a 'mental disorder' or are 'mentally vulnerable' (Code C, Note for Guidance 1G). *In England and Wales*, 'mental disorder' means 'the range of clinically recognised conditions' described at p. 26, para. 2.5 in the MHA 1983 Code of Practice (PACE Code C, Note for Guidance 1GB) and *in Northern Ireland* it means 'any disorder or disability of the mind' (MCA(NI), s 305), mental vulnerability or communication difficulties. *In England and Wales*, PACE Code C 1.13(d) states that 'vulnerable' applies to any person who, because of a mental health condition or mental disorder:

(i) may have difficulty understanding or communicating effectively about the full implications for them of any procedures and processes connected with:
- their arrest and detention; or (as the case may be)
- their voluntary attendance at a police station or their presence elsewhere, for the purpose of a voluntary interview; and
- the exercise of their rights and entitlements.

(ii) does not appear to understand the significance of what they are told, of questions they are asked or of their replies;

(iii) appears to be particularly prone to:
- becoming confused and unclear about their position;
- providing unreliable, misleading or incriminating information without knowing or wishing to do so;
- accepting or acting on suggestions from others without consciously knowing or wishing to do so; or
- readily agreeing to suggestions or proposals without any protest or question.

Code C of the Manx Codes makes similar provisions for those with 'mental disorder', defined in the Mental Health Act 1998, s 1(2) as 'mental illness, arrested or incomplete development of mind, psychopathic disorder and any other disorder or disability of mind'.

Mental vulnerability probably includes states of extreme emotion and distress (*R v Souter* [1994] 11 WLUK 101). Gudjonsson *et al.* (1993) found that a third of suspects were not in a normal mental state while in police custody due to extreme distress or mental disorder which could impair their capacity for rational decision-making or coping effectively with interview and they have suggested that even detainees whose mental health or psychological problems do not amount to actual mental illness or mental disorder are potentially vulnerable to giving misleading or unreliable statements.

In England and Wales, Code C 11.15 provides that '[a] . . . vulnerable person must not be interviewed . . . in the absence of the appropriate adult' unless delay might give rise to certain risks (set out in C 11.1) and the interview would not significantly harm the detainee's physical or mental state (C 11.18). The role of the appropriate adult is to safeguard the rights, entitlements and welfare of the detainee. Code C, 11.15, 11.18 of the Northern Ireland and Manx Codes have a similar provision.

In Ireland, there is a general provision (Criminal Justice Act 1984, (Treatment of Persons in Custody in Garda Síochána Stations) Regulations 1987, reg 3) that members of the Gardaí should have regard for the special needs of any detainees who may be under a 'mental disability' and there is a requirement (reg 12) that the interview must be conducted in a fair and humane manner. The Children Act 2001, s 55 requires the Gardaí to act 'with due respect for the personal rights of the children and their dignity as human persons, for their vulnerability owing to their age and level of maturity and for the special needs of any of them who may be under a physical or mental disability'. In *The People (DPP) v Diver* [2005] 3 IR 270, the Supreme Court suggested that if there was a breach of the Regulations the issue was whether it prejudiced the fairness of the accused's trial.

In England and Wales, *Northern Ireland* and *the Isle of Man*, Code C 1.7b states that 'appropriate adult', in the case of a mentally disordered or mentally vulnerable person, means:

(i) a relative, guardian or other person responsible for their care or custody;
(ii) someone experienced in dealing with mentally disordered or mentally vulnerable persons . . .
(iii) failing these, some other responsible adult aged 18 or over, but not a police officer or police employee etc.

In England and Wales and *Northern Ireland*, in the case of a juvenile who is estranged from their parent, the parent should not act as the appropriate adult if the juvenile expressly and specifically objects (Note for Guidance 1B). Also, *in Northern Ireland*, a person who appears to be mentally disordered or otherwise mentally vulnerable should not be an appropriate adult (Note for Guidance 1B). *In Northern Ireland*, the police are required to provide the appropriate adult with written guidance as to their role if they require it (Note for Guidance 1AA of Code C of the PCE(NI)O).

In Ireland, detainees suspected of being, or known to be, 'mentally handicapped' can only exceptionally be interviewed in the absence of a 'responsible adult' who cannot be a member of An Garda Síochána and who, where practicable, has 'experience in dealing with the mentally handicapped'. 'Mental handicap' is not defined and the expression has not been amended in any subsequent revisions of the custody regulations. At best, it must be taken to mean intellectual disability or impairment, as distinct from mental illness or any other form of mental disorder. Solicitors are advised that '[i]n circumstances where a client is labouring under a mental or psychiatric disability', they may request that a psychiatrist or psychologist is contacted to assess the detainee's fitness to be questioned by Gardaí (Law Society of Ireland 2016). However, there are no specific provisions in relation to fitness to be interviewed (FTBI).

Appropriate adult schemes also exist in Scotland and there is a similar requirement for an appropriate adult to attend if a police officer suspects that someone who is being interviewed has a mental disorder.

'[A]ny mental or personality abnormalities may be of relevance' (*R v Wilkinson* (Court of Appeal Criminal Division, unreported, 25 July 1996)) when considering mental disorder and mental vulnerability, including 'a personality disorder so severe as properly to be categorised as mental disorder' (*R v Ward (Judith)* [1993] 1 WLR 619). But this is not enough as 'the abnormal disorder must not only be of a type which might render a confession or evidence unreliable; there must also be a very significant deviation from the norm shown' (*R v O'Brien* [2000] All ER (D) 62).

Severe personality disorder was the basis of a prostitute's successful appeal against a robbery conviction (*R v Walker* [1997] 7 WLUK 689). A psychiatrist gave evidence that she might have elaborated inaccurately on events without understanding the implications of doing so. The conviction was quashed in *R v Lawless* [2009] EWCA Crim 1308, where psychological evidence showed that the appellant was emotionally unstable, had high levels of compliance and had a pathological dependency on others.

Where the case against an accused with intellectual disability depends wholly or substantially on their confession and the court is satisfied that they are 'mentally handicapped' and that the confession was not made in the presence of an independent person, the jury has to be warned to be cautious before convicting in reliance on the confession (PACE, s 77, PE(NI)O, art 78). 'Mentally handicapped' means having a state of arrested or incomplete development of mind which includes significant impairment of intelligence and social functioning. *R v Silcott* [1991] 12 WLUK 49 established that significant impairment of intelligence is not defined by a specific intelligence quotient (IQ) level as the court was 'not attracted to the concept that the judicial approach to the submissions under section 76(2)(b) should be governed by which side of an arbitrary line, whether at 69/70 or elsewhere, the IQ fell'.

In *R v Ali* [1999] 2 Archbold News, the appellant had an IQ between 66 and 72. His conviction for drug dealing was quashed on thc ground that his admissions and assertions were obviously exaggerated and likely to be unreliable as a result of his intellectual disability. *R v Steel* [2003] EWCA Crim 1640 is the case of a man convicted of murder in 1979 when a psychiatrist decided that his measured IQ of 67 was probably an underestimate and he was of 'dull normal intelligence'. The report was not put in evidence. Subsequently, on the basis of his IQ of 74 in 1996 (on the Wechsler Adult Intelligence Scale – Revised) and 65 in 2001 (on the Wechsler Adult Intelligence Scale – 3rd edn), and degrees of suggestibility and compliance 'near the borderline of abnormality', his conviction was quashed because 'his unforeseen abnormally low IQ rendered him particularly vulnerable to interrogation'.

Personality disorder, specifically psychopathic disorder, and 'low normal intelligence' together led to the successful appeal against a murder conviction in *R v Harvey* [1988] Crim LR 241. Harvey falsely confessed to the murder after hearing her lover's confession. Her admission was excluded as the prosecution could not prove beyond reasonable doubt that it was not made as a consequence of a child-like desire to protect him.

A combination of factors led to the exclusion of interview evidence under PACE, s 78 in *R v Aspinall* [1999] Crim LR 741. Aspinall informed the custody officer of his schizophrenia, but was considered fit to be interviewed. He declined a solicitor. He was eventually interviewed thirteen hours after arrest without an appropriate adult. He wanted to get home to his wife and children. Although his own psychiatrist testified that he would probably have been tired, under stress and worried and therefore possibly less able to cope with questions and might have given answers to effect an early release from custody, the interview was admitted. At his successful appeal, it was held that there had been a clear breach of Code C because there was no appropriate adult and:

> A vulnerable person who has been in custody for some 13 hours and who is more likely to be stressed than a normal person cannot be equated with a person lacking any disability ... the appropriate adult or legal advisor could have been expected to advise him to tell the truth at interview. If he had done that, his answers would have assisted the defence and not the police ...

There will continue to be cases in which expert evidence by psychiatrists and psychologists, as to reliability, will be necessary in order to avoid the mentally disordered and mentally vulnerable being wrongly convicted. The factors identified as relevant when determining the fairness of the interview in *Duncan* helpfully summarise the issues:

- the presence of mental disorder;
- the format of the interview;
- the degree of coercion used to obtain a confession;
- the interviewee's suggestibility;
- the interviewee's level of understanding and comprehension;
- if present, the competence of the appropriate adult acting within their role.

Reliability is essentially about the capacity of the detainee for truthfulness and for accuracy unimpaired by mental disorder or mental vulnerability or, where such dangers exist, the steps taken to negate their potential effect on the interview (Ventress *et al.* 2008). An internal element relates to the detainee and an external element to circumstances or things that are said or done that might affect the detainee. This is reflected in the three considerations in Annex G to Codes C of the PACE and the PCE(NI)O:

(a) how the detainee's physical or mental state might affect their ability to understand the nature and purpose of the interview, to comprehend what is being asked and to appreciate the significance of any answers given and make rational decisions about whether they want to say anything;
(b) the extent to which the detainee's replies may be affected by their physical or mental condition rather than representing a rational and accurate explanation of their involvement in the offence;
(c) how the nature of the interview, which could include particularly probing questions, might affect the detainee.

Assessment focuses not only on the detainee's mental state, but on what effect the circumstances and the things said or done by the police may have had. *R v Delaney* [1988] 8 WLUK 34 was the case of a man whose confession to indecently assaulting a child was the whole basis of the prosecution case. A psychologist gave evidence that he was 'educationally subnormal', had an IQ of 80 and his personality was such that he would be 'subject to quick emotional arousal which might lead him to wish to rid himself of the interview by bringing it to an end as rapidly as possible'. The interviewing police officers deliberately sought to play down the seriousness of the assault and to suggest that he needed psychiatric help. In quashing the conviction, the court found that he might have felt that it was easier to get away from his unpleasant state of arousal by confessing, particularly in the light of the suggestion that what was required was treatment rather than prison.

Box 7.7 is a framework for investigating such cases. One objective is to reconstruct the detainee's mental and physical state whilst in police custody (Gudjonsson 2003, p. 313) and then to determine the potential reliability or otherwise of the interview. It is advisable to work in tandem with a forensic psychologist.

Central to the assessment are the actual interviews and the circumstances in which they took place. There has to be an analysis of the interviews that demonstrates how the detainee's mental disorder or mental vulnerability appears to have given rise to unreliability. In *Ackerley v Her Majesty's Attorney General of the Isle of Man* [2013] UKPC 26, although expert evidence raised concerns about the procedural course of the investigation of a sexual assault by a man with autism, the court concluded that they did not affect the safety of the conviction. It is a 'functional test' and not a 'state' test. This is reflected in Annex G of Code C of the PACE and the PCE(NI)O: 'It is essential healthcare professionals who are consulted consider the functional ability of the detainee rather than simply relying on a medical diagnosis, e.g. it is possible for a person with severe mental illness to be fit for interview.'

Box 7.7 A Framework for the Investigation of a Case Where Psychological or Psychiatric Factors May Be Relevant to the Admissibility or Reliability of Police Interviews

- detailed psychiatric history from the accused;
- review of general, practice, psychiatric, prison, medical, social service records;
- review of witness statements and other evidence;
- review of the custody record and noting particularly:
    - disclosure by detainee on reception, or suspicion by police, of a history of mental disorder or anything suggesting mental vulnerability;
    - drugs in the possession of detainee;
    - findings of the forensic physician;
    - the detailed written notes of any psychiatric examination;
    - observations of behaviour by custody officers;
- examination of rest, sleep patterns, refreshments;
- examination of timings of interviews in relation to arrest and time of day;
- untoward events (e.g. collapse, hospital admissions, recall of forensic physician or nurse);
- listen to taped police interviews/watch videotaped police interviews;
- read the transcripts of police interview(s);
- understand and examine the role of the appropriate adult;
- understand and examine the nature of the police interview and questioning, with particular reference to interview style and the use of coercion;
- detailed examination of the detainee, noting mental state, functional intellectual ability, presence of mental disorder or mental distress or other vulnerabilities;
- arrange appropriate specialised psychological investigation (e.g. intellectual functioning, suggestibility and compliance testing, personality testing).

There has to be evidence in, or outside, the interviews themselves of things said or done, that can be demonstrated to question reliability: 'the real criterion must simply be whether the abnormal disorder [sic] might render the confession or evidence unreliable' (*O'Brien*); 'a causal link between what was said or done and the subsequent confession had to be shown' (*R v Goldenberg* [1988] 5 WLUK 173).

Where someone with a mental disorder or mental vulnerability has not been afforded the assistance of an appropriate adult, or where the appropriate adult has not intervened at all, or appears to have failed to intervene when they should, it will be necessary to say how the interview would have been different, had they intervened.

Work with complete transcripts and an audiotape or videotape of the interview. Pauses, tension, shouting or distress may be evident. The police's edited transcript does not always fully convey the way in which the accused communicates. Determining whether rather jumbled comments by the accused represent a clinical phenomenon, such as thought disorder, may be assisted by listening to the recording. The beginning of the interview and the caution may be omitted. Difficulties in explaining the caution and sometimes the detainee's complete failure to understand it may be important clues to the nature of their difficulties and an important ground for a submission to exclude the interview. In *R v McGovern* (1990) 92 Cr App Rep 228, where a 19-year-old pregnant woman with an IQ of 73 was charged with murder, it was part of her successful appeal against conviction for manslaughter that her confession was made in the absence of a solicitor when she was 'physically ill, emotionally distressed and unable to understand the caution until it was explained in simple language'.

Box 7.8 lists aspects of the interview that may have a bearing on their reliability.

Whether a suspect was suffering from a mental disorder at the time of the interviews is an objective test. In *R v Everett* [1988] Crim LR 826, the medical evidence was that the detainee had an IQ of 61. The Court of Appeal held that it did not matter what the police officers thought; the test was the detainee's actual condition as subsequently diagnosed by the doctor. *R v Beattie* [2018] NICA 1 has established that suspicion may be dispelled upon examination by a forensic physician.

It may be necessary to try and re-examine the basis for a judgement, by the doctors involved at the time of the interview, that the suspect was fit to be interviewed or did not need an appropriate adult. Gudjonnson (2003, p. 269) describes a case where the trial judge held that the two doctors had considered only potential harm rather than potential unreliability.

Box 7.8 Some Pointers to Possibly Unreliable Police Interviews

- failure to understand the police caution;
- failure by solicitor or appropriate adult to seek a break to consult with detainee who becomes distressed;
- failure by the solicitor or appropriate adult to seek a break if interview is lengthy or interrogation sustained and there is evidence of the detainee becoming confused, incoherent or rambling;
- failure by the police to respond appropriately to interventions by the solicitor or appropriate adult – for example, take a break, use shorter words, explain terminology (such as 'bail', 'custody');
- evidence of acquiescence when leading questions are put, especially when put with some force;
- 'yes' responses to questions which the detainee probably did not understand;
- evidence of the accused being led;
- the police minimising the gravity of the offences (*R v Delaney*);
- the police suggesting that treatment, not punishment, is the likely outcome (*R v Delaney*);
- the police shouting, using bad language, being rude or being discourteous (*R v Emmerson*);
- a desire by the detainee to obtain release from detention as quickly as possible (*R v Delaney, R v Crampton, R v Aspinall*);
- misunderstanding of, or failure to understand, questions or what is being put to the detainee;
- changing answers in response to negative feedback (interrogative suggestibility);
- confessing to crimes that could not possibly have been committed (false confessions).

Under the PACE, s 76, the court must exclude the confession if it finds that it was obtained by 'oppression' or under circumstances likely to render it 'unreliable'. Oppression is subjective: 'What may be oppressive as regards a child, an invalid or an old man or somebody inexperienced in the ways of the world may turn out not to be oppressive when one finds that the accused is of tough character and an experienced man of the world' (*R v Priestley* (1965) 51 Cr App R 1).

In *R v Emmerson* [1990] 11 WLUK 266, the court did not accept that the police's rude and discourteous questioning, with some shouting and bad language, was oppressive, but it might be so in someone who could easily be overwhelmed by such behaviour. In *R v Miller* [1986] 1 WLR 1191, it was held that it might be oppressive to put questions to someone known to be mentally ill so as 'skilfully and deliberately' to induce a 'delusionary' state. While an 'experienced professional criminal' might expect a vigorous interrogation (*R v Gowan* [1982] 6 WLUK 123), it was held that there had been oppression in the case of *R v Hudson* [1980] 10 WLUK 280, where a middle-aged man of previous good character had been subjected to a lengthy and, in some respects unlawful, interrogation.

In Ireland, the test is one of fairness. *The People (DPP) v Shaw* [1982] IR 1 established that what was technically a voluntary statement could be 'excluded if, by reason of the manner or circumstances in which it was obtained, it falls below the standard of fairness'.

An Irish case helpfully defines oppression: 'Questioning which by its nature, duration or other attendant circumstances (including defective custody) excites hopes (such as the hope of release) or fears, or so affects the mind of the subject that his will crumbles and he speaks when otherwise he would have remained silent' (*The People (DPP) v McNally and Breathnach* [1981] 2 Frewen 43).

What interviewing techniques may be oppressive or render the suspect's evidence unreliable is a specialised area (Gudjonsson 2003, pp. 75–114). Not all of the 'oppressive' tactics identified by Gudjonsson are unacceptable and, even when they are used, their identification is not in itself sufficient to submit that the evidence elicited may be unreliable. Furthermore, not all impropriety necessarily involves oppression. What matters is whether reliability is compromised. However, when reporting, it is of critical importance to state not that there is unreliability, but why there might be unreliability (see Chapter 6, 'Treading on the Judge's Toes', for details of *Pora*).

In *R v Paris* (1993) 97 Crim App R 99, where the detainee was on the borderline of 'mental handicap', the Court of Appeal identified an interview in which he was 'bullied and hectored' as oppressive and said that it should have been excluded. It also pointed out that it would have been oppressive even with a detainee of normal intelligence. However, in *R v L* [1994] Crim LR 839, similar tactics seem to have been regarded as acceptable as long as they did not affect the reliability of the confession. In *L & R v R* [2011] EWCA Crim 649, there was evidence that L, who showed signs of autistic spectrum disorder, was 'suggestible particularly when under pressure and when required to respond to complex statements or questions'. A confrontational style of questioning, far from eliciting the truth, might make erroneous answers more likely. There was a risk that under pressure he would give answers in which he did not believe. It was ruled that the admission of the interview, conducted in the absence of an appropriate adult and a solicitor, would be unfairly prejudicial to him.

It is not just 'oppressive' interviewing which needs to be identified. In *R v Waters* [1988] 7 WLUK 374, it was sufficient to have identified merely 'improper' questioning which had resulted in ambiguous and potentially unreliable answers. In *R v Blackburn* [2005] EWCA Crim 1349, the issue was the effect of prolonged questioning on a 15-year-old boy who suffered from no mental disorder, but was described as 'a vulnerable individual'. Expert evidence was admitted as to whether someone, after prolonged questioning, might make a false confession in the form of a 'coerced compliant confession'.

It will often be advisable to have a formal assessment of IQ by a psychologist because clinical impressions by prison medical officers and psychiatrists about intelligence are often misleading (Gudjonsson 2003, pp. 322, 469). Also, in *R v Kenny* [1993] 7 WLUK 202, it was held that it is not appropriate to take IQ test results from one case and apply them slavishly to another case because every case has its individual features.

Psychological test results, even in the absence of a mental disorder, may be evidence of mental vulnerability which is relevant and important in rendering evidence unreliable. It used to be the law that a mental abnormality had to fall into a recognised category of mental disorder for expert evidence to be properly admissible (*Ward*), but in *O'Brien* the court questioned this and indicated that the operative consideration was simply whether the abnormality might render the confession unreliable. It also needs to be established that there was evidence of these vulnerabilities prior to police interview.

Abnormal suggestibility and abnormal compliance are vulnerabilities of particular importance. In *R v Smith* [2003] EWCA Crim 927, convictions for attempted rape and burglary with intent to rape were quashed upon receipt of evidence from psychologists to the effect that the appellant produced abnormally high confabulation scores, both on immediate and delayed recall, and according to the defence psychologist he was 'abnormally suggestible and compliant on testing'. In *Roberts*, expert evidence was admitted to show that the accused had a 'compliant and unreliable' personality.

Suggestibility may be particularly important in people with an intellectual disability who have a greater tendency to go along with a story that is put to them and the more so if they are under pressure. In *R v King* [1999] 12 WLUK 333, the appellant's unsuccessful defence to a charge of murder was that his confession had been obtained under pressure as a result of accepting suggestions put to him by the interviewing officers. At his successful appeal, a psychologist gave evidence that his IQ was 78 and his scores for suggestibility and compliance were in the abnormal range. The court held that he was 'more vulnerable than was understood at the time, and abnormally ready to accept what was put to him'.

When you prepare the report, be familiar with all of the other evidence and be prepared to place your findings within the context of the totality of the case (Gudjonsson 2003, p. 328). Do not to fall into the trap of assuming that, because there is evidence that a confession is true, there is no issue of reliability. In *R v Cox* [1990] 11 WLUK 165, where the accused had an IQ of 58, at the *voir dire* (a trial within a trial at which the judge decides an issue in the absence of the jury), he admitted one of the offences with which he was charged. The trial judge admitted this confession, but was held to have been wrong to do so. Likewise, in *R v Crampton* [1990] 11 WLUK 258, it was held that, if acts were done or words were spoken which were likely to induce unreliable confessions, then an admission was inadmissible, whether or not true. As to whether a confession is unreliable, the issue of whether the confession is true is strictly irrelevant.

If the accused gives evidence on a *voir dire*, you should be in court to observe this. In *R v Weeks* [1995] Crim LR 52, it was held that the demeanour of the accused when giving evidence on the *voir dire* could assist the prosecution in showing that he was not affected by the threats allegedly made at the interview.

The presence of an appropriate adult is meant to provide safeguards for the detainee, but their mere presence may not be sufficient. Paragraph 11.17 of the Codes of *England and*

Wales, Northern Ireland and *the Isle of Man* makes it clear that the appropriate adult is not expected to act simply as an observer. The role is an active one: to advise the detainee, to observe whether the interview is being conducted properly and fairly, and to facilitate communication. *In Northern Ireland*, there is also a discretion for the police to provide a 'registered intermediary' where a detainee with a mental disorder or significant impairment of intelligence and social functioning is unable to participate effectively (Notes for Guidance 1GG of Code C). Their role includes advising interviewing officers about appropriate communication strategies and if present they, not the appropriate adult, are responsible for facilitating communication.

The transcripts of the interviews may reveal a failure to advise the person being interviewed, improper or unfair interviewing about which the appropriate adult (or registered intermediary) is silent or a failure to facilitate communication so that misunderstandings are apparent. It may be clear from the custody record that the appropriate adult did not consult with the detainee in private before the interview. In *R v Dutton* (Central Criminal Court, unreported, 1987), the court concluded that an appropriate adult 'would, before the police interview, have ascertained from Mr. Dutton, quietly and without any pressure, what he wished to say; and/or . . . ensured that Mr. Dutton had the advice of a solicitor before he was interviewed'.

In a case which was dismissed after magistrates heard the evidence of a psychologist that the accused was someone who needed an appropriate adult (*DPP v Cornish* [1997] 1 WLUK 250), an appeal by the prosecution led the court to set out the approach which ought to be adopted in such cases, including receiving prosecution evidence about the interviews. This was identified as: '. . . who was there at the time of the interview and how the interview went, so that the court could form some impression of the effect of the absence of the appropriate adult upon the conduct of the interview and other matters of that kind'.

The psychiatrist or psychologist needs to study the interview records and decide what the effect was of the absence of the appropriate adult, or what the effect was of an appropriate adult being present but not providing the safeguards expected or being an inappropriate appropriate adult (see Box 7.9).

The appropriate adult 'cannot . . . be a person with whom the juvenile has no empathy' (*DPP v Blake* [1989] 1 WLR 432). In *Blake*, the appropriate adult was a juvenile's estranged father whom she did not wish to see. It has been argued that '*any person* to whom the suspect expressly objects is *per se* inappropriate' (Mirfield 1997, p. 289, emphasis in the original).

Box 7.9 Possible Reasons for Seeking to Disqualify the Appropriate Adult

- detainee has no empathy with the appropriate adult;
- detainee expressly objected to the appropriate adult;
- appropriate adult incapable of fulfilling the functions as a result of being intellectually disabled or mentally disordered;
- appropriate adult has some involvement in the offence (e.g. as a victim or witness);
- appropriate adult is involved in the investigation;
- appropriate adult has already received admissions from the detainee.

Although case law supports the exclusion of an intellectually disabled or mentally disordered person from being an appropriate adult, as happened in *R v Morse* [1990] 11 WLUK 237, where the father of the juvenile detainee, acting as appropriate adult, had an IQ of between 60 and 70, was virtually illiterate and was probably incapable of appreciating the gravity of his son's situation, the test is whether the appropriate adult is capable of fulfilling their functions. Thus, in *Ward*, where the detainee's mother was almost certainly psychotic when acting as appropriate adult and had an IQ of 76, the trial judge accepted the psychiatric evidence that she was capable of fulfilling her functions and ruled that she did qualify as an appropriate adult. Her psychosis concerned her neighbours and so, arguably, it did not affect her perception of what was happening to her daughter. The Court of Appeal did not overturn the trial judge on either his description of her as having 'some intellectual deficit as a result of her chronic psychosis' or on his judgement of her overall capability of functioning as an appropriate adult.

An appropriate adult is not rendered inappropriate just because they are a 'somewhat critical observer and participant', for example, the father of a 15-year-old boy who 'intervened robustly from time to time, sometimes joining in the questioning of his son and challenging his exculpatory account of certain incidents' (*R v Jefferson* [1994] 1 All ER 270).

Failings of the appropriate adult which may render an interview inadmissible or lead to a challenge to reliability are set out in Box 7.10.

Although FTBI is to be distinguished from, and not confused with, FTP (see below), in *R v B* [2012] EWCA Crim 1799, the Court of Appeal found it very difficult to understand how the judge, having found that the appellant was unfit to plead, could have found that the appellant would understand the caution and have sufficient understanding to be interviewed. It therefore went on to say that it could not understand how his police interview could have been admitted for the trial of the facts (see below) to decide if he had done the act charged.

Box 7.10 Potential Failings of the Appropriate Adult

- failure to understand role;
- failure to make sure that the detainee understands the caution and can explain it in their own words;
- failure to ascertain that detainee understands legal rights:
  - right to silence (i.e. the caution);
  - right to free, independent legal advice;
  - right to consult the Codes of Practice;
  - right to have another person informed of detention;
- failure to advise the detainee:
  - for example, to obtain legal representation, tell the truth;
- adopts a purely passive role;
- overlooks detainee's failure to understand questions;
- overlooks detainee's incoherent answers;
- takes on role of interrogator and/or sides with police;
- fails to stop interview when detainee becomes too distressed.

Out-of-Court Silence

In England and Wales, a detainee who does not answer questions put to him by the police will be at risk of the court allowing an adverse inference to be drawn from his silence (Criminal Justice and Public Order Act 1994 (CJPOA), ss. 34, 36 and 37). However, the courts have made special allowances for the mentally disordered or otherwise mentally vulnerable. In *R v Argent* [1996] 12 WLUK 323, the court established a subjective test to be applied to a detainee who did not answer the questions put by the police, taking into account such matters as the time of day, the detainee's age, experience, mental capacity, state of health, sobriety, tiredness, knowledge and personality. *R v Howell* [2003] EWCA Crim 1 confirmed that 'the suspect's ill-health, in particular mental disability', was relevant.

In such a case, a psychiatrist may be instructed in order to decide if, when interviewed, one or more of these conditions applied. In such a case, and where the solicitor has advised the detainee not to answer questions, a request should be made for access to what should be her full and comprehensive record of all the factors that she has taken into consideration. The solicitor will be aware that, if relied upon by the psychiatrist, this information will no longer be legally privileged. See Rix (1998) for a case in which the accused's personality disorder was accepted as a condition relevant to drawing an inference from his out-of-court silence.

Fitness to Plead and Stand Trial

At the York Spring Assizes in 1831, Esther Dyson, who was 'deaf and dumb', was indicted for the murder of her illegitimate child (*R v Dyson* (1831) 7 Car & P 303) (Rix 2012). A sign language interpreter testified that it was impossible to make her understand that she could challenge jury members and that she could not put words together. Her incapacity to understand the mode of her trial or to conduct her defence was proved. She was ordered to be kept in strict custody until His Majesty's pleasure was known.

When Pritchard, who was also 'deaf and dumb', was indicted for the capital offence of bestiality a few years later, the court followed the procedure in *Dyson* (*R v Pritchard* (1836) 7 Car & P 303), but the adoption of the *Pritchard* jury direction (Box 7.11) in *R v Podola* [1960] 1 QB 325 has made *Pritchard* the leading case.

In England and Wales, the procedure for determining whether an accused is 'under a disability' is governed by the Criminal Procedure (Insanity) Act 1964 (CP(I)A), the Criminal Procedure (Insanity and Unfitness to Plead) Act 1991 (CP(IUP)A) and the Domestic Violence, Crime and Victims Act 2004 (DVCVA). If raised by the defence, it bears the burden of establishing unfitness on a balance of probability; if raised by the

Box 7.11 The *Pritchard* Test (*R v Pritchard* (1836) 7 Car & P 303)

[Is the accused] of sufficient intellect to comprehend the course of proceedings on the trial, so as to make a proper defence – to know that he might challenge [any jurors] to whom he may object – and to comprehend the details of the evidence, which in a case of this nature must constitute a minute investigation ... if you think that there is no certain mode of communicating the details of the trial to the prisoner, so that he can clearly understand them, and be able properly to make his defence to the charge; you ought to find that he is not of sane mind.

prosecution, it bears the burden of proving unfitness beyond reasonable doubt. If raised by the court, *Halsbury's Laws* suggest that the burden lies on the prosecution to disprove the accused's unfitness. It is usually raised by the defence.

The CP(I)A does not apply to summary proceedings where the usual course, if there is evidence of unfitness, is to determine whether the accused did the act or made the omission charged and, if so, make a hospital order under the MHA 1983, s 37(3) or make no order at all. So, when the accused is charged with a summary offence and the court is satisfied that he did the act or made the omission, if the court does not have sufficient medical evidence to decide on an order under s 37(3), the Powers of the Criminal Courts (Sentencing) Act 2000, s 11(1)(a) gives the court the power to remand the accused in custody or on bail for a medical report and, if remanding on bail, to impose a condition that the accused cooperates. The power to order medical reports depends merely on the court being satisfied that the accused committed the *actus reus* of the offence. The report's focus is narrow – the criteria for a hospital order under the MHA 1983, s 37, but including a risk assessment that informs the recommendation and sets out the proposed treatment, particularly if there is to be no recommendation of a hospital order and it is proposed to care for the accused in the community.

In Jersey, there is no mechanism or direction for FTP to be determined by the lower, magistrate's court. Where the magistrate's court has doubt as to a person's fitness to enter a plea, the court must immediately refer the case to the Royal Court for determination, no matter how minor the alleged offence, although it is open to the Attorney General to consider whether or not the criminal law should be engaged if it is a relatively trivial offence (*Attorney-General v O'Driscoll* [2003] JRC 117).

In England and Wales, in the youth court, where also the CP(I)A does not apply, the test is of 'effective participation'. In *SC v United Kingdom* [2004] 6 WLUK 252, an 11-year-old boy of limited intellectual ability and with a poor attention span had been convicted of robbery. The European Court of Human Rights ruled that:

> In the case of a child, it was essential that the proceedings take full account of his age, level of maturity and intellectual and emotional capacities, and that steps [are] taken to promote his ability to understand and participate, including conducting the hearing in such a way as to reduce as far as possible his feelings of intimidation and inhibition.

SC v United Kingdom was considered in *R (P) v West London Youth Court* [2005] EWHC 2583 (Admin). The accused was aged 15 years, had an IQ of 63 and on appeal it was argued that he could not effectively participate in the proceedings. The court held that neither youth nor limited intellectual capacity necessarily led to a breach of the European Convention on Human Rights (ECHR), art 6 (the right to a fair trial). It found that crucially the district judge had taken into account how the youth court was designed and adapted to deal 'with the kind of problems presented by the claimant and other youngsters whose intellectual capacity falls at the lower end of the scale'. The court identified a number of steps that could be taken (Box 7.12).

The issue is decided by a judge alone on the evidence (written or oral) of two or more RMPs, at least one of whom must be an AMP (CP(I)A, s 4(6)), but this does not apply to summary proceedings (see above). Where the medical evidence is unanimous, it may be read, but the judge is entitled to reject it and, in which case, as where it is contested, oral

Box 7.12 Steps to Be Taken to Ensure the Fair Trial of a Youth with a Mild Learning Disability

- keeping the claimant's level of cognitive functioning in mind;
- using concise and simple language;
- having regular breaks;
- taking additional time to explain court proceedings;
- being proactive in ensuring the claimant has access to support;
- explaining and ensuring the claimant understands the ingredients of the charge;
- explaining the possible outcomes and sentences;
- ensuring that cross-examination is carefully controlled so that questions are short and clear and frustration is minimised.

R (P) v West London Youth Court [2005] EWHC 2583 (Admin)

Box 7.13 The *Pritchard* Test as Operationalised in *R v M (John)* [2003] EWCA Crim 3452

Are any of the following beyond the accused's capabilities?

- understanding the *nature and effect of the* charges;
- deciding whether to plead guilty or not;
- exercising his right to challenge jurors;
- instructing solicitors and counsel *so as to prepare and make a proper defence in this case including understanding the details of the evidence which can reasonably be expected to be given in his case and advising his solicitor and counsel in relation to that evidence – this applies to his ability to instruct his legal advisers before and/or during his trial*;
- following the course of the proceedings;
- giving evidence in his own defence.

Expansions in italics based on *R v Whitefield* (Leeds Crown Court, unreported, 1995) (Rix 1996a)

testimony will be necessary. *R v Walls* [2011] EWCA Crim 443 established that: 'Save in cases where the unfitness is clear, the fact that psychiatrists agree is not enough . . . a court would be failing in its duty to both the public and to an accused if it did not rigorously examine the evidence and reach its own conclusion.'

Box 7.13 shows how the test for FTP is operationalised. Note that 'the current test . . . is expressed as a single, indivisible test which must be met in its entirety. An accused will not be fit to plead or stand trial if any one or more of the specified competences is beyond his capability' (*Marcantonio v R* [2016] EWCA Crim 14).

Box 7.14 shows some common misunderstandings about FTP. The test has a high threshold.

The following explanations of the competences for FTP, taken from *R v M (John)* [2003] EWCA Crim 3452, and some of the requirements for effective participation established in *SC v United Kingdom* should be read in conjunction with Box 7.13.

The accused must have a broad understanding of the nature of the trial process and of what is at stake, including the significance of any potential penalty, the role of the jury and the importance of making a good impression on the jury.

Box 7.14 What Does Not Necessarily Amount to Unfitness to Plead and Stand Trial

- a complete loss of memory for the events at the material time (*Podola*);
- being unable to remember some of the matters giving rise to the charges (*M (John)*);
- not being capable of acting in one's best interests (*R v Robertson* [1968] 1 WLR 1767);
- being deluded as to the material facts (*Robertson*);
- having delusions that might lead to a wrong or unwise challenge of a juror (*Robertson*);
- having delusions about the punishment liable to be inflicted (*R v Moyle* [2008] EWCA Crim 3059);
- having a delusional belief that the jury were possessed (*Moyle*);
- having delusions that might at any moment interfere with a proper action (*Robertson*);
- a grossly abnormal mental state and being unable to view actions in any sort of sensible manner (*R v Berry* [1977] 6 WLUK 141);
- giving instructions that are implausible, unbelievable or unreliable or not being able to recognise them as such (*M (John)*);
- being unable to make valid or helpful comments on the evidence and counsels' speeches (*M (John)*);
- failing to see what is or is not a good point in his defence (*M (John)*);
- being unable to remember at the end of a court session all the points that may have occurred to the accused about what has been said (*M (John)*);
- being unable, in his own defence, to give answers that are plausible, believable or reliable or not being able to recognise them as such (*M (John)*).

Instructing solicitors and counsel involves being able to (1) understand the lawyer's questions, (2) apply the mind to answering them, (3) convey intelligibly the answers which they wish to give, (4) explain their version of events, (5) point out any statements with which they disagree and (6) point out any facts which should be put forward in their defence.

Following the course of the proceedings means being able to (1) understand and follow what is said by the witnesses and counsel in their speeches to the jury and (2) communicate intelligibly to their lawyers any comment they may wish to make on anything that is said by the witnesses or counsel – for example, that a witness is saying something that is not true. This does not mean understanding, or being capable of understanding, every point of law or evidential detail – only having 'a grasp of the essential issues' (*JD v R* [2013] EWCA Crim 465).

Giving evidence if they wish in their own defence means being able to (1) understand the questions asked, (2) apply their mind to answering them and (3) convey intelligibly to the jury the answers which they wish to give. It includes being cross-examined (*R. v Orr* [2016] EWCA Crim 889).

The test is case specific:

> [T]he court is required to undertake an assessment of the accused's capabilities in the context of the particular proceedings. An assessment of whether an accused has the capacity to participate effectively . . . should require the court to have regard to what that legal process will involve and what demands it will make on the accused. It should be addressed . . . in the context of the particular case . . . [considering], for example, the nature and complexity of the issues arising in the particular proceedings, [their] likely duration . . . and the number of parties. (*Marcantonio*)

Box 7.15 Statutory Criteria for Unfitness for Trial in Scotland

In determining unfitness for trial the court is to have regard to the ability of the person to:

- understand that nature of the charge;
- understand the requirement to tender a plea to the charge and the effect of such a plea;
- understand the purpose of, and follow the course of, the trial;
- understand the evidence that may be given against the person;
- instruct and otherwise communicate with the person's legal representative; and
- any other factor which the court considers relevant.

Criminal Procedure (Scotland) Act 1995, s 53F

For example, in *JD v R*, '[t]he evidence was not complicated. It was before the court in a readily comprehensible form . . . The Appellant was able to convey his defence to his legal team. He understood sufficiently that his potential involvement went beyond his own actions.'

Walls illustrates the difficulties in not addressing the *Pritchard* criteria. The court found the expert psychiatric witness somewhat unsatisfactory and rejected his evidence. He had not considered the appellant's police interview and at the appeal he reluctantly agreed that the appellant was able to give an explanation of what had happened and maintain a consistent account (as he did at trial). He suggested that the appellant could accept suggestions uncritically, but it was clear from his interview that this was not so. He could not provide satisfactory answers to questions exploring his dogmatic assertion that the appellant was unfit to plead or explain how his views related to the *Pritchard* criteria.

In Scotland, statutory criteria for unfitness for trial are contained in the CP(S)A, s 53F (Box 7.15). The standard of proof is the balance of probabilities. Medical or psychological evidence is needed. The test is whether the person is 'incapable, by reason of a mental or physical condition, of participating effectively in a trial'. Someone is not unfit for trial by reason only of being unable to recall whether the event which forms the basis of the charge occurred in the manner described in the charge.

In Northern Ireland, the procedure for determining fitness to be tried is set out in MCA(NI), s 204. It is a matter for the decision of the court without a jury. It requires evidence from two RMPs, including the oral evidence of an AMP. There are no statutory criteria for FTP, but the Northern Ireland Law Commission (2013) has recommended that the '*Pritchard* test' is updated to incorporate the language of capacity.

In Ireland, the Criminal Law (Insanity) Act 2006 (CL(I)A), s 4 governs fitness to be tried (Box 7.16). It may arise at the instance of the defence, the prosecution or the court. It is determined on the evidence of an 'approved medical officer' (AMO) (a consultant psychiatrist within the meaning of the MHA 2001) by the District Court where the person is charged with a summary offence and in all other cases by the trial judge.

In Jersey, the capacity to participate effectively takes into account the accused's ability 'to make rational decisions in relation to his participation in the proceedings (including whether or not to plead guilty) which reflect true and informed choices on his part' (*O'Driscoll*), although in *Harding v Attorney General* [2010] JCA 091, the court said that it did not regard this test as any different in principle from that which has been held to apply in England.

Box 7.16 Criteria for Unfitness to Be Tried in the Republic of Ireland

An accused person shall be deemed unfit to be tried if he or she is unable by reason of mental disorder to understand the nature or course of the proceedings so as to –

- plead to the charge;
- instruct a legal representative;
- in the case of an indictable offence which may be tried summarily, elect for a trial by jury;
- make a proper defence;
- in the case of a trial by jury, challenge a juror to whom it might be wished to object; or
- understand the evidence.

Criminal Law (Insanity) Act 2006, s 4(2)

Assessment is best approached, following a minimum of introduction, by asking the accused to explain his attendance. His response may indicate that he understands the adversarial criminal proceedings and the nature of the offence(s). Questions as to plea may reveal whether he understands the available pleas and their effects. If pleading not guilty, the accused can be asked to explain why, although, if the assessment is at the request of the prosecution, he may have been advised not to discuss his defence. Then it will be more difficult to decide whether or not he can give instructions. This is because 'where the assessment almost inevitably will entail questioning about the circumstances of the alleged offence', apart from the PACE, s 78, there seems to be no specific protection regarding the subsequent use of those statements either in a hearing under the CP(I)A (as amended by the CP(IUP)A), s 4A to ascertain if an unfit accused committed the act or omission in the charged offence, or in a trial if the accused is found fit to plead *(R (M) v Kingston Crown Court*). If two or more have been charged, the accused's relationship with them should be explored, as an accused's vulnerability might be such as to require consideration of special provisions, such as not sitting with the other accused persons or even a separate trial. To test his ability to give instructions and his understanding of the evidence, put some of the evidence to the accused and ask him to comment or explain. This will also assist as to the accused's ability to give evidence. The test of challenging a juror is satisfied if the accused is capable of understanding that he should tell his lawyers if he knows or recognises a juror and can tell them so. The case should not be considered in isolation: how the accused conducts the affairs of everyday life will shed light on the abilities needed to understand evidence, give instructions and give evidence. Witness statements, reports and medical records should be searched for evidence of the accused's everyday functioning. The police interview record may reveal what the accused has previously demonstrated as to his understanding of the allegations, his ability to understand evidence and explanations that may suggest what his instructions to his legal representatives might be. As FTP may change over time, re-examination on the day of the trial may be advisable; this is usually done on a joint basis with the other expert(s).

Borderline cases of intellectual disability can be problematic. Although it will often be advisable to have the evidence of a psychologist, the test is a legal test and not a matter of IQ or performance on some particular test. Cases involving dementia can be difficult, as impaired memory can affect the ability to follow the course of the proceedings. The most difficult cases involve depressive disorders. These often involve hitherto, or still, law-abiding professional or business people who are understandably unhappy when charged with an offence such as fraud and fear not just financial and professional ruin, but years of imprisonment to which they will be unaccustomed. But remember that many accused are unhappy at being prosecuted and fearful of the outcome, but are not under a disability. Memory and concentration impairments severe enough to interfere with understanding evidence, giving instructions or giving evidence are easy to assert and for some not difficult to represent. Careful forensic assessment is needed to assess genuineness. The recollection of a recent event can call into question alleged memory impairment. An admission to spending six hours a day going over statements and documentary exhibits with a solicitor calls into question impairment of concentration. Careful study of medical records and witness statements may reveal evidence inconsistent with the symptoms alleged.

Particularly in cases of depressive disorder, there are often concerns that the trial will make the accused suicidal. The courts are wary of such concerns. In *R v Lederman* [2015] EWCA Crim 1308, the trial judge referred to this as 'holding a gun at the court's head saying: don't you dare tip him over the edge'. He was upheld by the Court of Appeal: 'Concerns about suicidal ideation and mental fragility are not part of the *Pritchard* criteria for consideration of unfitness to plead.'

Allowance needs to be made for the adjustments that can reasonably be made to the trial to assist an accused and ensure their effective participation (see 'The vulnerable defendant', below). In *Walls*, the court stated that this includes the use of an intermediary.

Be prepared for the court seeking assistance as to the disposal of the case. If it is a case in which the court ought to consider imposing restrictions on discharge, make this clear in the report. Some judges take the opportunity to hear oral evidence on this issue, with the opportunity for cross-examination, during the enquiry into unfitness. It is then unnecessary to recall the psychiatrist to give evidence if the jury's finding is that the accused did the act(s) or made the omission alleged.

In England and Wales, if the accused is found to be 'under a disability', the court then conducts a trial of the facts under the CP(I)A, s 4A(2) and a jury decides whether the accused 'did the act or made the omission charged against him as the offence'. Although an accused found unfit to plead and stand trial may rarely be permitted to give evidence at the trial of the facts, the judge and counsel 'should always give careful consideration to whether it is right that the defendant should do so' (*R v Egan (Michael)* [1998] 1 Cr App R 121) and although an interview with an accused who has been found unfit to plead and stand trial can be introduced during the trial of the issue, 'the court will usually need to be persuaded by expert evidence that notwithstanding the finding of unfitness, the defendant understood the caution and generally it was safe to interview him' (*R v Swinbourne* [2013] EWCA Crim 2329).

If found to have done the act or made the omission alleged, the court must make: (1) a hospital order with or without a restriction order without limit of time; (2) a supervision order, which may include treatment by or under the direction of an RMP; or (3) an order for absolute discharge (DVCVA, s 24(1)). Before a supervision order can be made, there has to be evidence that such supervision is available and that the necessary arrangements are in place (*City and County of Swansea v Swansea Crown Court* [2016] EWHC 1389 (Admin)). Additionally, the CP(I)A, s 5A permits the making of orders under the MHA 1983, ss. 35, 36 and 38 prior to final disposal of the case where there has been a finding of disability (or insanity).

In Scotland, the CP(S)A, s 57 provides for the following disposals for a person found unfit for trial and found beyond reasonable doubt on an examination of the facts to have committed the act charged: a compulsion order, a compulsion order with a restriction order, an interim compulsion order, a guardianship order, a supervision and treatment order, and a discharge with no order.

In Ireland, if the accused is found to be unfit, the court may then allow evidence to be adduced as to whether or not the accused did the act alleged. If satisfied that there is reasonable doubt as to whether the accused did it, they must be discharged; once committed to a designated centre, further disposal is subject to the Mental Health (Criminal Law) Review Board.

In Northern Ireland, if following a finding of unfitness to be tried and a finding by a jury that the accused did the act or made the omission charged, the court has to make a public protection order (PPO), a public protection order with restrictions (PPOR), a supervision and assessment order or order an absolute discharge. If the offence charged is one for which the penalty is fixed by law, the only possible disposal is a PPOR (MCA(NI), s 207(b)) and it cannot be for a specified period (s 207(c)).

It can be a ground for appeal against conviction that the appellant was not FTP. In *R v Moyle* [2008] EWCA Crim 3059, the Court of Appeal had evidence from three psychiatrists to the effect that the appellant had been unfit to plead at the time of his trial, but the court was unable to accede to the submission that he was not FTP. The reasons given by the court illustrate matters that should be carefully considered in such cases at the time of the trial and where the issue arises on appeal. They included how the appellant gave evidence at his trial; he did so in a way which did not create doubts about his ability to understand questions put to him and to give the answers he saw fit to give; there was no indication that he failed to understand the evidence given or to respond to it with his own account, albeit an account which the jury disbelieved. He understood that the proceedings were serious proceedings, that he was being tried for a serious offence and that the aim of the trial was to determine his guilt or wrongdoing. He demonstrated a tactical awareness which was difficult to reconcile with unfitness to plead. His embarrassment at his predicament and his inability to accept that his conduct was the cause of death were reactions not uncommon in those charged with serious crime and certainly not supportive of unfitness to plead. He believed, the court hoped as a result of delusion, that the court was biased, but this cannot extinguish a person's right to be tried or the public's right to have that person tried. A false belief about the punishment liable to be inflicted does not impair the accused's ability to be tried. Not acting in his own best interests, in the evidence and instructions he gave, does not, in itself, create, or contribute to, a finding of unfitness. Although his condition had not changed substantially since his trial, his legal advisors for the appeal had sought specific instructions from him and appeared to have had no difficulty in obtaining them.

The Vulnerable Defendant

For England and Wales, the *Practice Direction (Criminal Proceedings: Further Directions)* [2007] 1 WLR 1790 sets out vulnerable defendant provisions applicable to defendants who suffer from a mental disorder under the MHA 1983 or who otherwise have any impairment of intelligence or social functioning (or learning disability). These provisions are now incorporated in CrPR CPD I 3G Vulnerable Defendants. The steps that should be taken are to be judged having regard to such matters as the age, maturity and development (intellectual, social and emotional) of the defendant and all other circumstances of the case. These directions also ensure compliance with the judgment in *SC v United Kingdom* (see above).

The court will decide what special measures, if any, should be implemented at a pre-trial 'ground rules hearing' (GRH) (CrPR 3.9(7)(b)). The psychiatrist should be prepared to provide a report for, and if required attend, the GRH. There, the judge may require the advocates to go through their cross-examination questions with the psychiatrist (Cooper and Grace 2016).

Special measures can include: visiting the courtroom in advance and out of court hours; the judge, counsel and court officers dispensing with wigs and robes and sitting on the same level as the defendant; extra time to go through papers with a defendant who cannot read and extra time to allow counsel to take instructions; the defendant sitting, if he wishes, and security considerations permitting, in the well of the court beside their solicitor or barrister or with members of his family or others in a like relationship and with a suitable supporting adult who can explain the proceedings as they unfold step by step; alternatively, being accompanied in the dock by someone such as a nurse; the number of members of public in court being limited; frequent and regular breaks, including short, non-adjourned breaks during which the court stays sitting, for those with impairments of attention or concentration and to allow the defendant's solicitor, or a supporting adult, to explain evidence, in language the defendant can understand, and take instructions; assistance in the dock to access or follow written evidence and, if so, consideration as to how this will be achieved; speaking slowly and in plain, simple language; questioning of prosecution witnesses in a manner that enables the defendant to understand and follow the trial; counsel and the judge putting short, clear, simple or even very simple questions to the defendant; the defendant giving his evidence by a live television link; the use of a facilitator or intermediary.

The use of a 'facilitator' was approved in *R v SH* [2003] EWCA Crim 1028. This was the case of a 'learning disabled' adult. Their role was to assist the defendant to communicate with the judge and counsel by putting into language they could understand the nature of the question that he was being asked. Approval was also given to two measures to assist a defendant who had a poor memory which was hampering his ability to give evidence: (1) reading the defendant's defence statement to the jury to assist in understanding his evidence; (2) allowing the defendant to refer to his proof of evidence or, if he could not read, allowing leading questions from such a document to be put to him.

This 'facilitator' role is similar to that of an 'intermediary' and the Youth Justice and Criminal Evidence Act 1999 (YJCEA), s 33BA permits the use of an intermediary in the case of defendants under the age of 18 years whose ability to participate effectively is compromised by their level of intellectual ability or social functioning and in the case of defendants over the age of 18 years who suffer from a mental disorder within the meaning of the MHA 1983 or are unable to participate effectively due to an impairment of intelligence and social functioning. This section has not yet been implemented, but CrPR CPD I 3D.2 requires the court to take 'every reasonable step' to encourage and facilitate the participation of any person, including the defendant, and this includes enabling a defendant to give their best evidence, to comprehend the proceedings and to engage fully with their defence.

R (OP) v The Secretary of State for Justice and Cheltenham Magistrates Court and Crown Prosecution Service. Just for Kids Law as Intervener [2014] EWHC 1944 (Admin) identified two roles in a trial for which an intermediary is fitted: (1) general support, reassurance and calm interpretation of unfolding events; and (2) skilled support and interpretation with the potential for intervention and on occasion suggestion to the Bench associated with the giving of the defendant's evidence. The latter includes communicating questions put to the defendant, communicating their answers to any person putting the questions and explaining such questions or answers so far as is necessary to ensure that they are understood by the defendant or the person in question. Specifically in *R (AS) v Great Yarmouth Youth Court* [2011] EWHC 2059 (Admin), the intermediary's role was identified as ensuring that questions were simple and that the defendant had adequate time to respond and was able to alert the court to the difficulties which he faced in answering them; in *R v Cox* [2012] EWCA Crim 549, the court cited with approval the assistance of intermediaries to the trial judge and counsel in establishing what types of question are likely to cause misunderstanding and how to avert them. In relation to a trial involving a young child, the intermediary was described as 'someone to befriend and help him, both during the trial itself and in preparation for it' (*R (C) v Sevenoaks Youth Court* [2009] EWHC 3088 (Admin)).

The role of the intermediary is illustrated in *JD v R*. JD had an IQ of between 68 and 71, a history of hyperactive conduct disorder and communication difficulties. Reference was made to how the intermediary's assistance contributed to the defendant's ability to participate meaningfully in his trial:

> She maintained a visual record to enable the Appellant to follow the evidence; she wrote simple sentences for him; and she held twice daily meetings with the Appellant outside court to summarise past and future events in the trial; she assisted him with a vocabulary folder to explain more difficult concepts; and she was eventually able to explain satisfactorily to him what the role of the jury was . . . Steps were taken by the intermediary to provide real assistance to the Appellant in explaining to him what was happening and simplifying the court process . . . actions taken by Ms Berriman to ensure that the Appellant could follow in simpler terms what was going on.

These provisions are particularly likely to apply to the young, the intellectually disabled and people with autistic spectrum disorder (see *R v Thompson* [2014] EWCA Crim 836). However, they need to be considered in any case where the psychiatrist is of the opinion that the defendant is not fit to plead and stand trial because otherwise the court or another expert may suggest that with certain such provisions, he will be able to plead and stand trial.

The court will decide whether the jury will be assisted by an explanation about a vulnerable defendant's condition and its effect on their behaviour so as to avoid that behaviour being misinterpreted (*Thompson*). The expert should therefore pay particular attention to their definition of the defendant's diagnosis or condition in their glossary. In such a circumstance, it may be advisable to provide a more detailed and extensive glossary entry from which the judge can derive an explanation without the need to return to the expert for clarification or further explanation.

In Northern Ireland, the Justice Act (Northern Ireland) 2011, s 12, by amending the Criminal Evidence (Northern Ireland) Order 1999, has made similar provisions for the use of intermediaries for persons aged under 18 years whose effective participation is compromised by their level of intellectual ability or social functioning (art 21BA(5)) and for adults with mental disorder or who otherwise have a significant impairment of intelligence and social functioning and are unable to participate effectively (art 21BA(6)). *In Ireland*, there are no particular statutory provisions dealing with vulnerable defendants (other than children). *In the Isle of Man*, there are no specific provisions for vulnerable defendants, but the courts have shown willingness to accommodate intermediaries and make adjustments.

Undesirability of Giving Evidence

In England and Wales, the CJPOA, s 35, and *in the Isle of Man* the Police Powers and Procedures Act, s 71(1), provide for the court to refrain from giving the adverse inference direction to the jury in respect of the accused's silence at trial if 'it appears to the court that the physical or mental condition of the accused makes it undesirable for him to give evidence', but '[t]he defendant must be suffering from a recognised mental disorder, the impact of which may affect his presentation in giving evidence' (*R v Mulwinda* [2017] EWCA Crim 416). *In Ireland*, inferences may not be drawn from an accused's silence at trial.

Grubin (1996) described a case in which the accused's 'personality was such that under the stress of cross-examination he was likely to become anxious, frustrated and confused, and ... this could cause him to behave in an inappropriate manner, with the risk of prejudicing the jury against him'. Although he did not suffer from a form of mental disorder, there was a risk that he might appear to do so to a lay individual. However, the subsequent ruling in *Mulwinda* casts doubt on the decision to accede to the application.

Orr makes it clear that the undesirability of giving evidence due to the risk of an adverse inference is to be distinguished from a disability which would fall to be considered under the *Pritchard* rules. Two psychiatrists had given evidence at the appellant's trial that he was 'unable to be responsive to cross examination' and 'unable to give evidence in his own defence'. The Court of Appeal regarded the CJPOA, s 35(1) provision as supporting the contention that a finding that an accused was unfit to give evidence in cross-examination did not necessarily determine the question of FTP.

For the application of the CJPOA, s 35(1), there is no requirement for medical evidence, but in such a case the psychiatrist should be prepared to give reasons for their opinion and by reference to the factors that it is within their expertise to identify and describe. These are likely to include, for example, inappropriate behaviour resulting from the accused, as in Grubin's case, becoming anxious, frustrated, confused, irrational, angry or flippant. But in *Dixon v R* [2013] EWCA Crim 465, where the accused had ADHD and an IQ of 68, the court held that having a mental condition that might merely cause some difficulty was insufficient. Even 'extreme difficulty' in giving evidence or the possibility (but put no higher than that) of an impact on the accused's mental health is not enough (*R v Ensor* [2010] 1 Cr App R 18). In *R v Tabbakh* [2009] EWCA Crim 464, there was psychiatric evidence that the accused, who had PTSD and a history of self-harm, might not do himself justice in the witness box, because he was unable to retain control of himself and might not remember some parts of his evidence. The judge's decision to refuse to accept that it would be 'undesirable' for him to give evidence was upheld. However, the judge did permit the psychiatrists to give evidence of the difficulties he faced in giving evidence. In *Mulwinda*, the accused had schizophrenia. The court upheld the trial judge's refusal to accept that it would be 'undesirable' for the accused to give evidence, but confirmed that, if he had elected to testify, expert evidence could have been given to the effect that signs that he might be responding to hallucinations were a feature of his mental condition.

R v S [2014] EWCA Crim 2648 concerns the potential impact on the jury of an accused's strange behaviour in court. The appellant was convicted of the rape and indecent assault of his wife. During her evidence, he was casually reading a book. The convictions were quashed on the basis that his then undiagnosed autism could explain what the jury might have thought was evidence of callous indifference.

Trial Issues

Self-Defence

Self-defence may be raised as a defence to an offence of force. There are two limbs: (1) were the facts as the accused believed them to be such that the use of force was necessary; and (2) was the degree of force used reasonable in the light of those perceived facts.

In *R v Oye* [2013] EWCA Crim 1725, the issue was whether 'an insanely held delusion on the part of the appellant that he was being attacked or threatened, causing him violently to respond, entitle[d] him to an acquittal on the basis of reasonable self-defence'. The jury had found him guilty. The Court of Appeal decided that: 'An insane person cannot set the standards of reasonableness as to the degree of force used by reference to his own insanity. In truth it makes . . . little sense to talk of the reasonable lunatic.' So he was not entitled to an acquittal based on self-defence. However, the court quashed the conviction and substituted a finding of insanity.

The court relied on *R v Martin* [2001] EWCA Crim 2245, where fresh medical evidence indicated that the accused suffered from a long-standing paranoid personality disorder (PPD) and also from depression. It was submitted that this caused him to perceive a much greater danger to his safety than would an average person, thereby contributing to his shooting the two burglars of his farmhouse. However, the Court of Appeal decided that it 'would not agree that it is appropriate, except in exceptional circumstances which would make the evidence especially probative, in deciding whether excessive force has been used to take into account whether the accused is suffering from some psychiatric condition'.

So far, no case has revealed what such exceptional circumstances might be, and other cases have followed *Martin*. In *R v Canns* [2005] EWCA Crim 2264, the appellant, who suffered from chronic paranoid schizophrenia, killed a male nurse in a secure hospital. He was convicted of manslaughter by reason of diminished responsibility. His defence had been self-defence, he believing, genuinely as a result of delusion, that the nurse was attacking him in order to rape him. It was submitted that it would be 'unjust and unrealistic' to deprive such an accused of a defence 'based on the reality, to him, of what was going on'. This was rejected and the court expressly stated, with regard to *Martin* and on the asserted existence of 'exceptional circumstances', that each member of the court 'has found it impossible to identify the sort of exceptional circumstances in which it would be appropriate to take a psychiatric condition from which an accused is suffering into account, when addressing the question of whether excessive force is used'.

Nevertheless, in *R v Press* [2013] EWCA Crim 1849, the trial judge was found to have correctly invited the jury to consider evidence that the defendant's PTSD, sustained during military service in Afghanistan, may have caused him to react over-sensitively to perceived threats, when resolving the question of whether he did only what he honestly believed was necessary in the circumstances. Thus, exceptionally, psychiatric evidence may also be admissible in relation to the second limb.

In *Ibrahim*, the court accepted that medical evidence was admissible as to a psychiatric condition which caused the accused to believe in a state of affairs which did not exist – that is, it is admissible in relation to the first limb of the defence in order to establish what state of affairs the defendant genuinely believed to exist. However, in this case, where the basis of the appeal was that the trial judge had erred in refusing to admit expert evidence as to the appellant's ADHD, that decision was upheld. One of the trial judge's reasons was that the evidence was not relevant to issues in the case. The expert medical evidence was to the effect that persons suffering from ADHD have poor impulse control and are more likely to act impulsively; they are likely to have an exaggerated response to threats; and they have a reduced capacity to evaluate current circumstances. The court found that this evidence would not have assisted the jury on the main issue in the case. However, if the complainant did slap or kick the appellant who then unnecessarily returned to the fray and punched the complainant, whereas for a normal person to act in that way it could not sensibly be characterised as self-defence, it was submitted that things were different because of the appellant's ADHD. It was submitted that the jury might have concluded that the act of punching was self-defence if the medical evidence had been admitted. But the court thought that such evidence could only have provided slender assistance at best; it gave little assistance in making out the defence case that the appellant then thought it necessary to return to the fray and knock the complainant to the ground.

In Ireland, the Non-Fatal Offences Against the Person Act 1997 (NFOAPA), s 18 provides that the use of force for a specified purpose, essentially self-protection, the protection of others, the protection of property from criminal acts or the prevention of crime or a breach of the peace, is not an offence 'if only such as is reasonable in the circumstances as he or she believes them to be'. As 'it is immaterial whether a belief is justified or not if it is honestly held but the presence or absence of reasonable grounds for the belief is a matter to which the court or the jury is to have regard, in conjunction with any other relevant matters, in considering whether the person honestly held the belief' (s 1(2)), it must follow that expert medical evidence as to an honestly held delusional belief as to the circumstances may support such a defence. Where the charge is murder, if, objectively, the degree of force was not reasonable, but the subjective view of the accused was that it was reasonable, the correct verdict is manslaughter. A margin of error must be afforded to a person in a self-defence situation (*The People (DPP) v Higgins* [2015] IECA 200).

Diminished Responsibility

In England and Wales, under the Homicide Act 1957, s 2, *in Northern Ireland* under the Criminal Justice Act (Northern Ireland) 1966 (CJA(NI)), s 5(1) as substituted by the Coroners and Justice Act 2009 (CJA 2009), s 52, and *in the Isle of Man* under the Criminal Code 1872, s 22A, the partial defence of 'diminished responsibility' is a statutory defence (Box 7.17) and, if successful, reduces the offence of murder to one of manslaughter on the grounds of diminished responsibility.

In Scotland, diminished responsibility has a statutory basis in the CP(S)A, s 51B: instead of being convicted of murder, a person can 'be convicted of culpable homicide on grounds of diminished responsibility if the person's ability to determine or control conduct for which the person would otherwise be convicted of murder was, at the time of the conduct, substantially impaired by reason of abnormality of mind'. However, *Galbraith v HM Advocate*, 2002 JC 1 has established that 'it is not the function of the witnesses lay, psychological, medical or psychiatric, to say whether an accused's responsibility can properly be regarded as diminished. Rather they give evidence as to the accused's mental state.' Abnormality of mind includes 'mental disorder' and 'a recognised abnormality caused by sexual or other abuse [but] the abuse must result in some recognised medical abnormality' (*Galbraith*). Being under the influence of alcohol, drugs or any other substance does not constitute an abnormality of mind, but does not prevent such abnormality from being established for the purpose of this section. Unlike the special defence of not criminally

Box 7.17 **Diminished Responsibility as Substituted by the Coroners and Justice Act 2009, s 52**

(1) A person ('D') who kills or is a party to the killing of another is not to be convicted if D was suffering from an abnormality of mental functioning which –

(a) arose from a recognised medical condition,

(b) substantially impaired D's ability to do one or more of the things mentioned in subsection (1A), and

(c) provides an explanation for D's acts or omissions in being a party to the killing.

(1A) Those things are –

(a) to understand the nature of D's conduct;

(b) to form a rational judgment;

(c) to exercise self-control.

(1B) For the purposes of subsection (1)(c) an abnormality of mental functioning provides an explanation for D's conduct if it causes, or is a significant contributory factor in causing, D to carry out that conduct.

responsible by reason of mental disorder (see below), there is no exclusion of a personality disorder which is characterised solely or principally by abnormally aggressive or seriously irresponsible conduct. However, *Kalyanjee v HM Advocate* [2014] HCJAC 44 illustrates some of the difficulties in basing a defence of diminished responsibility on a diagnosis of personality disorder. Here, the diagnosis was PPD, but the court observed that this was:

> ... by no means clear given the absence of any longstanding symptoms or a current diagnosis by his treating psychiatrist. However, many persons functioning in society have such a disorder yet they do not commit crimes of extreme violence. Its existence is not at all determinative of the critical issue of causality ... despite any PPD, [he had] not behaved in this type of way before and his PPD could thus be seen as essentially under control ... the jury, in assessing the effects of the PPD at the time of the killings, would have been bound to take into account the length of time during which the appellant carried out his preparations in advance of killing his sons.

In Ireland, under the CL(I)A, s 6, where a person is tried for murder and the jury or the Special Criminal Court finds that the person who did the act alleged was at the time suffering from a mental disorder, and it was not such as to justify a verdict of not guilty by reason of insanity (NGRI), but was such as to diminish substantially their responsibility for the act, the court must find the person not guilty of murder but guilty of manslaughter on the ground of diminished responsibility. The burden of proof is on the defence, subject to the prosecution being allowed to adduce evidence tending to prove insanity in the alternative. 'Mental disorder', in this context, 'includes mental illness, mental disability, dementia or any other disease of the mind', but does not include intoxication (CL(I)A, s 1). Personality disorder is excluded from the definition of 'mental disorder' in the MHA 2001, but not the CL(I)A. The standard of proof is the balance of probabilities; it is not sufficient merely to raise a reasonable doubt as to a liability to be convicted of murder. Real engagement in setting out the nature of the mental illness and the dynamic of the impairment as it unfolded in the context of homicide is necessary. Mere doubt as to the major handicap of mental illness so severe as to substantially diminish responsibility for killing another person is insufficient (*The People (DPP) v Heffernan* [2015] IECA 310). *Heffernan* has confirmed that the evidence has to be from a consultant psychiatrist. Evidence of premeditation may negative the defence of provocation, but is not necessarily inconsistent with diminished responsibility (*The People (DPP) v Tomkins* [2012] IECCA 82).

In Jersey, the law on diminished responsibility is set out in the Homicide (Jersey) Law 1986, art 3:

> Where a person kills or is party to the killing of another, the person shall not be convicted of murder if the person was suffering from such abnormality of mind (whether arising from a condition of arrested or incomplete development of mind or any inherent causes or induced by disease or injury) as substantially impaired the person's mental responsibility for the person's acts and omissions in doing or being a party to the killing.

As this is based on that which previously applied in England and Wales under the Homicide Act 1957, there are many England and Wales cases that assist in its interpretation (see Rix 2011b).

Diminished responsibility is not a defence against any charge other than murder, including attempted murder (*R v Campbell* [1996] 10 WLUK 421) (*except in Scotland*, where it is a common law defence to a charge of attempted murder (*HM Advocate v Kerr* [2011] HCJAC 17, but, arguably, only for crimes committed before 25 June 2012).

The defence has four ingredients: (1) abnormality of mental functioning; (2) the cause of such in the form of a recognised medical condition; (3) substantial impairment of ability to do one or more of three defined things; and (4) an explanation for the killing.

'Abnormality of mental functioning' replaces 'abnormality of mind' in the Homicide Act 1957. Until case law provides a definition of 'abnormality of mental functioning', the definition in *R v Byrne* [1960] 2 QB 396 (Box 7.18) remains relevant. Nevertheless, insofar as 'mental functioning' is a psychiatric concept, Ormerod (2011) has suggested that the jury cannot have a sound grasp of the concept without expert assistance to decide how far the accused's mental functioning deviates from the norm. It is doubtful if they can be left with as open a direction as in *Byrne*. He also asked if there will be much for the jury to do if there is uncontradicted expert evidence as to the presence of abnormal mental functioning. The court made it clear in *Byrne* that, whereas 'medical evidence is of no doubt of importance' as to 'abnormality of mind', the jury is not bound to accept this evidence and the issue is 'in their good judgment', but this may not apply to 'abnormality of mental functioning'.

Box 7.18 The 'Abnormality of Mind' Test

> [A] state of mind so different from that of ordinary human beings that the reasonable man would term it abnormal. It appears to us to be wide enough to cover the mind's activities in all its aspects, not only the perception of physical acts and matters and the ability to form a rational judgement whether an act is right or wrong, but also the ability to exercise will-power to control physical acts in accordance with that rational judgement.

R v Byrne [1960] 2 QB 396

Indeed, in *R v Brennan* [2014] EWCA Crim 2387, a murder conviction was overturned because there was 'uncontroverted reputable medical evidence that all the elements of the defence were made out, including the substantial impairment of one or more of the abilities mentioned in s 2(1A)'.

In *R v Bunch* [2013] EWCA Crim 2498, where the trial judge accepted that the accused had the alcohol dependence syndrome, the Court of Appeal did not accept that the judge was wrong to refuse to leave diminished responsibility to the jury when there was 'no evidence on which the jury could find that the applicant was suffering from an abnormality of mental functioning which arose from that medical condition and which substantially impaired one of the three capacities mentioned in the Act'. There is a burden on the accused to prove each ingredient of the defence.

So far as the cause of any 'abnormality of mental functioning' is concerned, the jury is likely to be asked to accept the evidence of the psychiatric expert as to the 'medical condition' from which the abnormality arose, unless that evidence is questioned by other expert evidence. *Brennan* supports this suggestion.

The term 'recognised medical condition' has yet to be defined, but it is likely that, within reason, any mental disorder listed in *ICD-11 for Mortality and Morbidity Statistics* (ICD-11) (World Health Organization 2018) or the *Diagnostic and Statistical Manual of Mental Disorders* (5th edn) (DSM5) (American Psychiatric Association 2013) will be regarded as a 'medical condition'. What is meant by 'within reason' is illustrated by *R v Dowds* [2012] EWCA Crim 281. The court listed as conditions in the international classifications which the courts would be reluctant to recognise as giving rise to an abnormality of mind 'unhappiness', 'irritability' and 'paedophilia'. The court also acknowledged that although 'alcohol intoxication' may also be a recognised medical condition, it is not recognised for the purpose of the diminished responsibility defence because Parliament had not meant to 'reverse the well-established rule that voluntary acute intoxication is not capable of being relied upon'. In explaining why a great many more of the conditions listed in ICD and DSM raise important legal questions, when it is sought to invoke them in the legal context, the court in *Dowds* used the example of intermittent explosive disorder, observing that it:

> ... may well be a medically useful description of something which underlies the vast majority of violent offending, but any suggestion that it could give rise to a defence, whether because it amounted to an impairment of mental functioning or otherwise, would, to say the least, demand extremely careful attention. In other words, the medical classification begs the question whether the condition is simply a description of (often criminal) behaviour, or is capable of forming a defence to an allegation of such.

There is a warning here not just about relying on a diagnosis of intermittent explosive disorder in a murder case, but probably also some other forms of personality disorder.

Dowds perhaps hints at what types of medical conditions will qualify. It refers to how 'there may be genuine medical conditions, in no sense the fault of the accused and well recognised by doctors, which although temporary may indeed be within the ambit of the Act'. *R v Webb* [2011] EWCA Crim 152 and *R v Brown* [2011] EWCA Crim 2796 illustrate how, notwithstanding what might be regarded as the subthreshold status of adjustment disorder (Rix 2018), this condition may be accepted as a recognised medical condition for the purposes of the defence. In *Webb*, the accused killed his sick wife who believed, without medical evidence, that her cancer had recurred. The psychiatrists agreed that he had an adjustment disorder with prominent features of depression and in this state of subjective distress and emotional disturbance there was interference with social functioning and performance. However, it is a verdict which has been received with some scepticism: 'A plea of manslaughter by reason of diminished responsibility was accepted, based only on a diagnosis of "adjustment disorder", with the psychiatric report reading that the accused had not recognised his "emotional distress" in the circumstances' (Clough 2015).

The word 'only' suggests some difficulty accepting emotional distress and such a minor disorder as the basis for the defence. The outcome might have been quite different if there had been contested psychiatric evidence or if the accused had not attracted the sympathy that he probably did. The case of *Brown*, who killed his estranged wife, involved contested psychiatric evidence and is remarkable because the defence, that 'as a result of the pressures which the appellant was under his ability to exercise self-control at the time of the killing and his acts in disposing of the body were substantially impaired', was successful; there was evidence that he had prepared a grave and made other arrangements for the disposal of the body before killing his wife. In *R v Blackman* [2017] EWCA Crim 190, the case of a Marine sergeant who killed a severely wounded Taliban insurgent in Afghanistan, the Court of Appeal accepted unanimous psychiatric evidence that Blackman's moderately severe adjustment disorder substantially impaired his ability to form a rational judgement and exercise self-control.

In Scotland, adjustment disorder also successfully founded a defence of diminished responsibility under common law (*NYK v Secretary of State for the Home Department* [2013] CSOH 84), but it is not clear from the judgment, which concerned an appeal against sentence, how it was asserted that the adjustment disorder had the effect of diminishing responsibility and since then the common law defence has been replaced by statute.

The unsuccessful reliance on the diagnosis of adjustment disorder in *R v Douglas* [2014] EWCA Crim 2322, where the accused killed her 73-year-old mother, who was in failing health and suffering with emphysema and long-standing heart disease, is significant in that the psychiatrist instructed by the prosecution was of the opinion that the accused's distress about her mother's physical illness and decline was a normal emotion and not mental disorder.

In Ireland, adjustment disorder has not featured prominently in the jurisprudence: the accused was said to suffer from it in *Heffernan*, but was convicted of murder.

In *R v Reynolds* [2004] EWCA Crim 1834, a murder conviction was quashed on the basis of neuropsychiatric evidence that the appellant had been suffering from undiagnosed Asperger syndrome, which may have substantially diminished his responsibility for the killing. It is not clear how this might have been so and it was a conviction under previous legislation, but American cases (Weiss and Westphal 2015) where there has been 'an attempt by the defense to educate the judge or jury about the characteristics of these individuals [so as to establish] reasonable doubt as to criminal intent and culpability' suggest the possible relevance of deficits in social cognition, disability in social insight and alternative explanatory narratives based on impaired communication and social skills, circumscribed interests and deficits in abstract thought that undermine social adaptation. However, in *R v Conroy* [2017] EWCA Crim 81, Asperger syndrome was unsuccessfully raised as a diminished responsibility defence. The jury rejected evidence that as a result of an inability to appraise the social, emotional and intellectual dimensions of an action, the accused was unable to form a rational judgment or that his lack of a theory of mind and his very egocentric view of the world contributed to an inability to exercise self-control.

The term 'recognised medical condition' will also include non-psychiatric conditions such as epilepsy, thyroid disorders, sleep disorders and diabetes. It appears broader in scope than the 'bracketed causes' it replaces, but 'there is ironically a danger that – because it focuses exclusively on the need for a defined and demonstrable condition which is medically recognised – it may fail to include those "mercy killing" cases' (Mackay 2010a) which had hitherto qualified albeit on the basis that the wording of 'old diminished responsibility' was 'so obscure [that] the court and the experts [were] sometimes able to enter into a benign conspiracy thus permitting the psychiatric evidence to be stretched' to an extent that its terms did not really justify.

Acute alcohol intoxication is not, however, a 'recognised medical condition'. In rejecting this submission, based on the inclusion of 'acute intoxication' in *The ICD-10 Classification of Mental and Behavioural Disorders* (World Health Organization 1992), in an appeal against conviction for murder (*Dowds*), the court reiterated the axiomatic rule, as expressed in *R v Wood* [2008] EWCA Crim 1305, that: 'Public policy proceeds on the basis that a defendant who voluntarily takes alcohol and behaves in a way which he might not have behaved when sober is not normally entitled to be excused from the consequences of his actions.' That rule is illustrated in an Irish case where the issue was reducing the charge from murder to manslaughter:

> Drink is no defence if the only effect of the drink is to more readily to allow a man to give way to his passions. That is insufficient. The effect of drink has to go much further. It has to go so far as either to render him incapable of knowing what he is doing at all, or, if he appreciated that, of knowing the consequences or probable consequences of his actions. (*The People (Attorney General) v Manning* (1953) 89 ILTR 155)

The exclusion of substance-induced states from the meaning of a 'recognised medical condition' was extended in *R v Lindo* [2016] EWCA Crim 1940 to include drug-induced psychosis. The court held that 'drug-induced psychosis standing alone would not suffice and a drug-induced psychosis combined with a prodromal state does not seem to us to be sufficient to trigger the operation of this section'.

'Substantial impairment of ability' replaces 'substantial impairment of mental responsibility' (although paradoxically the title of the CJA 2009, s 52 still refers to 'Persons suffering from diminished responsibility'). Previously, psychiatrists often tried to avoid giving an opinion on 'mental responsibility'. The court held in *Byrne* that substantial impairment of mental responsibility was 'a question of degree and essentially one for the jury. Medical evidence is, of course, relevant ... but whether such an impairment can properly be called 'substantial', [is] a matter on which juries may quite legitimately differ from doctors'. Now that 'mental responsibility for acts or omissions' has been replaced with the 'ability' of the accused to (1) understand their own conduct, (2) form a rational judgment or (3) exercise self-control, it is likely that medical evidence will become more determinative. Ormerod (2011) has suggested that, as impairment of ability to do one of these three specified things is purely a psychiatric question, it would seem appropriate for the expert to offer an opinion on whether there is 'substantial' impairment. So, arguably, there could be greater influence from experts than previously. Although this may not be so because the degree of impairment will remain, both as a matter of fact and as to degree, an ultimate issue for the jury, the decision of the Court of Appeal to overturn the conviction for murder in *Brennan*, because there was uncontroverted reputable medical evidence of substantial impairment, illustrates how more weight may be given to the psychiatric evidence.

Although the term 'mental responsibility' has disappeared from the diminished responsibility legislation, it may still be an issue in appeals against convictions which took place before the implementation of the CJA 2009. It may therefore be helpful to note the definition of 'mental responsibility', adopted by the court in *R v Williams* [2013] EWCA Crim 2749: 'the extent to which a person's acts are the choice of a free and rational mind'.

The meaning of 'substantial impairment' has recently been subjected to analysis in *R v Golds* [2016] UKSC 61. The Supreme Court clarified that it is not usually necessary to direct the jury on the meaning of an ordinary word such as 'substantial' and attempts to offer alternative definitions risk complicating the jury's task. If, however, the need does arise, then the judge should avoid both a single synonym and the 'spectrum' approach mentioned in *R v Lloyd* [1967] 1 QB 175 (i.e. more than merely trivial, but less than total). The Supreme Court reflected on the ordinary usage of 'substantial' as either 'having some substance' and 'important or weighty', and suggested that the authorities have always held it to have been used in the second of these meanings.

Mackay (2010b) has observed that, although these three 'abilities' (or 'limbs') can be traced to *Byrne*, 'by specifying what abilities need to be impaired [this] means that "abnormality of mental functioning" now seems narrower than "abnormality of mind", as the only mind's activities which are included are the three specified things in subsection (1A)'. Thus, however widely 'abnormality of mental functioning' is defined and however wide the range of recognised medical conditions, the defence now appears to be narrower. It is possible, for example, that personality disorders will be more likely to be excluded by the new formulation unless the accused's ability to exercise self-control can be demonstrated to have been substantially impaired. Ormerod (2011) suggests that as 'ability' is more specific than 'mental responsibility', 'it leaves less moral elbow room for the jury and is arguably harder for [the accused] to prove'. He has also suggested that insofar as the ability of the accused to understand his own conduct and to form a rational judgment are akin to insanity, if these are construed narrowly, in many cases the accused might be better to plead the complete defence of insanity than the partial defence of diminished responsibility. In any event, there is almost never a reliance on the first 'limb' on its own (Mackay and Mitchell 2017).

Medical evidence is also likely to be crucial in persuading, or dissuading, a jury that the abnormality of mental functioning has caused, or made a significant contribution to the cause of, the conduct that has led to the killing. This is a stronger causal requirement than previously, although it is arguable whether, in view of the requirement for the three specified things in subsection (1A), subsection (1B) adds to the clear linkage between the relevant substantial impairment and the homicidal conduct (Mackay 2010b). It does, however, make clear what may not have previously been as clear that, even when there is undoubtedly a mental condition present, unless this condition has a material bearing on the killing, it does not provide a defence. Furthermore, the jury can take into account not only the effect of the abnormality of mental functioning at the time of the killing, but also 'all relevant circumstances preceding, and perhaps preceding over a very long period, the killing as well as any relevant circumstances following the killing' (*Conroy*). This happened in *R v Squelch* [2017] EWCA Crim 204. Paranoid personality disorder was unsuccessfully advanced as a diminished responsibility defence and the court held that 'consideration may very well, and indeed usually will, involve a consideration of aspects of the evidence relating to a period of time preceding the killing. In some cases, in fact, it may relate to a period of time going back over many years and even sometimes to a particular defendant's childhood.'

A psychiatrist preparing a report where there is an issue of 'diminished responsibility' should have in mind the questions set out in Box 7.19 and be aware that oral expert evidence

Box 7.19 Issues to Be Addressed by Psychiatric Examination in Relation to Diminished Responsibility

1. Presence of psychiatric disorder
   - Was there a recognised medical condition at the time of the incident?
   - If so, specify with reference to recognised diagnostic terms (e.g. ICD or DSM) and set out diagnostic criteria.
2. Presence of abnormality of mental functioning
   - At the material time, was there an abnormality of mental functioning that arose from the recognised medical condition?
   - If so, describe using accepted terms and definitions.
3. Effect of abnormality of mental functioning
   - Did the abnormality of mental functioning (that arose from the medical condition) substantially impair the individual's ability to understand the nature of his/her actions, to form a rational judgement or to exercise self-control?
   - If so, describe how (on the basis of relevant recognised mental processes) and, if possible, estimate the extent of the impairment.
4. Connection between abnormality of mental functioning and behaviour
   - Did the abnormality of mental functioning cause, or make a significant contribution to, the defendant's acts or omissions in being a party to the killing?
   - If so, describe the nature and extent of the connection (on the basis of relevant recognised mental processes) so as to provide an explanation for the defendant's acts or omissions in being a party to the killing.

Nathan and Medland 2016

will be more likely as the greater specificity of the defence will make it easier for the prosecution to contest the defence.

It is important to consider all of the evidence. If the psychiatric opinion is based solely on statements made to the psychiatrist by the accused alone, and so not entirely independent, and does not take into account the circumstances surrounding the killing, the defence may fail (*R v Eifinger* [2001] EWCA Crim 1855). Following *Walton v The Queen* [1978] AC 788, juries are directed to consider all the evidence in a 'broad, common sense way' and to examine both 'the medical evidence and the evidence on the whole facts and circumstances of the case'. *R v Khan* [2009] EWCA Crim 1569 is an example of a case in which, notwithstanding the evidence that the accused was in a schizophrenic state at the material time, the jury convicted him of murder. It was recognised at his unsuccessful appeal that the jury had 'to weigh much other evidence which suggested that, to a greater or lesser extent, [he] comprehended what physical acts he was doing in attacking the victim and that he had the power to exercise control over his actions'. This was a case which was governed by earlier diminished responsibility legislation. Under the present law, the psychiatrist would need to explain how someone who behaved as the defendant did could be said to be impaired in his ability to understand his own conduct, form a rational judgement or exercise self-control.

Homicides involving an alcohol-dependent defendant have been so problematic as to engage the Court of Appeal in issuing guidance on this issue (*R v Stewart* [2009] EWCA Crim 593). This appeal did not take account of the then proposed changes to the law on diminished responsibility, and what follows translates the guidance into the language of 'new' diminished responsibility. It was held that whether or not the alcohol dependence syndrome constituted an abnormality of mental functioning would depend on the nature and extent of the syndrome and whether, looking at the matter broadly, the accused's consumption of alcohol before the killing was fairly to be regarded as the involuntary result of an irresistible craving for, or compulsion to, drink. It was held that the second question, that of causation, would normally follow from the answer to the first, so, if the alcohol dependence syndrome amounted to an abnormality of mental functioning, it would be attributed to a medical condition. If the jury was satisfied that the defendant's alcohol dependence syndrome constituted an abnormality of mental functioning due to a medical condition, the issue of 'substantial impairment of ability is to be decided according to the conventional terms'. But it was pointed out that the jury might be invited to reflect on the difference between an accused who failed to resist his impulses to behave as he actually did and an inability, consequent upon his alcohol dependence syndrome, to resist his impulses to act as he did.

The issue of the voluntariness of the consumption of alcohol had very recently been addressed in *Wood*, where the court recognised that two of the four psychiatrists 'attempted to address head on some of the underlying difficulties of explaining how a true alcoholic may, on any particular occasion, be drinking voluntarily, and on another may be acting under the compulsion caused by his condition'. The court acknowledged that hitherto the bar might have been set too high and although it has established that 'the defence does not require proof that the alcohol dependent accused is subject to or acting under some form of automatism . . . when he is drinking', the bar remains high:

> [T]he jury should focus exclusively on the effect of alcohol consumed as a direct result of his illness or disease and ignore the effect of any alcohol consumed voluntarily . . . this . . . embraces questions such as whether the accused's craving for alcohol was . . . irresistible, and whether his consumption of alcohol in the period leading up to the killing was voluntary (and if so, to what extent).

Even if it is possible to distinguish voluntarily from involuntarily consumed alcohol, if the killing takes place before all of the involuntarily consumed alcohol has been metabolised, there is no scientific means of distinguishing between the effects of the voluntarily consumed alcohol and the effects of the involuntarily consumed alcohol.

Stewart also refers to the jury's consideration of the medical evidence. Box 7.20 lists the issues likely to arise and on which the jury should be invited to form their own judgement. These issues, at least, should be covered in the psychiatric report. Whether or not the expert can distinguish the effects of voluntarily consumed alcohol from the effects of involuntarily consumed alcohol is another matter and, unless asked to do so, the psychiatrist might be well advised to avoid this issue.

R v Dietschmann [2003] 1 AC 1209 HL deals with the related issue of an abnormality of mental functioning occurring along with alcohol intoxication. It is best illustrated by the appropriate judicial direction to the jury (emphasis in italics and bracketed clauses added to reflect 'new diminished responsibility'):

Box 7.20 **Issues for the Judgement of the Jury Where Alcohol Dependence Is Raised as a Defence to a Charge of Murder**

- the extent and seriousness of the accused's dependency, if any, on alcohol;
- the extent to which his ability to control his drinking, or to choose whether to drink or not, was reduced;
- whether he was capable of abstinence from alcohol and, if so:
  - for how long; and
  - whether he was choosing for some particular reason to decide to get drunk or to drink even more than usual;
- the accused's pattern of drinking on the days leading up to the day of the homicide and on the day of the homicide;
- notwithstanding the accused's consumption of alcohol, his ability, if any, to make apparently sensible and rational decisions about ordinary day-to-day matters at the material time.

> Assuming the defence have established that the defendant was suffering from *an abnormality of mental functioning* . . . the important question is 'Did that abnormality substantially impair his *ability* [to perform the] acts in doing the killing?' You know that he had a lot to drink. Drink cannot be taken into account as something which contributed to his *abnormality of mental functioning* and to any impairment of *ability* arising from that abnormality. But you may take the view that both the accused's *abnormality of mental functioning* and drink played a part in impairing his *ability* [in carrying out] the killing and that he might have killed if he had not taken drink. If you take that view then the question . . . to decide is this: 'Has the accused satisfied you that, despite the drink, his *abnormality of mental functioning* substantially impaired his *ability* [in carrying out] his fatal acts?'

However, 'even if the defendant would not have killed if he had not taken drink, the causative effect of the drink does not necessarily prevent *an abnormality of mental functioning* suffered by the defendant from substantially impairing his *ability*'. This is strictly a jury matter, but psychiatric experts are often asked to deal with it.

Infanticide

In England and Wales, the Isle of Man and *Northern Ireland*, infanticide is another partial defence to a charge of murder which, if successful, reduces the offence to one of manslaughter. It is also an alternative to manslaughter. However, it differs from 'diminished responsibility' in that it can be charged from the outset and so it can avoid a woman being charged with the murder of her own child.

It is defined by the Infanticide Act 1938, s 1, the Infanticide Act (Northern Ireland) 1939 (as amended by the CJA 2009, ss 57 and 58 respectively) and the Isle of Man's Infanticide and Infant Life (Preservation) Act 1938, s 2(1). It is thereby limited to a woman who is charged with, or would otherwise be convicted of, the murder or manslaughter of her child under the age of 12 months. It applies where the woman has caused her child's death by any wilful act or omission when 'the balance of her mind was disturbed by reason of her not having fully recovered from the effect of giving birth to the child or by reason of the effect of lactation consequent upon the birth of the child'. The 'lactation' limb is now redundant.

Although it is in some respects of more limited application than diminished responsibility, analysis of the successful cases suggests that it is an easier defence and, in a recent case in which the *mens rea* for infanticide was reviewed (*R v Gore* [2007] EWCA Crim 2789), the court recognised that the offence 'covers a wide range of cases . . . often a woman in severe distress', illustrating the 'resultant breadth of offence' that Ormerod and Perry (2019, para. B.100) describe 'as a good thing insofar as it avoids detailed examination or rehearsal of the often tragic circumstances where a distressed mother kills her young child'. It is probably also because in diminished responsibility the burden of proof is on the defence, whereas if the defence of infanticide is raised the prosecution carries the more difficult burden of proving beyond reasonable doubt that it is not infanticide.

The difficulty is that disturbance of the balance of the mind is not a psychiatric concept and case law has not defined it. Furthermore, in the cases reviewed by Mackay (1995), there was little analysis or discussion of it by the psychiatrists. The nearest definition is 'left the balance of your mind disturbed so as to prevent rational judgment and decision' (*R v Sainsbury* [1989] 11 WLUK 317).

Some case reports assist. Some of Mackay's (1993) cases were women with fairly obvious mental disorders such as 'puerperal depressive illness', 'clinical depression' and a manic-depressive psychosis manifesting in command hallucinations, but there was also a case of 'severe hysterical dissociation' and a case in which the only abnormality was 'emotional disturbances'. Consistent with this, a half of the women in the series reported by d'Orbán (1979) were not suffering from any identifiable mental disorder. Bluglass (1990) reported similar cases: a woman in whom no persisting psychiatric disorder was found other than her distressed state after the homicide; a woman who was depressed and distressed, but showed 'no underlying disorder'; and a woman who gave birth to a baby with Down syndrome and in which case nothing more abnormal is reported than her shock, inability to accept the appearance of the baby and her sense of hopelessness about its future. The cases reported by Mackay and Bluglass therefore confirm the impression of d'Orbán that for infanticide 'the degree of abnormality is much less than that required to substantiate "abnormality of mind" amounting to substantially diminished responsibility'.

This matter was addressed by the Royal College of Psychiatrists in its evidence to the Criminal Law Revision Committee (1978). The College submission identified four circumstances which might in practice justify an infanticide verdict, but might not be sufficient for a defence of diminished responsibility: (1) overwhelming stress from the social environment being highlighted by the birth of a baby, with the emphasis on the unsuitability of accommodation, etc.; (2) overwhelming stress from an additional member to a household struggling with poverty; (3) psychological injury and pressures and stress from a husband or other member of the family as a result of the mother's incapacity to arrange the demands of the extra member of the family; (4) failure of bonding between mother and child through illness or disability which impairs the mother's capacity to care for the infant.

One of Bluglass's cases is particularly illustrative:

> A 21 year old mother of a new baby, her first child, moved shortly after the child's birth to a new locality in another part of the country where she had no social contacts. She was left alone with her baby for long periods while her husband was establishing himself in a new job. She was a dull young woman (IQ 88) who became increasingly depressed and resentful

> in her attitude towards the child. One night in frustration and anger she threw the baby against the corner of his cot and killed him . . . The child was aged 11 months . . . and initially a defence of infanticide could not be supported as there appeared to be little connection between childbirth or lactation and her actions. There was widespread sympathy towards her by the court, which suggested that it could not be stated with certainty that there was no association with the effects of pregnancy and that a finding of infanticide was therefore appropriate. (Bluglass 1990)

The role of 'widespread sympathy' supports the view of Mackay that the criteria in the statute have been used to ensure that leniency can be meted out in appropriate cases. However, whereas sympathy may move a jury to conclude that the prosecution has not proved beyond reasonable doubt that it is not infanticide, sympathy may not be enough to persuade the Court of Appeal to quash a murder conviction and substitute one of infanticide. In *R v Kai-Whitewind* [2005] EWCA Crim 1092, the court acknowledged that this 'sad case' demonstrated the need for a re-examination of an unsatisfactory and outdated law, but upheld the murder conviction.

In the meantime, notwithstanding the limited amendments by the CJA 2009, this unsatisfactory and outdated law remains on the statute book. The best advice to the psychiatrist is to set out if possible: (1) how the woman's mental state has changed since childbirth, whether or not the changes could be regarded as amounting to an 'abnormality of mind' or recognisable mental disorder; (2) indicate how this amounts to a disturbance of the balance of mind, showing how it has affected rational judgement and decision-making; and (3) explain how this mental state can be attributed to the effects of childbirth.

R v Tunstill [2018] EWCA Crim 169, a case of a mother with Asperger syndrome, has established that 'by reason of' should not be read as if it said 'solely by reason of' and that as long as the effect of the birth is an 'operative or substantial cause' of the disturbance, that should be sufficient.

Although the maximum sentence for infanticide is life imprisonment, in fifty-nine cases between 1979 and 1988 there were no custodial sentences and all disposals were by way of probation, supervision and hospital orders (*Sainsbury*), so reports in such cases are likely to require careful consideration of issues related to sentencing.

In Ireland, the CL(I)A, s 22 amends the Infanticide Act 1949 by substituting 'by reason of mental disorder' within the meaning of the CL(I)A for 'by reason of the effect of lactation'. The act provides that, in the case of a woman who by any wilful act or omission has caused the death of her child under the age of 12 months and but for this provision the act or omission would have amounted to murder, she may be tried and punished as if she had been found guilty of manslaughter on the grounds of diminished responsibility.

Insanity and Related Mental Condition Defences

In England and Wales, the defence of insanity is governed by the M'Naghten Rules (*M'Naghten's Case* (1843) 10 Cl & F 200). The M'Naghten Rules state that:

> [T]he jurors ought to be told in all cases that every man is to be presumed to be sane, and to possess a sufficient degree of reason to be held responsible for his crimes, until the contrary be proved to their satisfaction; and that to establish a defence on the ground of insanity, it must be clearly proved that, at the time of committing the act, the party accused was labouring under such a defect of reason, from disease of the mind, as not to know the nature

> and quality of the act he was doing; or, if he did know it, that he did not know he was doing what was wrong.

The presumption of sanity means that the burden of proof is placed on the defence and the standard of proof is the balance of probabilities.

The reference to 'the time of committing the act' is extremely important as mental states can fluctuate and what matters is the material time rather than before or after the offence.

Central to the defence is a 'defect of reason'. If the terminology is strictly applied, this is not a defence that is likely to be successful when the act is carried out on impulse or in a state of so-called loss of control or in a highly disturbed emotional state. It is necessary to show the defective process of reasoning that has resulted in the accused either not knowing the nature and quality of the act he was doing (the first limb) or, if he did, not knowing that what he was doing was wrong (the second limb) or both. This is a narrow, cognitive test. Thus, in *R v Clarke* [1972] 1 All ER 219, it was held that the momentary confusion and absent-mindedness of a depressed 'shoplifter', who retained her ordinary powers of reason, fell far short of a 'defect of reason'.

It is also critically important to identify a 'disease of the mind' that has resulted in the defect of reasoning. Although medical evidence is required (CP(IUP)A, s 1), it is for the judge to decide what is a disease of the mind:

> . . . 'mind' in the M'Naghten Rules is used in the ordinary sense of the mental faculties of reason, memory and understanding. If the effect of a disease is to impair these faculties so severely as to have either of the consequences referred to in the latter part of the rules, it matters not whether the aetiology is organic . . . or functional, or whether the impairment is permanent or transient and intermittent, provided that it subsisted at the time of commission of the act. (*R v Sullivan* [1984] AC 156)

The role of the psychiatric expert is to show that the impairment of faculties did occur and what its cause was. The disease has to be 'internal'. Impairment of the faculties resulting from some external factor such as violence, drugs, including anaesthetics, alcohol and 'hypnotic influences' is held not to be due to disease (*R v Quick* [1973] QB 910). In more than a half of successful insanity defences, the diagnosis is schizophrenia (Mackay 1995).

It has been ruled that 'the nature and quality of the act' refers to the physical rather than the moral quality of the act. There are no published law reports which show how a successful defence based on the first limb operates. There are cases which show its unsuccessful operation (e.g. *R v Codère* (1917) 12 Cr App R 21). In fact, only about 25 per cent of successful insanity defences between 1975 and 1989 used the 'nature and quality' limb (Mackay 1995). The court in *Sullivan* said that for jurors in the 1980s it could be put in the terms: 'He did not know what he was doing.' Standard illustrations are of someone killing another under the delusion that he is breaking a jar, and a man cutting a woman's throat in the belief that he was cutting a loaf of bread.

It has been ruled that not to know 'he was doing what was wrong' means *legally* wrong, or contrary to the law; it does not mean *morally* wrong (*R v Johnson* [2007] EWCA Crim 1978). Thus, the defence was not available to Windle who thought that it was morally right to kill his suicidal wife and yet knew that it was legally wrong – 'I suppose they will hang me for this' (*R v Windle* [1952] 2 QB 826). In Mackay's study, 56 per cent of the cases relied on this second limb. The reason that 56 plus 25 does not make 100 is that in nineteen cases it was not possible to identify the basis for the defence in the psychiatric reports. Mackay is critical of the psychiatrists who approached the wrongness issue 'with little attempt made to distinguish between lack of knowledge of legal wrong ... as opposed to unawareness of moral wrong'. Our experience is of the defence being successful in cases of accused with particular religious delusions. An accused, whose forename was 'Leo', believed that he was 'Leo, the Lion of Judah', he believed that he was second only to God and he believed that God's law requiring him to kill his next-door neighbour, for refusing to hand him the keys to Jerusalem, gave him a legal right to kill him notwithstanding that this was against the law of the land.

The Law Commission (2013), contrary to *Codère*, regards the interpretation of the Court of Appeal as 'unwarrantedly narrow' (para. 4.20) and has argued that the nature of an act includes an appreciation of its moral qualities (para. 4.25). Rix (2015b, 2016) has argued that the appellate courts have erroneously restricted the meaning of 'wrong' to legal wrongness and has suggested that if psychiatrists apply the strict letter of the law, as established and confirmed in *Windle*, the insanity defence will remain beyond the reach of a multitude of mentally disordered people who would not otherwise be criminalised. He has suggested that in order for the issue of moral wrongfulness to be considered again by the Court of Appeal or by the Supreme Court, reports should address not only the questions that arise from a strict interpretation of the law, but other questions reflecting a wider interpretation of the law and its application in more progressive jurisdictions. Box 7.21 contains the suggested questions to be answered in an insanity case. The terms 'competent understanding' and 'appreciation' have been used in the sense of being able to think rationally of all the reasons that have a bearing on the rightness or wrongness of an action, to think calmly and rationally with some, or a moderate, degree of calmness, or sense of composure of the action's wrongfulness or to have the capacity to appreciate the wrongfulness of the act. It is also in the sense of 'appreciating' that, albeit that the conduct was in breach of legal or moral norms, there were reasons for believing that the action was right. It is unclear whether someone has to 'know' everything in that moment or only have a general 'appreciation' of it or 'know' it at some level.

Box 7.21 Suggested Questions to Be Answered in a Case Where the Insanity Defence Is Raised

- Is there evidence of a defect of reasoning?
- Is there evidence of disease of the mind?
- Did the defect of reasoning arise from a disease of the mind?
- Did the accused have a competent understanding or appreciation of the nature of the act?
- Did the accused have a competent understanding or appreciation of the quality of the act?
- Did the accused know that the act is contrary to the law of the land?
- Did the accused have a competent understanding or appreciation of whether the act was wrong, having regard to the commonly accepted standards of right and wrong or according to the moral standards of society?
- Did the accused act with calmness and composure and, if not, to what degree was this lacking?

Based on Rix 2016

The Law Commission (2013) has proposed that in England and Wales the present insanity defence is replaced by a defence of 'not criminally responsible by reason of a recognised medical condition'. This will go with a requirement that there must be expert evidence to the effect that:

> . . . the accused wholly lacked the capacity
>
> i. rationally to form a judgment about the relevant conduct or circumstances;
> ii. to understand the wrongfulness of what he or she is charged with having done; or
> iii. to control his or her physical acts in relation to the relevant conduct or circumstances
>
> as a result of a qualifying recognised medical condition.

Rix (2016) has criticised this proposal because 'wrongfulness' is not qualified with 'moral or legal', because there is no reference to 'composure' or 'calmness', and because the requirement for a total lack of capacity may considerably restrict the application of the defence.

In Jersey, insanity at the time of the commission of the offence derives from the Criminal Justice (Insane Persons) (Jersey) Law 1964, art 2(1):

> If on the trial before the Royal Court of any person charged with any act or omission punishable with death or imprisonment, the jury is satisfied that the accused did the act or made the omission charged against him or her but that the accused was insane at the time when the act was done or omission made so as not to be responsible according to law for his or her actions, the jury shall return a special verdict to the effect that the accused did the act or made the omission charged but is not guilty on the ground that he or she was insane so as not to be responsible according to law at the time.

In *Attorney General v Prior* [2001] JLR 146, the Royal Court held that the M'Naghten Rules were not part of Jersey law and it was clear that Jersey law required a volitional test of insanity. The test adopted was that 'a person is insane . . . if at the time of the commission of the offence, his unsoundness of mind affected his criminal behaviour to such a substantial degree that the jury consider that he ought not to be found criminally responsible'.

In Scotland, under the CP(S)A 1995, s 51A as amended by the Criminal Justice and Licensing (Scotland) Act 2010, there is a special defence of being not criminally responsible for conduct constituting an offence 'if the person was at the time of the conduct unable by reason of mental disorder to appreciate the nature or wrongfulness of the conduct'. However, the defence does not apply if 'the mental disorder in question consists only of a personality disorder which is characterised solely or principally by abnormally aggressive or seriously irresponsible conduct'. Here, mental disorder means mental illness, personality disorder or learning disability however manifested. However, not only is psychopathic personality disorder specifically excluded, but the 'appreciate' test is likely to keep this defence out of the reach of persons with other forms of personality disorder. The use of 'appreciate' instead of 'know' provides for a potential wider scope for the insanity defence in Scotland than in England and Wales.

In Ireland, under the CL(I)A, s 5 for a successful defence of NGRI, and where the jury finds that the accused committed the act alleged, the court has to hear evidence relating to their mental condition from a consultant psychiatrist. It has to establish that '(a) the accused person was suffering at the time from a mental disorder, and (b) the mental disorder was such that the accused person ought not to be held responsible for the act alleged by reason of the fact that he or she – (i) did not know the nature and quality of the act, or (ii) did not know that what he or she was doing was wrong, or (iii) was unable to refrain from committing the act'. Thus, the test is one of mental disorder, within the meaning of the Act. In addition, it encompasses the defence of 'irresistible impulse', which has long been part of the law in this area (*Attorney-General v O'Brien* [1936] IR 263, *Attorney-General v Hayes* (Central Criminal Court, unreported, 30 November 1967) and *Doyle v Wicklow County Council* [1974] IR 55). A verdict of NGRI is an acquittal, but where the court considers that the person is suffering from a mental disorder (within the meaning of the MHA 2001) and may be in need of in-patient care or treatment in a designated centre, it is empowered to commit the person to a specified designated centre (currently, the Central Mental Hospital (CMH)) and direct examination by an AMO at that centre. The consultant psychiatrist must report as to whether the person is suffering from a mental disorder within the meaning of the MHA 2001 and is in need of in-patient care or treatment in a designated centre. If the court accepts this opinion, it must commit that person to a specified designated centre (i.e. the CMH). Committal is mandatory in such circumstances and this is the sole disposal provided for. The legislative scheme is silent, however, on what is to happen if the report is to the effect that the person does not suffer from a mental disorder or does not require in-patient care or treatment in a designated centre. As the special verdict is, as a matter of law, an acquittal, logic suggests that no order other than discharge can be made. There is no express statutory provision for any other orders.

In Northern Ireland, the MCA(NI), s 206 allows the court to find a person NGRI on the evidence of two RMPs, including the oral evidence of one AMP (s 206(3)). The meaning of insanity is retained from the CJA(NI), which states at s 1 that:

> ... 'insane person' means a person who suffers from mental abnormality which prevents him –
>
> (a) from appreciating what he is doing; or
> (b) from appreciating that what he is doing is either wrong or contrary to law; or
> (c) from controlling his own conduct.

'Mental abnormality' means an abnormality of mind which arises from a condition of arrested or retarded development of mind or any inherent causes or is induced by disease or injury. This is also broader than the interpretation adopted by the Court of Appeal in England and Wales. Significantly, it uses the term 'appreciate' instead of 'know', as in Scotland, and it makes explicit that appreciating the wrongfulness of the conduct can found the defence even if there is appreciation of its unlawfulness.

In England and Wales, under the DVCVA, s 24(1), upon a finding of insanity the court must make (1) a hospital order with or without a restriction order without limit of time; (2) a supervision order, which may include treatment by or under the direction of an RMP; or (3) an order for absolute discharge. *In Northern Ireland*, the court must make a PPO, a PPOR or a supervision and assessment order, or order an absolute discharge. If the offence charged is one for which the penalty is fixed by law, the only disposal is a PPOR (MCA(NI), s 207(b)) and it cannot be for a specified period (s 207(c)).

Automatism

The essence of the defence of automatism is involuntariness: the alleged act was carried out involuntarily when the accused was not in control of his mind or body. According to Yannoulidis (2012): 'Automatism refers to an individual's lack of control for his or her conduct resulting in him or her acting in an unwilled fashion. It is an individual's lack of volition which gives rise to automatism.'

Automatism is defined by case law as follows:

> The state of a person who, though capable of action, is not conscious of what he is doing; this means unconscious, involuntary action, and it is a defence because the mind does not go with what is done . . . (*Bratty v Attorney General for Northern Ireland* [1963] AC 386)
>
> . . . action without any knowledge of acting, or action with no consciousness of doing what is being done . . . (*R v Cottle* [1958] NZLR 999)
>
> . . . total alienation of reason amounting to a complete absence of self-control . . . (*Ross v HM Advocate*, 1991 JC 210)
>
> . . . impairment of relevant capacities as distinct from total deprivation of these capacities [will not suffice] . . . It is fundamental to a defence of automatism that the actor has no control over his actions . . . (*R v Milloy* (1991) 54 A Crim R 340)

So, two features are recognised, not just involuntariness, or the absence of volition, but also the lack, or an altered state, of consciousness. Examples of automatism without loss of consciousness relevant to driving are a motor response accompanying sneezing or a reflex reaction to, for example, a sudden loud noise or being stung by a wasp.

The law distinguishes two forms of automatism: non-insane automatism (synonymous with sane automatism, *automatism simpliciter*) and insane automatism (i.e. automatism due to disease of the mind). The distinction is based on the cause of the automatism. Non-insane automatisms are caused by *external* factors such as drugs, hypnosis or concussion. Insane automatisms are regarded as arising from an *internal* factor such as epilepsy, cerebrovascular disease or diabetes. If the trial judge decides that the defence raised is 'insane automatism', he will direct the jury to decide whether the accused is guilty or NGRI. It is an important distinction. A successful defence of non-insane automatism results in acquittal. If it is a successful defence of insane automatism, disposal of the case will be under the DVCVA, s 24(1) which has amended the disposal options under the CP(IUP)A.

From a medical perspective, the legal classification is unsatisfactory if not nonsensical: 'For a violent act committed while the mind is disordered owing to an excess of insulin is a sane automatism if the insulin is injected, but an insane automatism if the insulin comes from an insulinoma of the pancreas' (Fenwick 1990).

The first stage is for the trial judge to decide if a proper evidential foundation has been laid. The judge will then decide if it is insane or non-insane automatism. If it is 'insane automatism', the defence has to prove its case on the balance of probabilities. If it is 'non-insane automatism', the prosecution carries the burden of proving beyond reasonable doubt that it was a voluntary act and not automatism, which is a high hurdle for the prosecution. It is sufficient for the defence to raise no more than a doubt as to the accused's guilt for the prosecution to be unable to prove its case beyond reasonable doubt.

Although the defence is ordinarily a defence to any criminal charge, including offences of strict liability, such as, in theory, driving over the prescribed limit (OPL), the defence is not open to those who have brought the state of automatism upon themselves – for example, by becoming exhausted or through consumption of alcohol or use of drugs. In the Irish case of *The People (DPP) v Reilly* [2005] 3 IR 111, where a killing occurred during a state of automatism brought about by a sleep disorder, the deep sleep arose as a result of consuming a very large quantiy of alcohol. Following the trial judge's direction in accordance with *DPP v Majewski* [1977] AC 443, he was convicted of manslaughter. The Court of Criminal Appeal considered that that direction was 'perfectly correct'.

Thus, in *R v Lipman* [1970] 1 QB 152, a conviction for manslaughter was upheld because it was self-induced intoxication with LSD which led to the automatism in the course of which the accused killed his girlfriend in the belief that she was a snake. However, self-induced automatism is a bar to the defence only if the accused was at fault. Thus, in *R v Bailey* [1983] 1 WLR 760, where the accused assaulted his victim during a period of loss of consciousness caused by hypoglycaemia because of his failure to take sufficient food following his last dose of insulin, the court held that:

> In cases of assault, if the accused knows that his actions or inaction are likely to make him aggressive, unpredictable or uncontrolled with the result that he may cause some injury to others and he persists in the action or takes no remedial action when he knows it is required, it will be open to the jury to find that he was reckless.

Box 7.22 lists psychiatric conditions potentially giving rise to an offence of automatism.

The leading English case on sleepwalking is *R v Burgess* [1991] 2 QB 92. Burgess had gone to the flat of a female friend and neighbour who was woken from sleep by blows to the head. She had been hit by a bottle and she saw Burgess, in a rage, holding a video player above his head. He then struck her with it causing a serious head injury. His defence was that he was asleep and in a state of automatism. The judge ruled that his sleep disorder was a disease of the mind and so it was a case of insane automatism.

Ebrahim and Fenwick (2008) have described a case of homicide in the course of confusional arousal. The accused, who had a personal and family history of sleepwalking, killed his father. The attack probably started in the accused's bedroom and continued downstairs where a cupboard was pulled from the wall and a chair broken. His father was dragged through the hallway and out of the front door where his head was banged on the

Box 7.22 Psychiatric Conditions Potentially Giving Rise to a Defence of Automatism

- sleep disorders
  - sleepwalking (somnambulism)
  - confusional arousal/sudden arousal disorders
  - sexsomnia (sexual behaviour in sleep)
- hysterical fugue
- personality disorder
- psychosis
- stress and PTSD

pavement and against a car. The accused took a shower, probably in his clothes, and made a very poor, disorganised attempt to mop up some blood with a towel. It was thought that the accused's father was likely to have aroused the accused from sleep either by a drunken attack or by shouting. Medical evidence was to the effect that the accused had responded with a confusional arousal that led to a sleepwalking episode. This was held legally to be a case of insane automatism.

Sexsomnia or sexual behaviour in sleep is a recognised parasomnia, but it differs from sleepwalking (Shapiro *et al.* 2003) in that it:

- originates in most cases from non-rapid eye movement sleep;
- occurs any time during sleep;
- involves widespread autonomic activation;
- is frequently associated with sexual arousal;
- possibly exceeds 30 minutes;
- only exceptionally involves violence or injurious behaviour;
- only exceptionally involves walking out of bed;
- occurs predominantly in adults.

In cases of sexsomnia, there is usually a history of parasomnias such as sleepwalking and a family history of arousal disorders. Often, there is a combination of trigger factors, in particular excess alcohol, too little sleep and stress. The proximity of a bed partner who may be a stimulus for arousal is another trigger factor. There may be an association with sleep apnoea.

Rix (2015a) has reported on a case in which sexsomnia was the basis for a defence to a charge of rape even though the accused was not disorientated on waking, there was evidence from the complainant of a conversation seemingly indicative of a high level of cognitive functioning and the accused had a partial recollection of events. The defence evidence was that there were both internal (genetic) and external factors (alcohol and proximity) operating and as the external factors were sufficient evidence for non-insane (sane) automatism to be left to the jury, the judge's direction was that, in order to convict, they had to be sure that the accused was not in an automatic state. This accorded with the approach in *R v Roach* [2001] EWCA Crim 2698, where it was decided that where there is a combination of internal and external factors, if the jury might conclude that the external causative factors were operative, a defence of non-insane automatism (which it is for the prosecution to disprove) should be left to them even if psychiatrists called by the defence had described the condition as insane automatism (and for which the burden of proof is on the accused). The accused was acquitted.

The defence of automatism was raised in *R v Isitt* [1977] 10 WLUK 148. It was put on the basis that the driver of a stolen vehicle was in a hysterical fugue so his subconscious mind was in control and he would not have appreciated what he was doing. However, the evidence of being able to circumvent a police road block was regarded as evidence of being in full voluntary control and the defence failed.

In *Roach*, where the accused was charged with wounding with intent to cause grievous bodily harm, there was contested psychiatric evidence. Two psychiatrists gave evidence that it was a case of 'insane automatism of psychogenic type', both basing their opinions on a diagnosis of personality disorder. The psychiatrist instructed by the prosecution disagreed and said that the accused's behaviour was entirely consistent with someone who had become increasingly anxious and lost his temper. The appellant appealed against conviction successfully because in his summing-up the trial judge had failed to draw attention to the evidence of two witnesses which provided some ambivalent support for the case that he had not realised what he was doing. However, the court did so reluctantly, observing that the case against the appellant was strong and that the jury had almost certainly rejected the defence on the basis of a strong preference for the prosecution psychiatrist's assessment and evidence. There was also evidence from what the accused said that he was conscious of what he was doing.

R v Coley [2013] EWCA Crim 223 is also illustrative of the effect of evidence as to the accused's behaviour at the material time. In this case, the accused had been convicted of attempted murder carried out during what was described as a brief psychotic episode resulting from the consumption of a great deal of cannabis. The Court of Appeal upheld the decision of the trial judge not to allow the defence of automatism to be put to the jury. However, it thought that there was an issue as to whether the appellant had been acting consciously. It accepted that the accused might have suffered a 'detachment from reality [which] might be described by some as an unconscious action', but held that this clearly fell short of involuntariness. The court observed: 'He must have made the decision to dress specifically for his intrusion next door, and to arm himself with his knife. He made the decision to find the keys and let himself in. That was not, as it seems to us, capable of being described as involuntary action.'

'Stress' is regarded as an external factor. It was held in *R v Rabey* [1980] SCR 513 that 'the ordinary stresses and disappointments of life which are the common lot of mankind do not constitute an external cause'. This is because they do not make everyone act like an automaton, so the real cause of the behaviour is 'internal'. However, in *R v Tate* [1990] Crim LR 256, where the defence was that the accused was in a state of automatism resulting from PTSD caused by rape when she took part in a robbery and an assault, the judge allowed the defence to go before the jury and ruled that it was sane automatism resulting from an external factor, the rape. This was on the basis that rape cannot be regarded as one of the 'ordinary stresses of life'. Nevertheless, the accused was convicted. There was evidence, as in the hysterical fugue, personality disorder and psychosis cases described above, that her mind went with her actions – for example, opening the blade of her penknife which the prosecution said required a controlled and positive action and which indicated that there was partial control.

In *Lederman*, the case of an 85-year-old man convicted of causing death by dangerous driving, two psychiatrists were called in his defence. His case was that the incident occurred because, at the relevant time, he was in 'a state of automatism relating to a medical episode', but the trial judge noted the accused's acknowledgement that his driving into a wall was deliberate and was effectively a safety manoeuvre. It was a ground for appeal that the trial judge should have acceded to a pre-trial request by the defence to dismiss the charges. The Court of Appeal did not accept this and said that there was ample evidence for the charge to go before the jury and for the jury to decide whether to convict.

Prescribed psychotropic drugs have figured in three automatism cases. In *R v Ball* [2007] EWCA Crim 3099, a psychiatrist attributed the behaviour of an off-duty police officer, charged with interfering with traffic equipment, to 'the taking of a sleeping pill with alcohol' which had caused 'a blackout and [caused him] to behave as an automaton'. However, this defence was abandoned in favour of a guilty plea when the psychiatrist agreed with a second doctor whose evidence was that the behaviour 'suggested the results of alcohol exaggerated by the sleeping tablet'. In *R v Smallshire* [2008] EWCA Crim 3217, the accused, who was prescribed citalopram, was convicted of causing grievous bodily harm with intent. On his own admission, he 'just went absolutely berserk', made a 'split second decision' to arm himself with a knife and then decided that he had to 'get the upper hand' and 'get the situation under control'. On appeal against conviction, this was not accepted as automatism. In *R v McGhee* [2013] EWCA Crim 223, the appellant was convicted of assault and wounding with intent following an incident outside an off-licence. A psychopharmacologist said that the combined effects of alcohol and temazepam might have resulted in paradoxical disinhibition. A psychiatrist gave evidence that the appellant was clearly aware and in control of his actions even if his judgement was impaired. The trial judge refused to allow the defence of automatism to go before the jury. In rejecting his appeal against conviction, the court took into account videotape evidence of his 'clearly voluntary behaviour in the shop and outside over quite an extended period' and added: 'Disinhibition is exactly not automatism.'

The psychiatrist is rather more likely to be instructed in a case of automatism caused by a physical condition, such as epilepsy, multiple sclerosis, migraine, cerebrovascular disease, concussion, obstructive sleep apnoea/hypopnoea syndrome or diabetes, than in the case of automatism resulting from psychiatric disorder. This is because such cases are more common and the CP(IUP)A requires written or oral evidence from two RMPs of whom at least one must be an AMP, and few neurologists and other medical specialists are AMPs. Although the assessment and investigation of such cases will be led by the appropriate medical expert (see Rix 2015a) and the psychiatrist will ride 'piggy-back' on the appropriate medical expert, it is important to look carefully at their opinion and the reasons for reaching it.

Thus, in a case of epilepsy, although the psychiatrist is likely to be heavily reliant on neurological opinion, often provided by the neurologist who has been instructed first, it is important that the psychiatrist heeds the advice of Fenwick (1990) as to the six points upon which to be satisfied before going to court to substantiate the diagnosis of epileptic automatism (Box 7.23). Indeed, this advice is of more general application and not limited to cases of epilepsy.

In Scotland, the law on automatism is similar. *Sorley v HM Advocate*, 1992 JC 102 has set out the requirements for a defence of sane automatism: (1) the automatic behaviour was caused by an external factor that was not self-induced; (2) this factor was not foreseeable (i.e.

Box 7.23 **Fenwick's Six Points upon Which the Psychiatrist Is to Be Satisfied before Going to Court to Substantiate a Defence of Epileptic Automatism**

1. The patient should be known to suffer from epilepsy.
2. The act should be out of character for the individual and inappropriate for the circumstances.
3. There must be no evidence of premeditation or concealment.
4. If witnesses are available, they should report a disorder of consciousness at the time of the act (e.g. staring eyes, glassy look, stereotyped movements, confusion and evidence that the person was out of touch with his surroundings).
5. A disorder of memory is the rule (but no loss of memory antedating the event).
6. The diagnosis of epilepsy can be substantiated on clinical grounds alone.

Fenwick 1990, p. 279

there was no prior fault); and (3) the effect of this factor was a total alienation of reason leading to a complete loss of self-control. Intoxication can be accepted as a cause of automatism if it is not self-induced. In *Ross*, where the accused had LSD and other drugs slipped into his beer and made a violent attack on others in the public house, it was established that intoxication can be a defence if it can be proved on evidence given that the intoxication was not self-induced and that the accused was as a result incapable of forming an intention, i.e. acting in a state of non-insane automatism.

It follows that in a case where the defence of automatism is at issue, the psychiatrist should: (1) analyse the evidence as to the state of mind of the accused at the material time so that, having regard to the legal definitions of automatism, paying particular attention to whether the accused's mind went with their action, the trial judge can decide whether or not the evidential foundation is laid; and (2) identify the likely cause or causes for the abnormal state of mind, distinguishing where appropriate between internal and external factors. In the event that the judge decides that it is an insane automatism, the psychiatric expert should be prepared to assist the court as to the disposal of the case.

Box 7.24 sets out a framework for assessment in cases of possible automatism. Particular attention should be paid to the evidence of witnesses who may report that the accused said that they were hungry or appeared anxious, pallid, sweaty or tremulous. There may be descriptions of the accused looking and acting as though intoxicated, appearing bewildered, seeming to be in shock, acting like a robot or an automaton, wandering aimlessly or lacking appropriate facial expressions. Terms used may include 'paranoid', 'fidgety' and 'out of it'. Conversation may be irrelevant or inappropriate to the circumstances.

Box 7.24 Assessment in a Case of Possible Automatism

History

- family history (e.g. sleepwalking, arousal disorders, sexsomnia);
- childhood history of sleepwalking;
- sleep history:
    - o time of onset of episodes during sleep;
    - o presence of confusional behaviour;
    - o amnesia/partial amnesia for episode;
    - o mentation on waking – non-narrative and non-dream-like experiences with only vague visual content, consisting mostly of thoughts and feelings;
- triggers for sleepwalking and/or sleep arousal disorders and/or sexsomnia (e.g. snoring, sleep apnoea, alcohol, drugs, fatigue, sleep deprivation, stressful life events and circumstances, strong emotions, intense physical activity).
- psychiatric history – major depressive disorder, obsessive-compulsive disorder and alcohol misuse/dependence increase the risk of sleepwalking; treatment with antidepressants or tranquillisers which may cause sleepwalking as side effect.
- general medical history – increased risk of sleepwalking and sexsomnia in sleep apnoea/hypopnoea syndrome; an association between sleep apnoea and depression; head injury and febrile illness can cause onset of sleepwalking in adulthood.

- History of episode:
  - events, symptoms, experiences leading up to and following the episode, such as disorientation, bewilderment, uncooperativeness;
  - recall of episode (e.g. complete amnesia, partial amnesia with fragments or distorted memories).
- Examination:
  - physical examination determined by nature of medical condition and medical assessment already carried out;
  - mental state examination (n.b.: abnormalities may support diagnosis, but may not assist as to mental state at material time).
- Investigations:
  - obtain medical records, importantly any created following alleged offence;
  - consider witness statements, CCTV recordings, police custody and interview records, police accident report and independent accident report, including provocation studies.

The case of *Bailey* (see above) is illustrative of the importance of analysing evidence as to the mental state of the accused at the material time as other evidence about the circumstances at that time and subsequent to it may not support the defence. Whilst holding that the jury had been misdirected, the court also found that it was:

> . . . very doubtful whether the appellant laid a sufficient basis for the defence . . . Although an episode of sudden transient loss of consciousness or awareness was theoretically possible, it was quite inconsistent with the graphic description that the appellant gave to the police both orally and in his written statement. There was abundant evidence that he had armed himself with the iron bar and gone to Harrison's house for the purpose of attacking him, because he wanted to teach him a lesson and because he was in the way.
>
> Moreover, the doctor's evidence to which we have referred showed it was extremely unlikely that such an episode could follow some five minutes after taking sugar and water.

For these reasons, the court found that there had been no miscarriage of justice and the appeal was dismissed.

The Law Commission (2013) is proposing a change to the law on automatism in England and Wales. The defence of insane automatism will be replaced by a defence of 'not criminally responsible by reason of a recognised medical condition'. The defence of non-insane automatism will be replaced by a defence of automatism where, at the material time, the accused suffered a total loss of capacity to control his or her actions which was not caused by a recognised medical condition.

Intent, *Mens Rea*, Motivation and Propensity

Except for offences of so-called strict liability, which do not require proof of fault, such as driving OPL, in order to convict a person of a criminal offence, it is necessary for the prosecution to prove beyond reasonable doubt two elements of the crime (Ormerod 2011). The first is that the person has caused something to happen, or is responsible for a certain state of affairs, that is forbidden by the criminal law (the *actus reus*). The second is that the person had a specific state of mind in relation to the causing of the event or the existence of the state of affairs (the *mens rea*); this is the mental element required by the definition of the particular crime. Usually, this means the intention to cause the *actus reus*.

Psychiatric evidence is not admissible on the issue of whether an accused had the *mens rea* for a particular offence. This is an ultimate issue for the jury. Psychiatric evidence may, however, be admissible as to whether the accused had a condition that could affect their capacity to form the particular intent required to prove the offence.

The most common circumstance in which psychiatric evidence may be sought as to the ability to form an intent is in cases where there is evidence that an accused person was intoxicated with alcohol or drugs at the material time.

There is a general rule that voluntary intoxication is not a defence. This is usually expressed as: 'A drunken intent is still intent.' It does not matter that it is an intent that the accused would not have formed if not intoxicated; it does not matter that the accused was so intoxicated that he does not recall what his intent was or what he did (*Majewski*). Majewski appealed against his conviction of four offences of occasioning actual bodily harm and three of assaulting a police constable in the execution of his duty. On appeal, his conviction was upheld as his crimes were of 'basic intent' and therefore his intoxication could not be relied on as a defence. *R v Taj* [2018] EWCA Crim 1743, where the accused suffered an episode of paranoia which led him to mistake an innocent man as a terrorist as a direct result of his earlier drink and drug-taking in the previous days and weeks, has established that this principle can extend to the more remote effects of drug or alcohol use even if the person is not intoxicated at the time. However, the court distinguished this from long-standing mental illness which might at some stage have been triggered by misuse of alcohol or drug misuse.

Voluntary intoxication is, however, a defence to crimes requiring 'specific intent'. As the Irish Court of Criminal Appeal noted in *The People (DPP) v Reilly* [2005] 3 IR 111, there is a 'general principle that intoxication is not a defence except in the rare cases where a specific intent is required'. As the distinction is one of policy rather than principle, it is necessary to base the classification on the decisions of the courts. Thus, the following have been identified as crimes of specific intent: murder, rape, wounding or causing grievous bodily harm with intent, theft, robbery, burglary with intent to steal, handling stolen goods, endeavouring to obtain money on a forged cheque, causing criminal damage where only intention to cause damage or endanger life is alleged and an *attempt* to commit any of these crimes of specific intent. The following are regarded as crimes of basic intent: manslaughter, malicious wounding or inflicting grievous bodily harm, kidnapping and false imprisonment, assault occasioning actual bodily harm, assault on a constable in execution of his duty, common assault, taking a vehicle without the owner's consent, criminal damage where recklessness, or only recklessness, is alleged and possibly an attempt to commit an offence where recklessness is a sufficient element in the *mens rea*, as in attempted rape.

R v Heard [2008] QB 43 seems to have established that, whereas the offence of sexual assault requires intentional rather than reckless touching, it is not an offence of specific intent. This adds to the difficulty in distinguishing crimes of specific and basic intent.

Instructed in such a case, first ascertain from the indictment, and if necessary by reference to the relevant act itself or a legal textbook, what the *mens rea* is for the offence. For example, it may be an allegation of burglary with intent; the particulars being that the accused entered, as a trespasser, a dwelling with intent to steal therein. The prosecution will need to prove that the accused entered with intent to steal. Second, ascertain from the witness statements what the evidence is that the accused was intoxicated and to what degree. There has to be evidence of consumption of a quantity sufficient to have affected the accused's state of mind (*R v Alden* [2001] 5 Archbold News 3). Third, the witness statements should be analysed for the presence or absence of evidence of the accused being able to act with forethought, form intentions and act on those intentions. To quote a typical summing-up to the jury: 'You look at his actions before, at the time of and, indeed, after the offence alleged. All these things, clearly, are capable you may think, of shedding a great deal of light upon what was on his mind at the time' (Rix and Clarkson 1994). For example, if there is evidence from the householder and from fingerprint evidence that the accused has moved aside a vase from the sill of the window by which he has entered the property, it may be difficult to argue that he was so intoxicated that he could not form the intent to steal. This means considering the evidence of witnesses as to what the accused said and did before, at and after the material time. If the accused has a recollection of what happened, or gave an account to the police or gives evidence at his trial, take into account what he told you or the police or says in evidence.

Pre-trial analysis usually allows cases to be identified as belonging to one of three categories.

First, there are those in which there is such ample evidence of the accused acting intentionally and with forethought that, notwithstanding his intoxication, it will not be possible to persuade a jury that he was so intoxicated that he lacked the specific intent for the offence. Second, there are those in which there is no evidence of the accused acting on intentions and with forethought and there is also evidence of behaviour that appears purposeless, pointless or confused. In such cases, the psychiatric evidence may lead the prosecution to offer to accept a plea of guilty to a lesser offence, for example, offering to accept a plea to unlawful wounding under the Offences Against the Person Act 1861 (OAPA), s 20 instead of trying to prove the more serious s 18 offence of wounding with intent to cause grievous bodily harm with the risk that the accused may be acquitted. Third, there are cases in which the evidence does not point one way or the other. In such cases, be prepared to go to court and base your opinion not on the evidence as set out in the witness statements, but on the evidence that these and perhaps other witnesses give in court.

Psychiatrists may be asked to comment on the effects of illicit substances, but many of these cases turn on the actual evidence from which the jury will infer intent rather than the pharmacology of the drug in question.

Psychiatric states particularly likely to give rise to issues as to the ability to form an intent are depressive states, where there may be impairment of attention and concentration, such as 'the depressed shoplifter' (see above, 'Insanity and Related Mental Condition Defences'), dissociation and depersonalisation.

Expert opinion needs to include an analysis of the psychopathology as well as consideration of the evidence. A man was charged with causing his estranged wife grievous bodily harm with intent with a ratchet spanner that he had fetched from the bottom of a cantilever tool box in the garage at 4 a.m. and in the course of which attack he struck between twenty and twenty-five blows, causing injuries that required eighty-six sutures, dislodged two teeth and fractured her jaw (Rix and Clarkson 1994). His defence was that he was in a state of severe depersonalisation and derealisation in which his actions appeared to be elaborate, but were not planned. The prosecution called a psychiatrist who explained the psychopathology of depersonalisation. His opinion was summarised as: 'A depersonalised intent is nevertheless an intent', although arguably he should not have commented on this because it is a legal issue or a legal point to be made by the prosecution. By a majority verdict, the accused was convicted of causing grievous bodily harm with intent. The case illustrates the approach recommended in cases where dissociation is raised as a defence:

> The courts should eschew any effort to discourage the defence of dissociation by interpreting it as evidence of insanity, or by withholding psychiatric evidence from the jury. The defence, if supported by medical evidence, should be adjudicated upon by the triers of fact, and if successful should result in an ordinary acquittal. But what is urgently needed is that the psychiatrist who deposes to dissociation in improbable circumstances should be subjected to skilled and deeply sceptical cross-examination, and that the Crown should, where possible, call counter-evidence. (Williams 1983)

There have been several intent cases in which there has been successful reliance on a diagnosis of Asperger syndrome. Convictions for sexual assault were quashed on the admission of expert evidence that as a result of the appellant's Asperger syndrome he 'might behave in a socially inappropriate but innocent manner towards children without having the comprehension that his actions could be misconstrued' (*Thompson*). In *R (Bavi) v Snaresbrook Crown Court v Thames Valley Police* [2013] EWHC 4015 (Admin), it was held that the appellant's Asperger syndrome, social phobia and obsessive-compulsive disorder, which manifested in compulsive saving and a tendency to fantasise, provided an explanation for his otherwise implausible explanation for being in possession of £18,500 on his way to the Reading Festival and which sum he had been ordered to forfeit as proceeds of crime.

The *mens rea* of many offences is 'wilfulness'. This was an issue in *R v Sheppard* [1981] AC 394. Parents of low intelligence were convicted of the wilful neglect of their child who died of hypothermia following severe gastroenteritis. They succeeded in their appeal against conviction because they had not appreciated the seriousness of his condition. This subjective aspect of wilfulness is reflected in the observation that 'a parent, who has genuinely failed to appreciate that his child needs medical care, through personal inadequacy or stupidity or both, is not guilty'.

The *mens rea* of some offences includes 'reasonable belief'. To prove the *mens rea* for rape, there must be evidence that the accused reasonably believed that the complainant was consenting at the time of penetration. This requires consideration of the effect of mental disorder on the accused's capacity to understand the true nature of the situation. This means taking into account the accused's relevant characteristics, such as extreme youth or an intellectual disability. However, in *R v B (MA)* [2013] EWCA Crim 3, the court held that psychotic thinking could never be considered reasonable, so, unless the accused's state of mind amounted to legal insanity, beliefs in consent resulting from delusions or personality disorder had to be judged by objective standards of reasonableness. This has been confirmed in *Oye* (see above, 'Self-Defence').

The court did recognise that there could be cases, such as that of an accused with less than ordinary intelligence, in which an impaired ability to read subtle social signals could be relevant to the reasonableness of their belief as to consent. Such cases might include those of people with Asperger syndrome. In *R v Sultan* [2008] EWCA Crim 6, where the appellant was convicted of rape (under the law prior to the Sexual Offences Act 2003 (SOA)), the court accepted that expert evidence would have been admissible to show that the appellant was suffering from a condition such as Asperger syndrome which might have affected his ability to judge a person's intentions, beliefs or desires in ambiguous situations.

The case of *R v Harris* [2013] EWCA Crim 223 illustrates how psychosis, insufficient to found a defence of insanity, may be associated with a lack of the subjective recklessness that is required for an offence of aggravated arson (i.e. arson being reckless as to the endangerment of life under the Criminal Damage Act 1971, s 1(2)). In the course of an alcohol withdrawal psychosis, Harris experienced voices telling him to burn his house down. He set fire to his semi-detached house, endangering the lives of his neighbours. The Court of Appeal quashed his conviction on the grounds that he 'was entitled to have tried the question of whether, in the condition in which he was, he was actually aware of the risk which he created for his neighbours', that is, he could have defended himself by way of a simple plea of lack of *mens rea*. This is similar to *R v Stephenson* [1979] QB 695, where a man had his conviction for arson quashed on the ground that he might not have foreseen the risk of the fire spreading. The fire had occurred after he made a hollow in a hayrick for the purposes of sleep and then lit a fire to warm himself.

An unsuccessful attempt to use evidence of adjustment disorder to overturn a conviction for fraud illustrates how difficult it is to admit medical evidence in respect of the issue of dishonesty and illustrates the need to show how the psychopathology may explain the person's behaviour (*R v Hayes* [2015] EWCA Crim 1944). On appeal, the argument was abandoned that medical evidence was relevant and admissible in respect of the dishonesty. It was a further ground for appeal that the trial judge had been wrong to rule inadmissible evidence of the appellant's adjustment disorder. It was argued that it was relevant to his state of mind and understanding when he entered into a formal agreement in which he admitted that he had acted dishonestly. However, the Court of Appeal accepted the trial judge's finding that there was no evidence that the appellant did not understand the process into which he entered or that his depressed emotional state impacted on his comprehension. It added that the jury did not need medical evidence to understand the pressure, and consequent distress, that the appellant must have been under.

R v Henry [2005] EWCA Crim 1681 is important in illustrating the general approach of the courts to the admissibility of evidence as to IQ (and to be distinguished from the approach in cases involving the reliability of confession evidence – see above, 'Fitness to Be Interviewed and Reliability of Police Interviews'). This was an appeal against convictions for soliciting murder and conspiracy to murder. The Court of Appeal refused to admit evidence from psychologists as to his intention. One assessed his IQ as 75 and the other as 72. The court held that their reports did not contain admissible evidence on the issue of intention and it relied on *R v Masih* [1986] Crim LR 395 as authority for adopting a cut-off point of 69, which it recognised had sometimes been criticised as arbitrary, but had psychological significance and had the advantage of being, according to the commentator, 'a clean rule', even if 'a rather stringent one':

> Generally speaking, if an accused is mentally defective, or otherwise comes in the last class, '69 and below mental defective', then in so far as that defectiveness is relevant . . . to the particular case – it may be that expert evidence should be admitted about it. That is in order to enlighten the jury upon a matter which is abnormal, and therefore *ex hypothesi*, presumably, outside their own experience. If it is admitted it should be confined to the assessment of the accused's Intelligence Quotient, and to an explanation of any relevant abnormal characteristics which such an assessment involves . . . Where the accused however is within the scale of normality, albeit, as this man was, at the lower end of that scale, expert evidence, in our judgment, is not as a rule, necessary and should be excluded.

Given the exclusion in *Turner* of psychiatric evidence as to 'how ordinary folk who are not suffering from any mental illness are likely to react to the stresses and strains of life', the judgment in *The People (DPP) v Abdi* [2005] 1 ILRM 382 is worth noting. The accused had killed his infant son and raised the defence of insanity. The prosecution psychiatrist was permitted to give evidence, not merely that the accused was not legally insane, but that he had been motivated by the inability to accept that he would not be able to rear his child in his own faith and might lose custody of him. The defence contended that this evidence was inadmissible, as the psychiatrist was in no better a position to express a view on motive than anyone else. The Court of Criminal Appeal held that where insanity was positively alleged, and the defence had called expert evidence which implied that a 'normal' person could not have carried out the act in question, the prosecution was 'plainly' entitled to counter it by reference to a sane, if perverted, attitude on the part of the accused. On the facts of the case, the evidence was admissible in principle.

In England and Wales, under the CJA 2003 and *in the Isle of Man*, under the Criminal Evidence Act 2019 (CEA), evidence of the accused's bad character is admissible if 'it is relevant to an important matter in issue between the accused and the prosecution' (CJA 2003, s 101(1)(d); CEA, s 7(d)). Such matters include 'the question whether the accused has a propensity to commit offences of the kind with which he is charged' (CJA 2003, s 103(1)(a); CEA, s 9(1)(a)). This means the propensity to act in a particular way. Thus, evidence of previous convictions, which would usually be withheld from the jury, may be admitted. In *Lowery v R* [1974] AC 85, a psychologist, who had tested two co-defendants with the Rorschach Test and the Thematic Apperception Test, was allowed to give evidence to the effect that one of them had a personality marked by aggressiveness and the other a personality which suggested that he would be led and dominated by someone who was aggressive. This evidence was admitted on the basis that it appeared probative of the issue of which co-defendant was more likely to have committed the offence of murder. However, in *R v Neale* (1977) 65 Cr App R 304, the court refused to admit evidence that one co-defendant had a propensity for arson and, in *R v Rimmer* [1983] Crim LR 250, the court refused to admit expert evidence in rebuttal of an accusation that one co-defendant had a history of mental illness, specifically 'fits' or 'brainstorms', and this was upheld on appeal because it 'would have served to confuse the jury and blur the crucial issues'.

In the case of an accused with a psychiatric history, a psychiatric expert might be instructed to consider their psychiatric and other records to identify any evidence which might indicate a propensity to commit the offence with which they are charged. Such a case requires a careful analysis of the evidence relating to the alleged offence as any evidence obtained by the psychiatrist from the records will have to be compared with the facts of the alleged offence.

Thus, in a case of alleged murder, there may be evidence of similar but non-fatal violence in the form of attacks on fellow patients or staff in psychiatric institutions. In a case of alleged murder, where the defendant was under the influence of certain intoxicants, the records may contain evidence of his behaviour previously when similarly intoxicated. It may be relatively easy to pick out episodes in the defendant's history that bear a similarity to the alleged offence, but, in order to address propensity, it is also necessary to take careful note of evidence that may be inconsistent; cross-examination will be likely to focus on this to argue, on behalf of the defendant, that there was no such propensity.

It is important to restrict opinion to propensity. Do not offer an opinion as to whether, in the light of the evidence subjected to psychiatric analysis, the accused was responsible for the offence alleged. This is for the court.

In Ireland, questions of propensity, as distinct from bad character, do not arise perhaps other than in the parole context, given the difficulty of any analysis of, and adjudication on, propensity.

Loss of Control

In England and Wales and *Northern Ireland*, instead of provocation there is, as a partial defence to a charge of murder, loss of self-control, which, if successful, reduces the offence to one of manslaughter (CJA 2009, s 54(1)). However, the new law generates a great deal of confusion and the old problems of the provocation defence remain. It may be but a rose by another name.

It does not apply where the accused acted in a considered desire for revenge 'whether performed calmly or in anger' (*R v Clinton* [2012] EWCA Crim 2). This is partly because having time to think and to reflect, so-called 'thinking time', is inconsistent with loss of self-control.

The defence bears the burden of proving loss of self-control. If, however, the judge finds that there is sufficient evidence to raise the issue, and upon which a jury properly directed could conclude that the defence might apply, the jury must assume that the defence is satisfied unless the prosecution proves otherwise beyond reasonable doubt.

The CJA 2009, s 54(1) states:

> Where a person ('D') kills or is party to the killing of another ('V'), D is not to be convicted of murder if –
>
> (a) D's acts and omissions in doing or being a party to the killing resulted from D's loss of self-control,
> (b) the loss of self-control had a qualifying trigger, and
> (c) a person of D's sex and age, with a normal degree of tolerance and self-restraint and in the circumstances of D, might have reacted in the same or in a similar way to D.

Section 54(2) provides that it does not matter whether the loss of self-control was sudden. This will assist, in particular, victims of domestic violence who previously had to prove a 'sudden and temporary' loss of control and were in difficulty in persuading the court that their 'slow burn' reaction to repeated violence brought them within the scope of provocation (Rix 2001).

For the psychiatric expert, the important provisions relate to the accused's circumstances and the qualifying triggers. Subsection 3 states that 'circumstances' is a reference to all of the accused's 'circumstances other than those whose only relevance' is that they bear on the capacity for tolerance or self-restraint. Ormerod (2011) has suggested that this opens up a broader range of subjective considerations than was previously allowed. He has also observed that there is now no positive requirement that the accused's individual circumstances have to affect the gravity of the triggering conduct in order for them to be included in the jury's assessment of what the person of the accused's age and sex might have done. He gives the example of an accused with a learning disability who is subjected to provocative taunts. His disability will be relevant event if the taunts relate to something completely different.

R v Gregson [2006] EWCA Crim 3364 also illustrates the relevance of the accused's sensitivity:

> It was open to the jury . . . to consider the appellant's illnesses when assessing the gravity of the provocation . . . [they] were potentially relevant because [he] could well have had a heightened sense of grievance about the insults because he felt that, due to his depression and epilepsy, it was not his fault he was out of work.

The meaning of 'qualifying trigger' is set out in the CJA 2009, s 55. First, it can be the accused's 'fear of serious violence from V against D or another identified person' (s 55(3)) (the fear trigger). Again, this is an accommodation for victims of domestic violence who kill violent and abusive partners. Second, it can be a thing or things done or said (or both) which (1) constituted circumstances of an extremely grave character and (2) caused the accused to have a justifiable sense of being seriously wronged (s 55(4)) (the anger trigger). Ormerod and Perry (2019, para. B1.26) observe that these requirements are designed to make the defence much more limited than the previous common law defence. Third, it can be a combination of these two triggers (s 55(5)).

Three triggers are excluded (s 55(6)). First, it is not a qualifying trigger if it is serious violence that the accused has caused by incitement in order to have an excuse to use violence. Second, it is not a qualifying trigger if the accused has incited the victim to do what has seriously wronged the accused in order to provide an excuse for violence. Third, sexual infidelity does not qualify as a trigger.

Psychiatric evidence was relevant and admissible in some cases where the defence of provocation was raised and it is likely that it will be so in some cases where it is one of loss of self-control. Insofar as the new law puts on a statutory footing the majority decisions on provocation of the Privy Council in *Attorney-General for Jersey v Holley* [2005] UKPC 23 and *Luc Thiet Thuan v The Queen* [1997] AC 131 and the House of Lords in *R v Camplin* [1978] AC 705, these cases are likely to continue to assist the psychiatric expert.

The new law appears to perpetuate, for loss of self-control, the requirement, for the defence of provocation, that the defence has to make out two conditions: (1) the 'subjective' condition that the accused was actually triggered to lose self-control; and (2) the 'objective' condition that a person of the accused's sex and age with a normal degree of tolerance and self-restraint, in the circumstances of the accused, might have done so (these two conditions being re-stated here in the language of loss of self-control).

Camplin's importance was that the characteristics of the accused could not be excluded, thus qualifying what, under the defence of provocation, the 'reasonable man' would have done, and what under the new law, a person of normal tolerance and reasonable restraint would have done. There is no reference to 'characteristics' in the new law, but mental disorders may form part of the 'circumstances'. Thus, where *Clinton* was charged with the murder of his wife and arson, the court recognised that the effect of his 'depressed state' would have meant that he was 'more likely to lose self-control following his wife's graphic account of sexual activity with other men and her taunts that he lacked the courage to commit suicide'. *R v Kelly* [2015] EWCA Crim 500 provides further support. It was argued at trial that the accused's PTSD was not only relevant to his capacity for tolerance and self-restraint, but also to his circumstances as a whole because it was part of his character. However, this was not re-argued on appeal and in *R v Rejmanski* [2017] EWCA Crim 2061, although PTSD attributable to military service was found to have affected the gravity of the qualifying trigger, which was taunts about that military service, it was held that it could not be taken into account in relation to the degree of tolerance and self-restraint expected. Furthermore, 'a personality disorder which made him unusually likely to be angry and aggressive at the slightest provocation' (*R v Wilcocks* [2016] EWCA Crim 2043) or an emotionally unstable personality disorder (*R v Gassman* [2017] EWCA Crim 2061) cannot be included in the accused's circumstances, although in *Wilcocks* his suicide attempt was admissible as 'circumstances', as it related to loss of self-restraint. The following is an adaptation of *Camplin* reflecting the terminology of the new law:

> ... the gravity of the trigger may well depend upon the particular circumstances of the person to whom a taunt or insult is addressed or to whom any other trigger is directed. To taunt a person because of his race, his physical infirmities or some shameful incident in his past may well be considered by the jury to be more offensive to the person, however equable his temperament, if the facts on which the taunt is founded are true than it would be if they were not ...
>
> ... a proper direction to a jury ... [would be to] explain to them that the person with a normal degree of tolerance and self-restraint ... is a person having the degree of tolerance and self-restraint to be expected of an ordinary person of the sex and age of the accused, but in other respects sharing such of the accused's circumstances as they think bear on how he might have reacted; and that the question is not merely whether such a person would in like circumstances be triggered to lose self-control but also whether he would react to the trigger as the accused did.

Subsequently, there were cases that blurred the distinction between the gravity of the provocation question and the powers of self-control test: *R v Humphreys* [1995] 4 All ER 1008, *R v Dryden* [1995] 4 All ER 987, *R v Thornton (No. 2)* [1996] 1 WLR 1174 and *R v Smith (Morgan)* [2001] 1 AC 146. They are now regarded as erroneous or wrongly decided. However, they shed light on the attempts to liberalise 'the reasonable man' test, reflecting that 'compassion to human frailty' which led Lord Diplock to take account of youth in *Camplin*. Insofar as there may be now more difficult attempts to liberalise the test within the strait-jacket of the new law, these may remain important cases. Also, as observed in Murphy (1999), these cases, along with *R v Parker* [1997] Crim LR 760, suggest that the characteristics with which the reasonable man was (wrongly, as subsequently decided) invested could still be relevant because they affect the gravity of the provocation (trigger):

> Thus an instance of abuse of a woman with battered woman syndrome can be regarded as more provocative than abuse of one not suffering from such a syndrome and a threat to evict a person who is possessive about his land (Dryden) may be more provocative than it would be to an ordinary person, even though each person would be expected to exercise the same level of self-control to a given level of gravity of provocation.

In *Luc Thiet Thuan*, the Privy Council ruled that the appellant's brain damage was not relevant to the objective test; it merely affected his powers of self-control rather than the gravity of the provocation. There was thus a direct conflict between the Privy Council in *Luc Thiet Thuan* and the House of Lords in *Smith (Morgan)*, where it was held that a characteristic such as Smith's severe depression was relevant not only to the gravity of the provocation, but also to the standard of self-control expected. *Holley* provided the Privy Council with the opportunity to resolve the conflict and clarify the law. It was resolved in favour of *Luc Thiet Thuan*. It was held that 'the sufficiency of the provocation ("whether the provocation was enough to make a reasonable man do as [the accused] did") is to be judged by one standard and not a standard which varies from one accused to another'.

The distinction is now between circumstances that bear only on the accused's general capacity for tolerance or self-restraint, which have to be excluded, and all other circumstances of the accused which bear on how he might have reacted (instead of relevant factors affecting the gravity of the trigger).

Voluntary intoxication with alcohol is not to be included in the accused's circumstances (*R v Asmelash* [2013] EWCA Crim 157). However, the court added the rider that this:

> . . . does not mean that the accused who has been drinking is deprived of any possible loss of control defence . . . If a sober individual in the accused's circumstances, with normal levels of tolerance and self-restraint might have behaved in the same way as the accused confronted by the relevant qualifying trigger, he would not be deprived of the loss of self control defence just because he was not sober.

Until the new defence has been deployed and there have been more appeals, it is difficult to know what psychiatric evidence will be relevant and admissible. There may be less reliance on psychiatric evidence if, as Norrie (2010) suggests: 'Under the new law, defendants . . . will be encouraged to portray themselves as ordinary people grievously harmed and acting out of a legitimate sense of anger at what has been done to them' or the defences of diminished responsibility and loss of control will be presented as alternatives now that 'the amended section 2 applies where a mental disorder substantially impairs the ability of the defendant to exercise self-control' (*Rejmanski*). *R v Foye* [2013] EWCA Crim 475 helpfully distinguishes them: 'Diminished Responsibility depends on the internal mental condition of the defendant. Loss of control depends on an objective judgment of his actions as a reaction to external circumstances.'

In England and Wales, the best advice meanwhile is to consider whether the accused has any psychiatric disorder or syndrome, such as so-called battered woman syndrome (BWS), and, if so, to set out how it has a bearing on how the accused might have reacted, in particular how, for example, it would result in the accused having a justifiable sense of being seriously wronged. For example, a particular look in the eye may be a qualifying trigger for the victim of domestic violence whose experience is that it has always been the precursor of serious violence. Again, in relation to domestic violence, there may be evidence of shameful incidents which may contribute to the accused believing, or being more sensitive to, some of the hurtful things said by the abusive partner and which might not otherwise be accepted as a qualifying trigger. Alternatively, psychiatric assessment may reveal a psychiatric condition that is associated with, or results in, an impairment of the accused's general capacity for tolerance or self-restraint, in which case the prosecution will rely on it to argue that the defence is not open to the accused. Finally, beware offering an opinion as to whether there was a loss of control.

In Ireland, the test of the common law defence of provocation is treated as entirely subjective, one which must be negatived by the prosecution once it is raised (*The People (DPP) v Lynch* [2015] IECCA 6). It is a defence of only partial excuse. The question is not whether a normal or reasonable person would have been so provoked as totally to lose self-control, but whether the particular accused, with his peculiar history and personality, was so provoked (*The People (DPP) v Kelly* [2000] 2 IR 1). In *The People (DPP) v MacEoin* [1978] IR 27, the Court of Criminal Appeal stated that the trial judge should examine whether there is any evidence of provocation 'which having regard to the accused's temperament, character and circumstances might have caused him to lose control of himself at the time of the wrongful act and whether the provocation bears a reasonable relation to the amount of force used by the accused'. *Lynch* has established that: 'The loss of control must be total and reaction must come suddenly and before time for emotions to cool. There must be a sudden and temporary loss of self-control rendering the accused so subject to passion as to make him or her for the moment not the master of his (or her) mind. Extreme anger and murderous rage are not themselves enough.'

In the Irish case of *(DPP) v Kehoe* [1992] ILRM 481 (SC), psychiatric evidence to support a defence of provocation was adduced, but it was the subject of adverse comment by the trial judge in charging the jury. The conviction was upheld, with the Court of Criminal Appeal ruling that the doctor could not give any relevant, admissible evidence as to the state of mind of the accused that the accused could not give himself. The robustness of the language in *Kehoe* does not really leave any uncertainty, but Charleton, McDermott and Bolger (1999; para. 14.38) comment: 'In the event that an accused person was less able to explain their own reaction to provocation, as in the case of a very young or mentally infirm accused, it is possible that medical evidence would be admissible as to the nature of the condition which caused this infirmity.'

In Jersey and *in the Isle of Man*, the law on provocation follows that in the Homicide Act 1957 of England and Wales. Article 4 of the Homicide (Jersey) Law 1986 and the Isle of Man's Criminal Code 1872, s 21A, state that:

> Where on a charge of murder there is evidence on which the jury can find that the person charged was provoked (whether by things done or by things said or by both together) to lose the person's self-control, the question of whether the provocation was enough to make the reasonable person do as he or she did shall be left to be determined by the jury; and in determining that question the jury shall take into account everything both done and said according to the effect which, in their opinion, it would have on a reasonable person.

The interpretation of this statute, however, is now governed by the Privy Council ruling in *Holley* (see above).

In Scotland, expert evidence is inadmissible with regard to the mental state of the accused because the test is how the ordinary person would react and this is an objective assessment to be made by the court. There is no subjective component. In practice, where mental disorder affects self-control, the basis for seeking a reduction from murder to culpable homicide is to advance a plea of diminished responsibility.

Duress, Coercion and Compulsion

It may be a defence to a criminal charge, which if successful results in acquittal, to plead duress because 'threats of immediate death or serious personal violence so great as to overbear the ordinary powers of human resistance should be accepted as a justification for acts which would otherwise be criminal' (*Attorney-General v Whelan* [1934] IR 518).

Psychiatric evidence may be relevant and admissible because the mental state of the accused, specifically 'the weak, immature or disabled person', may mean that they find the threats more compelling than 'a normal healthy person', but this defence does not apply if the defendant's will has been eroded by the voluntary consumption of alcohol or drugs (*R v Graham* [1982] 1 WLR 294). This is reflected in the direction given to the jury which was to require it to be 'sure that a sober person of reasonable firmness, *sharing the characteristics of* [the defendant], would not have responded' (emphasis added) as he did. Two problems emerge. The first is that characteristics that identify the accused as not being 'of reasonable firmness' are problematic because, whatever the effects of such characteristics, the standard is the person of reasonable firmness ('the objective test'). Second, the psychiatrist needs to know what the law will admit as characteristics.

R v Emery [1992] 11 WLUK 22 perpetuates the problem. The Court of Appeal could find 'no scope for attributing to that hypothetical person one of the characteristics of the accused a pre-existing mental condition of being "emotionally unstable" or in a "grossly elevated neurotic state"', but was prepared to admit PTSD as an admissible characteristic because it was a 'comparatively recent development ... complex and ... not known by the public at large'. Also, PTSD was accepted as a relevant characteristic in *R v Sewell* [2004] EWCA Crim 2322.

Thus, in *R v Horne* [1994] 2 WLUK 12, the Court of Appeal upheld the trial judge's refusal to admit psychiatric evidence as characteristics such as inherent weakness, vulnerability and susceptibility to threats were inconsistent with the requirements of the objective test because it 'would be a contradiction in terms to ask ... them to take into account, as one of the characteristics, that he was pliant or vulnerable'. This contradiction in terms was also recognised in *R v Hurst* [1994] 1 WLUK 539, where the court found it hard to see how 'the person of reasonable firmness can be invested with the characteristics of a personality which lacks reasonable firmness'.

Long-accepted judicial guidance comes from *R v Bowen* [1997] 1 WLR 372 (Box 7.25). Even though the appellant had, or may have had, a low IQ of 68, which inhibited his ability to seek the protection of the police, and been abnormally suggestible and vulnerable, the court held that: 'We do not see how low I.Q., short of mental impairment or mental

Box 7.25 Principles to Be Applied in a Case of Alleged Duress

1. The mere fact that the accused is more pliable, vulnerable, timid or susceptible to threats than a normal person are not characteristics with which it is legitimate to invest the reasonable/ordinary person for the purpose of considering the objective test.
2. The defendant may be in a category of person who the jury think are less able to resist pressure than people not within that category ... recognised mental illness or psychiatric condition, such as post-traumatic stress disorder leading to learned helplessness.
3. Characteristics which may be relevant in considering provocation, because they relate to the nature of the provocation, itself will not necessarily be relevant in cases of duress ...
4. Characteristics due to self-induced abuse, such as alcohol, drugs or glue-sniffing, cannot be relevant.
5. Psychiatric evidence may be admissible to show that the accused is suffering from some mental illness, mental impairment or recognised psychiatric condition provided persons generally suffering from such conditions may be more susceptible to pressure and threats and thus to assist the jury in deciding whether a reasonable person suffering from such a condition might have been impelled to act as the accused did. It is not admissible simply to show that in the doctor's opinion an accused, who is not suffering from such illness or condition, is especially timid, suggestible or vulnerable to pressure and threats.

R v Bowen [1997] 1 WLR 372

defectiveness, can be said to be a characteristic that makes those who have it less courageous and less able to withstand threats and pressure.'

This case seems to suggest that 'mental impairment' or 'mental defectiveness' is an admissible characteristic, but more than a bare IQ is needed to make such a diagnosis. It also makes it clear that, notwithstanding the problem for people who are more pliable, vulnerable, timid or susceptible to threats than an ordinary person, 'medical evidence is admissible if the mental condition or abnormality of the accused is relevant and the condition or abnormality and its effects lie outwith the knowledge and experience of laymen', as was held in *R v Hegarty* [1994] 1 WLUK 146.

This case also perpetuates the conflict between the fifth principle (Box 7.26), which refers to conditions that render a person 'more susceptible to pressure and threats', and the objective test of a person of reasonable firmness.

In *R v Antar* [2004] EWCA Crim 2708, the conviction for conspiracy to rob of an 18-year -old with a mild to moderate learning disability was overturned because the trial judge should have admitted the evidence of the psychologist as to his impairment and suggestibility, although it was a matter for the jury to decide on all the evidence whether he fell into a category of persons who were less able to resist pressure than the sober person of reasonable firmness.

Bowen was recently reasserted in *R v Coats* [2013] EWCA Crim 1472. It was an unsuccessful appeal against a conviction for importing drugs, because the court was not persuaded that the appellant had truly suffered abuse of a nature and degree sufficient to reach the high threshold required for the defence of duress and 'an accused would have to be suffering from battered woman syndrome in a severe form to be in a position to claim their will was overborne'. However, it does demonstrate that BWS may be accepted as the basis for a defence of duress. In particular, there appears to be acceptance of the relevance of two of its features: 'Learned helplessness would be of particular relevance to a possible defence of duress. Traumatic bonding . . . may mean a victim will stay with their abuser through a variety of emotions but particularly through fear.' The court also made a number of observations which experts will usefully consider not just in cases of alleged duress and BWS, but in BWS cases in general:

> [N]ot every woman who suffers from domestic violence goes on to suffer from Battered Woman's Syndrome. Not every woman who suffers from BWS can claim the defence of duress. It is essential to analyse, with some care, the extent and timing of the domestic violence, the impact upon the person concerned and their presentation at the relevant time. This may not be an easy task . . .
>
> Stereotypical images of how one would expect a battered woman or man to behave or present may be counter intuitive. The court and the expert advising the court must bear very much in mind that battered women may be inconsistent in their complaints of abuse, they make complaints and wrongly withdraw them, they make no complaints at all. Their feelings for their abuser may range between anger, hatred, forgiveness, loyalty and love. They may not seek sanctuary when they should and could. They may perform acts which are out of character because they feel they have no options, albeit the objective observer might consider their options obvious. They may also put the safety of the children they love at risk. They may not react to a traumatic situation as an objective observer might react.

Assuming that the mental state of the accused is relevant, it follows that psychiatric evidence is likely to be admitted if it satisfies the general test of falling outside the knowledge and experience of the lay person. *Emery* also assists as to what might be expected in the psychiatric report: 'the causes of the condition of learned helplessness, the circumstances in which it might arise and what level of abuse would be required to produce it; what degree of isolation of the person one would expect to find before it appeared and what sort of personality factors might be involved'.

Although this judgment focuses on 'learned helplessness', it gives an indication of the detailed evidence the court expects from psychiatrists. Until the law's seeming inconsistencies are resolved, best advice in possible duress cases is as far as possible to provide detailed evidence as to the mental condition and personality of the accused and explain how these assist in understanding the ability of the accused to resist threats of immediate death or serious violence and leave the court to decide on the admissibility of such evidence.

Mere acquiescence to the wishes of others is not duress. In *R v Jackson-Mason* [2014] EWCA Crim 1993, a woman with a borderline learning disability was one of a number of vulnerable people who were approached and asked to cash high quality counterfeit benefit cheques at post offices. She was convicted of fraud. She unsuccessfully appealed on the grounds that the trial judge wrongly excluded a psychologist's expert evidence:

> ... that her intellectual function was low and thus she was vulnerable to exploitation. The results of the 'Gudjonnson' test found her suggestibility level was high, making it likely that if requested to act in a certain way by people who may have power over her, she would acquiesce. However her intellectual disability was not so profound that she would have no understanding of the notion of dishonesty.

The Court of Appeal accepted that people who were suggestible would be within the experience of the jury and they did not require expert evidence to that effect. It was not satisfied that the principles in *Antar* could be extended to cases which do not involve the defence of duress or in circumstances where suggestibility might otherwise be in issue. It held that the question was not how easily she allowed herself to be drawn into the plan to cash the cheques, but what her state of mind at the time was and the expert evidence was not to the effect that she was unable to distinguish between acts deemed socially acceptable and those not so and it was common ground that she would know that dishonesty and fraud would be deemed unacceptable and, in relation to fraud, possibly illegal.

Section 45 of the Modern Slavery Act 2015 provides a defence for trafficked victims who commit certain offences because they are compelled to do so where the compulsion is attributable to slavery or to relevant exploitation and 'a reasonable person in the same situation as the person and having the person's relevant characteristics would do the act'. As the defence is predicated on the reasonable person, thus mirroring the objective test in the law of duress, the defence may replicate its deficiencies. Nevertheless, it may be that 'relevant characteristics' will include the psychiatric condition of the trafficked victim and permit the admission of psychiatric evidence.

In Ireland, the Supreme Court summarised the elements of duress (*The People (DPP) v Gleeson* [2018] IESC 53):

> In essence, duress excuses criminal conduct where unwished for constraint compels an accused of reasonable firmness, of the age, sex and other relevant fixed and permanent characteristics of the accused, into criminal conduct. That coercion, on a reasonable view, should be so serious as to overcome the resistance of the person seeking to assert the defence. Duress is a defence but only provided that person genuinely feels under threat of death or serious physical violence from a threat directed against the accused or the

accused's immediate family or someone close to him or her, or someone for whose safety the accused reasonably considers himself or herself responsible.

Failure to Provide a Specimen of Breath or Blood

In England and Wales, under the Road Traffic Act 1988 (RTA), s 7(6) and *in the Isle of Man* under the Road Traffic Act 1985, s 6(6), it is a defence to have had a reasonable excuse for failure to provide a required specimen of breath or blood. Medical (Marks 1995) and specifically psychiatric evidence (Rix 1996b) may be admitted as to a physical or mental incapacity to provide a specimen. Such evidence is usually needed not just to establish the reasonable excuse, but also to demonstrate the necessary causal link between the incapacity and the failure to provide. Under s 3(a), a requirement for a specimen of blood or urine cannot be made at a police station unless the constable making the requirement has reasonable cause to believe that for medical reasons a specimen of breath cannot be provided or should not be required.

A psychiatrist is likely to be instructed in cases involving failure to provide a specimen of breath when the accused claims that anxiety or a panic attack prevented them activating the breath-testing equipment. This is an easy excuse to make, but a difficult one to prove, and courts take some convincing that it is a reasonable excuse. To be accepted as a reasonable excuse, the courts are unlikely to accept a condition that is not of 'an extreme nature' (Marks 1995).

Post-accident stress, unaccompanied by a mental or physical disability, does not constitute a reasonable excuse (*DPP v Eddowes* [1990] 1 WLUK 591). However, intoxication alone (*Young v DPP* [1992] 3 WLUK 327), intoxication combined with 'a distraught, deeply emotional state' (*DPP v Pearman* [1992] 3 WLUK 308), breathlessness caused by pre-existing depression (*DPP v Crofton* [1994] 2 WLUK 333), being upset, shaken, intoxicated and distressed (*Webb v DPP* [1992] 3 WLUK 75) and the taking of prescribed medication (*Wade v DPP* [1995] 2 WLUK 78) have all been accepted as medical reasons amounting to a reasonable excuse. In *R v Beech* [1991] 7 WLUK 52 and *DPP v Camp* [2017] EWHC 3119, self-induced intoxication was rejected as a reasonable excuse. This may appear inconsistent, but as noted in *Camp*:

> . . . it is important to distinguish between, on the one hand, the concept of 'medical reasons' in section 7(3) and, on the other, the concept of a 'reasonable excuse' in section 7(6). The two concepts are not the same, nor should they be confused. The judgment required of a constable under section 7(3)(a) as to whether there are 'medical reasons' why a specimen of breath cannot be provided, or should not be required, is a different exercise from that involved in a court's exercise of judgment, on the evidence before it, as to whether the reason for the failure to provide a specimen of breath was such as to constitute, in the circumstances, a 'reasonable excuse'.

Cardiovascular or respiratory disease is sometimes also an issue. In such cases, the psychiatrist may report in tandem with a cardiologist or respiratory physician. And bear in mind that panic-like symptoms can occur in various medical conditions, including cardiovascular and respiratory disorders, but also phaeochromocytoma and hyperthyroidism.

A phobia of needles (*Wade*), blood or AIDS (*De Freitas v DPP* [1992] 6 WLUK 311) is capable of being a medical reason for not supplying a specimen of blood. The police officer administering the procedure has the power to form a view on whether a medical issue has been raised at all, but does not have a power to rule upon a medical issue that has been raised and if the medical practitioner who is asked to take the specimen, or whose opinion is considered by the registered healthcare professional (HCP) who is asked to take it, is of the opinion that for medical reasons it cannot or should not be taken, there can be no requirement to provide a specimen. If the police officer fails to apply his mind at all to whether the accused's claim of a phobia of needles raises a medical issue, this amounts to a breach of the statutory procedure (*Wade*). Alternatively, if the police officer decides for himself that what the accused says about a phobia of needles does not amount to a medical reason, the police officer is usurping the function of the doctor or HCP, which is also a statutory breach (*DPP v Wythe* [1995] 7 WLUK 261). If the police officer did not recount the facts of what the accused had said to them about the phobia fully and fairly to the HCP before they took the specimen of blood, the result of the specimen's analysis should be excluded under the PACE, s 78 (*Andrews v DPP* [1991] 5 WLUK 10).

In *Johnson v West Yorkshire Metropolitan Police* [1985] 7 WLUK 360, the court found that a repugnance to the taking of a specimen was capable of being a 'reasonable excuse' for the failure to provide a specimen, but only if it makes the suspect 'not merely unwilling, but unable to comply with the request'. It also ruled that such repugnance had to amount to 'a phobia recognised by medical science'. A phobia so serious that it manifests in symptoms such as light-headedness or fainting may be regarded as more compelling evidence of a 'medical reason' than a less serious one (*Sykes v White* [1982] 6 WLUK 136). The role of the medical expert is to give an opinion as to the 'medical reason'. Whether it amounts to a reasonable excuse is for the court. It is important, however, to consider the test of 'reasonableness': 'In our judgment no excuse can be adjudged a reasonable one unless the person from whom the specimen is required is physically or mentally unable to provide it or the provision of it would entail a substantial risk to his health' (*R v Lennard* [1973] 1 WLR 483). It is reasonable to draw attention to the risks of injury to arteries and veins, even by a doctor experienced in taking blood, and especially if the veins constrict as a result of anxiety or the suspect struggles to resist the needle. However, it is important to consider alternative approaches to obtaining a specimen. In *DPP v Mukandiwa* [2005] EWHC 2977 (Admin), where a district judge had accepted as the basis for reasonable excuse evidence that the accused could go into a potentially dangerous trance state on the sight of blood, the prosecution appeal succeeded because such a state could have been avoided by looking away, as many people do when a specimen of blood is taken.

Investigation includes careful analysis of the accused's medical records. A needle or blood phobia to which there is no reference in the medical records or an anxiety or panic disorder that seems to have occurred for the first time when confronted by a police officer demanding a breath specimen is to be viewed with some suspicion. Medical records may indicate that blood tests have been taken, drugs administered by injection, advice given about overseas travel for which sometimes injections are needed and there may even be a history of intravenous drug misuse. There may be a comment from a doctor to the effect that they would not attempt to take blood again unless absolutely necessary. The medical records may not reveal a history of a panic disorder or some other psychiatric disorder of which panic is a symptom, but the absence of such a documented history can be overcome if there is convincing evidence from the accused and witnesses.

Study police RTA documentation carefully. The police should record what the suspect says when they refuse to provide a specimen. Particularly important is a statement by the suspect that should or might have given the police officer 'reasonable cause to believe' that there is a specimen that cannot or should not be provided for medical reasons (*Davies v DPP* [1989] 6 WLUK 321) because the validity of the apparent medical reason has to be determined by a medical practitioner and the failure of a police officer to call one to investigate the purported difficulty can be fatal to the prosecution case.

There will usually be witness statements from police officers, and perhaps entries in the custody record, referring not only to what the suspect said, but also their demeanour. If a forensic physician has attended, their statement should be studied, along with any original notes.

A careful history should be taken of the condition which it is claimed prevents the accused supplying the specimen and they should be asked to describe exactly what happened when they were asked for the specimen of blood or when they tried to blow into the breath-testing device. Care should be taken to distinguish what the accused spontaneously reports and what symptomatology had to be elicited by specific enquiry. Either as part of a physical examination or mental state examination it is important to look for tattoos.

In Ireland, the Road Traffic Act 2010, s 22 provides that in a prosecution for an offence of refusing or failing to provide specimens of breath or blood, it is a defence to demonstrate that there 'was a special and substantial reason' for the refusal or failure and that, as soon as practicable afterwards, the person complied, or offered, but was not called upon, to comply, with a requirement in relation to the taking of a different specimen, whether of blood or urine. As to the meaning of the cognate provision, in *DPP (Keoghan) v Cagney* [2013] IESC 13, the trial judge had concluded that, as a matter of fact, the accused was (on medical evidence) unable, because of a transient medical condition (respiratory tract infection), to give the required samples of breath. The Supreme Court was satisfied that this constituted a 'special and substantial reason' and continued: 'If a person genuinely cannot provide the relevant samples then it is hard to see how those circumstances could not provide an appropriate basis for compliance with the first leg of the test set out . . . save where the person concerned has contrived to artificially create those circumstances.' It is difficult to contemplate how the defence might be maintained absent expert evidence. It is, ultimately, a question of fact for the trial judge to determine. An accused who satisfies the court that they have a special and substantial reason for failure or refusal to provide a breath sample is entitled to an acquittal where there is no warning that a failure to offer a blood or urine sample will preclude the defence of 'special and substantial reason'. The absence of warning does not, however, entitle an accused to an acquittal unless they have first satisfied the court of the existence of the 'special and substantial reason' for the failure or refusal.

Sentencing Issues

The Courts' Requirements

For England and Wales, *Good Practice Guidance* sets out the courts' requirements of psychiatrists preparing reports for sentencing purposes.

The guidance specifies a preference for report length: two to four pages for a 'summary report' and up to eight pages for a 'full report'. Only a brief summary is needed of the accused's personal background and of the psychiatrist's understanding of the event or events giving rise to the offence. Information is needed concerning relevant psychiatric history, relevant family history and current mental condition, including a mental state examination. 'Too much information' is identified as a common problem because '[g]iven the time constraints and focused nature of the sentencing context, only information relevant to the decisions at hand can be of practical value to the court'. The court does not generally need an extended history and collation of previous medical records in the report should be avoided. However, especially in more serious cases, such as where an indeterminate sentence is passed, a restriction order imposed or a hospital limitation direction made, a very detailed report can provide an essential baseline for those considering eventual release on licence or discharge from hospital many years later.

Box 7.26 Issues to Be Addressed in a Report for Sentencing

Diagnosis

- Presence or absence of mental disorder as defined in law

Mental state at material time

- Whether any mental disorder affected the behaviour giving rise to the offence

Treatment considerations

- Consent
- What treatment will involve
- What the components of treatment are
- Length of treatment
- Whether treatment should be under any particular order
- Availability of treatment/arrangements made
    - In-patient or out-patient/where the treatment will take place
    - Availability of bed
    - Under whose care will the person be
- Whether treatment will make a difference and, if so, how much
    - Distinguishing treatment which contains risk, prevents deterioration and reduces risk
- In the case of inpatient treatment, the likely circumstances of discharge

Prognosis considerations

- Effect of a custodial sentence on the disorder
- Effect of a custodial sentence on any possible treatment for the disorder
- Risk assessment
    - The kind(s) of violence the person is capable of perpetrating
    - The likely level of physical or psychological harm
    - The situation(s) in which the person is most likely to be violent
    - The likely victim(s) of that violence (e.g. self, public, known individuals, children, staff and fellow prisoners/patients)
    - The warning signs that the person may be at risk of being violent
    - The management strategies that need to be put into place to manage the risk of violence in the short term

- o The least restrictive environment in which the person's violence can easily be managed
- o Protective factors
- o Dynamic factors capable of change
- o The psychological, psychiatric or social treatments that may be given to help decrease the person's risk of violence in the long-term
- o Risk of reconviction

Risk assessment based on *Mental Health (Care and Treatment) (Scotland) Act 2003, Code of Practice*, Vol. 3: *Compulsory Powers in Relation to Mentally Disordered Offenders* (Scottish Executive 2005), ch. 5, para. 71.

The guidance continues: 'The court sentences; a psychiatrist can provide advice.' Such advice assists the sentencer to take into account treatment needs and balance the needs of the accused with the management of risk to the public.

Box 7.26 suggests a framework for the Opinion section.

There are various relevant statutory provisions, applicable guidelines and case law. *In England and Wales*, they include sentencing guidelines which must be applied under the CJA 2009, s 125, but they do not restrict the court when dealing with a mentally disordered offender in the manner it considers most appropriate in the circumstances. *In Scotland*, judges have a wide discretion when sentencing. The Criminal Justice and Licensing (Scotland) Act 2010 established the Scottish Sentencing Council and one guideline, *Principles and purposes of sentencing*, has been approved as of March 2019. *R v Rahman* [2013] EWCA Crim 887 illustrates how important it is not to be too speculative when giving an opinion on the effect of a custodial sentence on the defendant's mental disorder which was in this case an adjustment disorder.

Hospital Treatment Order Considerations

R v Vowles [2015] EWCA Crim 45 sets out that, even when there is medical evidence supporting a hospital order (MHA 2003, s 37), the court must not feel circumscribed by that evidence. In deciding between a hospital order with restrictions (ss 37/41), a hospital and limitation direction (s 45A) or a prison sentence, account should be taken of:

- the extent to which the offending is attributable to the mental disorder;
- the extent to which punishment is required;
- the extent to which treatment for the mental disorder is needed; and
- protection of the public, which includes consideration of the process of, and regime after, release.

Consideration also needs to be given to the *Vowles* criteria for a hospital order with restrictions in a case where an alternative is a life sentence:

- the mental disorder is treatable;
- once treated there is no evidence he would be in any way dangerous; and
- the offending is entirely due to that mental disorder.

However, the last criterion may be difficult to satisfy as, except perhaps in the case of automatism, it may not be possible to say that an offence is *entirely* due to a mental disorder.

As well as the psychiatric evidence, the court has to examine broader issues, including the culpability attributable to the mental disorder. However, culpability is a legal rather than a medical concept and an ultimate issue for the court; experts should not comment on it explicitly (Hallett 2020). Psychiatric training and experience do not provide a basis for a psychiatrist to opine as to whether a person deserves punishment. Nevertheless, psychiatric evidence may have a bearing on it. *R v Edwards* [2018] EWCA Crim 595 established that failure to take medication may not increase culpability if it is part of the disorder, but in other instances it could increase culpability. Psychiatrists might reasonably give an opinion on whether failure to take prescribed medication is part of the mental disorder itself. *Edwards* also clarifies that, although consideration of a s 45A order must come before making a hospital order (because the court must have 'sound reasons' for deviating from the usual approach of imposing a penal sentence and s 45A includes a penal element), imprisonment is not the default. In a case of psychopathic disorder (*R v Kitchener* [2017] EWCA Crim 937), a hospital order was substituted for a life sentence on the basis that the First-tier Tribunal was better placed to assess risk than the Parole Board. In *R v Ahmed* [2016] EWCA Crim 670, the Court of Appeal said that those responsible for monitoring a patient in the community following discharge from a hospital order had a higher level of expertise and resources than the probation service and would therefore provide better public protection. The court held in *Edwards* that this comment was not of general application, but the expert psychiatric witness should be in a position to assist the court in comparing the release regimes under ss 37/41 and s 45A.

With regard to hospital orders *in England and Wales*, there does not have to be a link between the mental disorder and the offence and a hospital order can be made even though the mental disorder has developed subsequent to the offence (*R v McBride* [1972] 1 WLUK 389; *R v Birch* [1989] 5 WLUK 26). With regard to restriction orders, which can only be attached in England and Wales to a hospital order and in Scotland to a compulsion order, the critical point is the risk of serious harm to the public in the event of a further offence being committed. It is not a serious risk of harm: 'serious' qualifies 'harm' and not 'risk' (Rix and Agarwal 1999). *In England and Wales*, the court has to have regard to: (1) the nature of the offence; (2) the antecedents of the offender; and (3) the risk of his committing further offences if set at large. 'Antecedents' is not limited to 'previous convictions'; it is appropriate to draw attention to such matters as violence in institutional settings that has not resulted in criminal convictions. Although the court will consider the psychiatrist's risk assessment, the court makes the ultimate assessment of the risk of serious harm. It can make a restriction order where the medical recommendations have been for no restriction order and vice versa. A restriction order can be made where there is no previous history of violence. In *R v Golding* [2006] EWCA Crim 1965, where the appellant had been repeatedly convicted of burglary, he was considered to be at risk of causing serious harm because his psychosis was uncontrolled and he had a predilection for drugs that could lead him to react violently to confrontation by a householder. 'Serious harm' has not been defined, but in *MJJAB(AP) v The Scottish Ministers* [2010] ScotCS CSIH 31, a case relating to a restriction order, the court endorsed the approach of the sheriff at the court of first instance and held that the test 'might be made good by commission of a very serious crime falling short of homicide, which, when considered with the mental disorder in question, gave rise to a significant risk of future commission of a very serious crime'. The court further held that 'satisfaction of the serious harm test cannot be divorced from the protective measure under consideration'; the test must require 'significantly serious harm and a serious risk of future commission of a crime of that nature'.

Even if you have not specifically been asked for an opinion on a restriction order, it is helpful if you indicate whether the court should consider one. No judge will object to an opinion being offered on this point and, where there is a requirement for the judge to hear oral evidence, it will assist to have advance notice.

In Scotland, a report in such a case should address the role of special restrictions in facilitating future management and this is a point of general application.

Sentencing in Cases of Manslaughter by Diminished Responsibility

In England and Wales, when sentencing offenders convicted of manslaughter by reason of diminished responsibility, there are now sentencing guidelines which require the sentencing judge first to determine whether the level of retained responsibility was 'high', 'medium' or 'lower' in order to identify the starting point for the length of the custodial sentence.

This means taking into account 'the extent to which the offender's responsibility was diminished by the mental disorder at the time of the offence with reference to the medical evidence and all the relevant information available to the court'. Other relevant considerations include the degree to which the offender's acts or omissions contributed to the seriousness of the mental disorder at the time of the offence. Voluntary misuse of alcohol or drugs may have exacerbated the mental disorder. Voluntary failure to follow medical advice may increase responsibility. A mental disorder that reduces the offender's ability to exercise self-control or to engage with medical services may reduce responsibility. Responsibility may be reduced where the mental disorder was undiagnosed or untreated or where the offender had sought but not received appropriate treatment.

From this starting point, the judge then adjusts the term upwards or downwards having regard to factors increasing seriousness and reducing seriousness or reflecting personal mitigation. The former include commission of the offence whilst under the influence of alcohol or drugs, but taking into account the extent to which a mental disorder has an effect on the offender's ability to make informed judgements or exercise self-control in deciding how much weight to attach to this factor. The latter factors include remorse, whether the offender made genuine and sustained efforts to seek treatment for the mental disorder, age and lack of maturity.

The court is also required to have regard to the regime on release. This is relevant in choosing between a hospital and limitation direction under s 45A and a hospital order with restrictions under the MHA 1983, ss 37/41.

In Ireland, in *The People (DPP) v Mahon* [2019] IESC 24, the Supreme Court, observing that manslaughter covers a broad band of conduct, gave the most recent guidance on sentencing for manslaughter in four bands: the worst cases, high culpability, medium culpability and lower culpability cases. Diminished responsibility or extreme provocation cases, the court considered, may fall into this lowest category.

Criminal Justice Act 2003 Provisions for England and Wales

In any case where the defendant is or appears to be mentally disordered, the CJA 2003, s 157 requires that a medical report, prepared by a person approved as having special experience in the diagnosis or treatment of mental disorder, must be obtained before passing a custodial sentence other than one that is fixed by law (i.e. for murder). Then, paradoxically, it allows the court to dispense with such a report if it is not necessary. This seems somewhat confusing, but at least it means that probably the sentencer has to make a conscious decision to dispense with the medical report and perhaps also give reasons. There is also a requirement to consider any other information on the accused's mental condition, the likely effect of a custodial sentence on it and on any possible treatment for it. It is recognised that 'custody can exacerbate mental ill health, heighten vulnerability and increase the risk of self-harm and suicide' (Bradley 2009).

Mitigation

In England and Wales, the CJA 2003, s 166(1) and (5) provides 'savings for powers to mitigate sentences and deal appropriately with mentally disordered offenders', allowing the court, where appropriate, flexibility in their sentencing. Furthermore, the Sentencing Guidelines Council (SGC) recognises 'mental illness or disability' as a mitigating factor (i.e. one indicating lower culpability), and refers specifically to mental disorder being a mitigating factor in certain types of case. In the case of assaults on children and cruelty to a child, mental illness, specifically depression, is identified as a relevant area of personal mitigation; so are 'indifference or apathy resulting from low intelligence . . . immaturity or social deprivation resulting in an inability to cope with the pressures of caring for children [and] psychiatric illness'. Mental disorder or mental disability is a specific mitigating factor for attempted murder. A 'lower level of understanding due to mental health issues or learning difficulties' can mitigate breach of an antisocial behaviour disorder. In the sentencing of children and young people, where the court is required under the Children and Young Persons Act 1933, s 44 to consider their welfare, the courts are alerted to the high rate of mental health problems and learning disabilities in young people in the criminal justice system, the impact of any speech or language difficulties on communication and their vulnerability to self-harm, especially in custody. The SGC also suggests that a psychiatric report may be appropriate when sentencing for a sexual offence, but in such cases the mental disorder may constitute an aggravating factor. This does not apply just to sexual offences. In *R v Johnson* [2007] 1 WLR 585, the inadequacy, suggestibility or vulnerability of the defendants were characteristics capable of leading to, or reinforcing, the conclusion that they were dangerous.

R v McFly [2013] EWCA Crim 729 illustrates the double-edged effect of including personality disorder in a plea of mitigation. McFly was convicted of murder after unsuccessfully pleading diminished responsibility on the basis of antisocial personality disorder that had manifested in impulsivity and aggression. His very troubled childhood was put to the judge and acknowledged as mitigating. However, when he imposed life imprisonment with a minimum term of twenty-four years, he left out the personality disorder. On appeal, the court substituted a minimum term of twenty-one years, having regard to the personality disorder attributable to his appalling childhood, but added that 'the fact the personality disorder was of relevance to what happened, and has been described as untreatable, can only increase the concern as to when if ever the appellant may be safely released'.

Two cases illustrate the relevance of expert neuropsychiatric evidence for mitigation. In *R v Hayes* [2013] EWCA Crim 897, an indeterminate sentence of imprisonment for public protection was imposed for offences of violence. It was subsequently found that the appellant had a meningioma extending from the middle of the frontal lobe into the parietal lobe. A neuropsychiatrist opined that the appellant was 'suffering from a mental abnormality arising from the tumour which did substantially impair his ability to form a rational judgment and to exercise self-control'. As this indicated a reduction in culpability, but there still being some remaining culpability, a determinate sentence of eleven years was substituted. *R v Bourne* [1994] 6 WLUK 324 is a diminished responsibility case where evidence of brain damage was used to argue successfully for a reduction in the custodial sentence.

Expert psychiatric evidence by child or adolescent psychiatrists can assist the court where not just the youth but the immaturity of the offender requires consideration. *R v N* [2010] EWCA Crim 941 illustrates how the offender's maturity will be at least as important as their chronological age. In *R v W* [2009] EWCA Crim 153, where the appellant, albeit a 20-year-old adult, had been convicted of three counts of the rape of a child under 13, and abuse of trust had been taken into account as an aggravating feature, the Court of Appeal held that this was inappropriate having regard to their learning difficulties and serious immaturity.

In Ireland, the Court of Criminal Appeal has accepted that if it is shown that the accused's offending behaviour has been significantly caused or affected by his psychiatric condition, that is, depending on all the circumstances, capable of mitigating:

> Where the act has been significantly the result of a psychiatric condition, the moral guilt of the accused may be less, depending on the circumstances. That qualification is important. The sentencing court will have to take account of all the circumstances, which will include the extent to which the accused is aware of or responsible for his condition or careless in regard to its treatment. (*The People (DPP) v C* [2013] IECCA 91)

Arson Cases

In cases of arson, the courts usually follow the advice in *R v Calladine* [1975] 1 WLUK 411, that it would be unwise to sentence without a psychiatric report.

Community Orders with Specified Requirements

In England and Wales, the CJA 2003, s 177 makes provision for a mental health treatment requirement (s 207), a drug rehabilitation requirement (s 209) or an alcohol treatment requirement (s 212) to be added to a community order. Such an order should be considered for a defendant who does not, or does not any longer, need treatment as an in-patient, although it can include provision for in-patient treatment other than in a high security hospital. Taylor and Krish (2010) set out the further circumstances in which such an order may be made:

> Such a disposal may be appropriate in a case where the custody threshold has been passed (as well as those cases in which it has not, but where the accused's culpability is substantially mitigated by his mental state at the time of the commission of the offence, and where the public interest is served by ensuring he continues to receive treatment for his mental disorder). It is usually not suitable for an accused who is unlikely to comply with treatment or who has a very chaotic lifestyle.

To make such an order with a mental health treatment requirement, the court must be satisfied that the accused's condition is such as requires and may be susceptible to treatment, but not such as to merit a hospital or guardianship order. The report should indicate where it is proposed that the accused should be admitted or where they will attend as a non-resident patient or the RMP or chartered psychologist by or under whose direction treatment will be provided. This may mean getting the express agreement of another doctor or psychologist to provide the treatment.

In Scotland, the CP(S)A 1995, s 227A provides for a similar community payback order with a mental health treatment requirement and there is a provision for in-patient treatment. *In Ireland*, under the Probation of Offenders Act 1907, a probation order can be made with a requirement of compliance with certain conditions, potentially including medical treatment or treatment for an alcohol addiction.

In order to make an order with a drug rehabilitation requirement, which includes drug treatment and testing in England and Wales, or a drug treatment and testing order in Scotland (CP(S)A, ss 234B–234K), various criteria have to be met. The offender has to be dependent on, or have a propensity to misuse, a controlled drug. The propensity has to be such as requires and may be susceptible to treatment. Specifically, there has to be a realistic prospect of reducing the drug dependence (*Attorney-General's Reference (No. 64 of 2003)* [2004] 2 Cr App R (S) 38 (106)). The court has to be satisfied that arrangements have been made or can be made for the proposed treatment. *In England and Wales*, a probation officer needs to have recommended the requirement and *in Scotland* there has to be a report from an officer of the local authority about the offender and his circumstances and as to the criteria being satisfied. *In England and Wales*, the offender must express a willingness to comply; indeed, there has to be clear evidence of the offender having a determination to free himself from drugs (*Attorney-General's Reference (No. 64 of 2003)*). The treatment can be as a resident in a specified institution or at a place of treatment as a non-resident. The treatment has to be by or under the direction of a specified person having the necessary qualifications or experience. *Attorney-General's Reference (No. 64 of 2003)* indicates that such an order would generally be appropriate for an acquisitive offence committed to obtain money for drugs, but rarely for an offence involving serious violence or threat of violence with a lethal weapon.

An alcohol treatment requirement requires the offender's submission to treatment, for a specified period, by, or under the direction of, a specified person having the necessary qualifications or experience, with a view to the reduction or elimination of the offender's alcohol dependence. The court has to be satisfied that the offender is dependent on alcohol and that his dependency is such as requires and may be susceptible to treatment. The court has to be satisfied that arrangements have been, or can be, made for the proposed treatment. The offender must express a willingness to comply. The treatment can be as a resident or as a non-resident by or under the direction of such person having the necessary qualification or experience. Such requirements can be for up to the three years' maximum length of a community order. Under the CJA 2003, s 212A, there is also provision for an alcohol abstinence and monitoring requirement (subject to a pilot scheme operating until April 2019). Such an order can be made where the consumption of alcohol is an element of the offence, the offender is *not* dependent on alcohol and an alcohol treatment requirement is not also imposed. Involvement with drug and alcohol services in England and Wales could also be part of a probation-led rehabilitation activity requirement under the CJA 2003, s 200A, which gives probation more flexibility.

There are similar provisions for defendants aged under 18 years under the Criminal Justice and Immigration Act 2008, s 1(1)(k) and Sch 1. However, instead of an alcohol treatment requirement, there is provision for an intoxicating substance treatment requirement which includes alcohol as well as any other substance or product (but not a controlled drug) capable of being inhaled or otherwise used for the purpose of causing intoxication. It is similar in other respects to the alcohol treatment requirement for adults.

In Northern Ireland, the MCA(NI), Sch 7 provides for a supervision and assessment order. It can include a residence element, but this will not enforce residence as a hospital in-patient or in a care home. To make such an order, four conditions have to be met: (1) the presence or reasonable suspicion that the person has a disorder; (2) medical evidence to the effect that examination of the person is necessary or desirable to assess (a) whether the disorder requires treatment and/or (b) whether consent will be given or such treatment can be given under Part 2 of the Act ('Lack of capacity: protection from liability, safeguards'); (3) supervision is desirable in the interests of securing the rehabilitation of the person or protecting the public from harm by them or preventing the commission of offences; and (4) this is the most suitable way of dealing with the person. If it is a mental disorder, there has to be medical evidence from two RMPs, including oral evidence from an AMP. For the supervision element, there has to be supervision by a social worker or probation officer for between six months and three years. For the assessment element, the person has to submit to assessment by an RMP as to their condition and either the need for treatment or their capacity to consent to treatment. However, there is no obligation that the supervised person accepts treatment. This requires either consent or an authorisation under Part 2. It will be possible for the assessment period to be the whole or any part of the supervision period. Where the supervised person breaches the conditions of the supervision and assessment order, the court will be able to revoke the order and revisit alternative disposal options, such as a PPO with or without restrictions or an absolute discharge (Sch 7, para. 13).

In Ireland, there is no provision for the making of community orders, other than community service orders and the imposition of conditions with regard to, *inter alia*, abstinence from intoxicating liquor 'and any other matters, as the court may, having regard to the particular circumstances of the case, consider necessary for preventing a repetition of the same offence or the commission of other offences' (Probation of Offenders Act 1907, s 2(2) as substituted by the Criminal Justice Administration Act 1914, s 8).

Suspended Sentences with Specific Requirements

In England and Wales, under the CJA 2003, s 189, when passing a suspended sentence, the court can make it a requirement to comply with a mental health treatment, alcohol treatment or drug rehabilitation order in terms identical to those applicable to a community order. However, the requirement cannot be for longer than two years and it cannot be longer than the period of time for which the sentence is suspended. *In Ireland*, conditions may also be imposed as part of suspending a sentence.

Assessment of Dangerousness

In England and Wales, the CJA 2003 provides for the imposition of discretionary life sentences (ss 225(1), 226(1)) and extended sentences (ss 226A, 226B) when the accused is convicted of one of a number of specified violent or sexual offences and, in the opinion of the court, there is a 'significant risk to members of the public of serious harm occasioned by the commission by him of further specified offences'. Harm is defined as 'death or personal injury whether physical or psychological' (CJA 2003, s 224(3)). 'Significant' means more than a possibility – it must be 'noteworthy, of considerable amount or importance' (*R v Lang* [2006] 1 WLR 2509). 'Members of the public' is a general term and should not be construed so as to exclude any particular group such as prison officers or mental hospital staff (*Lang*). It can apply to a small group of individuals and to just one potential victim (*R v Laverick* [2015] EWCA Crim 1059). In the case of young offenders, the courts are advised to take into account the possibility of change and development in a shorter time than in an adult and to consider level of maturity when assessing future conduct and whether this may give rise to a significant risk of harm (*Lang*).

It is still the expectation that in most of these cases the courts will rely on the pre-sentence report, but *Lang* established that in a small number of cases where 'the circumstances of the current offence or the history of the offender suggests mental abnormality', a medical report should usually be obtained. *Good Practice Guidance* recognises that: 'Expert psychiatric evidence has an important role in supporting or challenging a presumption of dangerousness', so a report in such a case should be clearly directed to the issue of dangerousness. Psychiatric assessment and consideration of psychiatric and other records may reveal information concerning aggressive or violent behaviour that has not been subjected to adversarial judicial proceedings and 'information' in the CJA 2003, s 229 is not restricted to 'evidence'; it can include relevant information having a bearing on the offender's dangerousness which has not been proved by criminal conviction (*R v Considine* [2007] EWCA Crim. 1166).

The accused needs to know that their assessment may lead to a longer than normal sentence. 'Characteristics such as inadequacy, suggestibility or vulnerability of the offender might serve to mitigate the offender's culpability but they might also serve to produce or reinforce the conclusion that the offender was dangerous' (*Attorney General's Reference (No. 64 of 2006)*, Times, 2 November 2006). Doing no harm may clash with justice. College guidelines may assist (Royal College of Psychiatrists 2004). As the court is required to 'have in mind all the alternative and cumulative methods of providing the necessary public protection against the risk posed by the individual offender' (*Attorney General's Reference (No. 55 of 2008)* [2009] 2 Cr App R (S) 142), address what treatment, if any, may be available in the community as part of what is termed 'the overall sentencing package'. *Attorney General's Reference (No. 91 of 2014) (Williams)* [2014] EWCA Crim 2891 illustrates how an extended sentence was imposed as a result of dangerousness that took into account personality traits in addition to already diagnosed depression and schizophrenia.

In Scotland, upon conviction for similarly serious offences, the CP(S)A 1995, ss 210B–210E provide for the making of a risk assessment order and the preparation of a risk assessment report by a person accredited by the Risk Management Authority dealing with risk to the safety of the public at large. The assessor has to indicate whether the risk is high, medium or low. Section 210E sets out the risk criteria:

> . . . the nature of, or the circumstances of the commission of, the offence of which the convicted person has been found guilty either in themselves or as part of a pattern of behaviour are such as to demonstrate that there is a likelihood that he, if at liberty, will seriously endanger the lives, or physical or psychological well-being, of members of the public at large.

The offender can also commission a report. Having regard to the results of the assessment, the court can impose a lifelong restriction order (s 210F) which results in indeterminate imprisonment or detention, or, if mental disorder is diagnosed, a compulsion order (s 57A). The decision whether the risk criteria, made on the balance of probabilities, are met, is for the judge, although the views of the expert risk assessor must be given particular attention.

In Ireland, a court does not have power to impose an open-ended detention on the grounds of anticipated future risk of harm.

In the Isle of Man, there is a power to impose an extended sentence to prevent the commission of further offences and secure the offender's rehabilitation when it is proposed to impose a custodial sentence for a sexual or violent offence (Criminal Justice Act 2001, s 38).

Structured clinical or professional judgement is preferable to actuarial approaches in risk assessment, not least because actuarial risk assessments inform only as to the population to which the individual belongs and not to the individual, but either way be prepared to explain and defend your approach. There is an expectation that instruments will 'have proven validity for the category of people that the assessed person falls into (e.g. mentally disordered offenders, prisoners, sex offenders)' (*Mental Health (Care and Treatment) (Scotland) Act 2003, Code of Practice*, Vol. 3: *Compulsory Powers in Relation to Mentally Disordered Offenders* (Scottish Executive 2005), ch. 5, para. 68). Also, in Scotland, it is recommended best practice, and we suggest of general application, that the assessment should attempt to place the risk the person presents in the context of their past history and current offending.

If the accused is not suffering from any mental disorder, it is arguable that you should offer no opinion as to risk. It is also arguable that a formal training in risk assessment may qualify you to do so, but, if so, it must be clear that this is the basis of the opinion.

It is not enough to categorise risk as, for example, 'high'. Set out the relevant information in a risk formulation so as to identify the most likely risk scenario (the kind of violence, the severity of the harm, the situation in which the violence is most likely to occur, the likely victims and the warning signs), to permit recognition of the imminence of violence by warning signs, to manage the risk in the short term, including an appropriate environment, and to provide treatments aimed at reducing the risk of violence in the long term.

Treatment Recommended

The section on treatment has to be crystal clear with unambiguous and clearly justified recommendations. It has to be an actionable opinion. If you are not going to be responsible for the treatment, you must liaise closely with the person who is going to provide the treatment and ensure that you properly represent what they have to offer. This is vital. Your report will otherwise be of limited practical value. If you are recommending a community order, you must liaise with the probation officer and preferably before finalising your report.

Witness Issues

Vulnerable Witnesses

In England and Wales, the YJCEA, ss 23–30 and in accordance with CrPR Part 18, special measures can be made available to provide effective support and assistance to vulnerable witnesses (Cooper and Grace 2016) (Box 7.27). Box 7.28 sets out the issues to be addressed in reports on such witnesses.

As in the case of vulnerable defendants (see above, 'The Vulnerable Defendant'), decisions about special measures, along with additional measures and other reasonable adjustments, are made at a GRH. This is expected 'in every case involving a vulnerable witness, save in very exceptional circumstances. If there are any doubts on how to proceed,

Box 7.27 Special Measures for Witnesses

- Preventing a witness from seeing the accused
- Allowing a witness to give evidence by live link
- Having a supporter to provide emotional support, help reduce their anxiety and stress and contribute to their ability to give best evidence
- Hearing a witness's evidence in private
- Dispensing with wigs and gowns
- Admitting video-recorded evidence
- Questioning a witness through an intermediary
- Using a device to help a witness communicate

CrPR Pt 18

Box 7.28 Issues to Be Addressed in a Report on a Potentially Vulnerable Witness

- competence to give evidence;
- the eligibility criteria which are whether or not they have:
  - mental disorder (as defined in the MHA 1983 or equivalent); or
  - 'significant impairment of intelligence and social functioning';
- the risk of emotional or psychological harm resulting from the trial process;
- how the nature or extent of the witness's condition might affect their ability to give evidence, particularly with reference to their:
  - response to questioning;
  - concentration and attention;
  - ability to communicate; and
  - interaction with other people.
- any relevant effects of prescribed psychotropic or other medication;
- any measures which can be taken to support the witness, maximise so far as practicable the quality of the evidence and ensure questioning does not cause further distress and/or exacerbate their condition;
- explain why special or additional measures would be likely to improve the quality of the witness's evidence.

guidance should be sought from those who have the responsibility for looking after the witness and or an expert' (*R v Lubemba; R v JP* [2014] EWCA Crim 2064).

The GRH 'should cover ... the general care of the witness, if, when and where the witness is to be shown their video interview, when, where and how the parties (and the judge if identified) intend to introduce themselves to the witness, the length of questioning and frequency of breaks and the nature of the questions to be asked' (*Lubemba*). In addition, ground rules may include directions about the manner of questioning, including how questions should be put to help the witness understand them, the need to restrict cross-examination to short, simple questions which put the essential elements of the

Box 7.29 Additional Adjustments that May Assist Mentally Disordered Witnesses

- Interviews and hearings taking place in rooms with natural light;
- Shorter sittings and/or the opportunity to take regular comfort breaks;
- Staying seated while giving evidence and during cross-examination;
- Permission to get up and walk around if this reduces discomfort, as some medication can cause restlessness;
- Allowing a supporter or carer to accompany the person at all times – including to stand alongside the witness box, where possible;
- Ensuring witnesses are comfortable with court procedures and environment, such as explaining why there are closed circuit television cameras present or switching them off;
- Asking police officers to remove hats and helmets to reduce distress caused by unfamiliarity or authority figures (as with wigs and gowns);
- Requesting the judiciary, clerks and defence to address the witness directly and display patience and sensitivity when explanation is necessary or distress becomes acute;
- Requests to clear the courtroom where sensitive medical information is raised for the first time and relevance needs to be determined. Mind

(Advocate's Gateway 2014)

accused's case to the witness, the duration of questioning, the number, frequency and nature of breaks (e.g. time to take medication), the topics that may or may not be covered, the use of communications aids, the use of screens and the use of live link (see also CrPR 3.9(7)). The court can dispense with the normal practice of, and impose restrictions on, the advocate regarding 'putting the case' where there is a risk of a vulnerable witness failing to understand, becoming distressed or acquiescing to leading questions. The decision may be taken that a witness's evidence should, for example, be given in the afternoon when the medication being taken for their mental disorder has had a chance to work and their mental state is at its most stable. The GRH may consider how the court will be enabled to access the person's non-verbal communication, for example, indicating, pointing, drawing, writing. The court can take into account the likely length of the witness's concentration span, which may be shorter than in an assessment situation because of the high-pressure environment of the court. The court can order examination of the witness through an intermediary.

Box 7.29 sets out reasonable adjustments identified by Mind (The Advocate's Gateway 2014) as of potential assistance in the case of witnesses with mental disorder.

The GRH itself can be held in the absence of the public and the expert should be in a position to advise this in an appropriate case.

A specific issue that may need to be addressed is whether a witness is competent to give evidence. They are said to be competent if they have the capacity to offer admissible evidence pertaining to an issue in the trial, but the threshold is low – an ability to understand questions and give intelligible answers on matters relevant to the trial issues. The test is generally satisfied if the witness is capable of understanding the oath and can convey their evidence in a manner which enables the jury and all concerned to follow it (*The People (DPP) v Campion* [2018] IESC 35).

Competence is defined in the YJCEA, s 53(3): A person is not competent to give evidence in criminal proceedings if it appears to the court that he is not a person who is able to –
(a) understand questions put to him as a witness, and

(b) give answers to them which can be understood.

In *R v Barker* [2010] EWCA Crim 4, the court held that: '[T]he witness need not understand every single question or give a readily understood answer to every question. Many competent adult witnesses would fail such a competency test.' There is provision in s 54 for the issue to be determined at a competency hearing at which expert evidence is admissible on the issue of competence as a witness. It is decided on the balance of probabilities.

As held in *Barker*:

> The statutory provisions ... apply to individuals of unsound mind. They apply to the infirm. The question in each case is whether the individual witness ... is competent to give evidence in the particular trial. The question is entirely witness ... specific. There are no presumptions or preconceptions. The witness need not understand the special importance that the truth should be told in court, and the witness need not understand every single question or give a readily understood answer to every question.

Another specific issue is whether, as a result of any aspect of the trial process, there is a risk of a vulnerable complainant suffering emotional or psychological harm. This is because the *EU Council Directive establishing minimum standards on the rights, support and protection of victims of crime* (2012), arts 3(2) and 18 require measures to be taken (without prejudice to the rights of the defence) to protect victims against the risk of emotional and psychological harm.

Further useful information is to be found on the Advocate's Gateway (www.theadvocatesgateway.org/), which 'provides free access to practical, evidence-based guidance on vulnerable witnesses and defendants'.

In Scotland, the CP(S)A, s 271 (as amended by the Victims and Witnesses (Scotland) Act 2014) defines a vulnerable witness as:

- a person under 18 on the date of the commencement of the proceedings in which the hearing is being or is to be held;
- any person if there is a significant risk that the quality of the evidence to be given by the person will be diminished by reason of (1) mental disorder within the meaning of the Mental Health (Care and Treatment) (Scotland) Act 2003, or (2) fear or distress in connection with giving evidence at the trial;
- a person deemed to be a vulnerable witness because of the nature of the complaint made by them – this involves allegations of sexual offences, people trafficking, domestic abuse and stalking;
- where there is considered to be a significant risk of harm to the person by reason only of the fact that the person is giving or is to give evidence in the proceedings.

The quality of the evidence means its completeness, coherence and accuracy (s 271(4)). Section 271A provides that child and deemed vulnerable witnesses are entitled to the benefit of one or more of the standard special measures (see below). Section 271B provides for special provisions for children under 12. Section 271C sets out the practicalities of making a vulnerable witness application. Section 271F provides for measures to be applied to an accused. The full range of special measures are the taking of evidence by a commissioner appointed by the court, a live television link, a screen, a supporter, giving evidence in chief in the form of a prior statement and excluding the public during the taking of evidence (s 271H).

In Northern Ireland, the Criminal Evidence (Northern Ireland) Order 1999, art 4 makes similar provisions for special measures in the case of witnesses whose 'quality of evidence ...

is likely to be diminished' as a result of mental disorder or a significant impairment of intelligence and social functioning. Here, the quality of a witness's evidence means its 'completeness, coherence and accuracy; and for this purpose "coherence" refers to a witness's ability in giving evidence to give answers which address the questions put to the witness and can be understood both individually and collectively'.

In Ireland, in cases of certain sexual and violent offences, there are special provisions under the Criminal Evidence Act 1992 relating to persons with a 'mental disorder' (defined as including 'mental illness, mental disability, dementia or any disease of the mind' under the Criminal Justice Act 1993, s 5) (previously a 'mental handicap'). A person with mental disorder, other than the accused, may be permitted to give evidence by a live television link (s 13(1)(a)). Where evidence is so given, the court can require questions to be put to the witness through an intermediary (s 14(1)(b)) appointed by the court and judged to be competent to act as such. There are also provisions for the use of screens and dispensing with wigs and gowns.

In deciding whether to permit a victim to give evidence through a live television link, the putting of questions to the victim through an intermediary or the screening of the accused from the victim, the court is required to have regard to the need to protect the victim from secondary and repeat victimisation, intimidation or retaliation, taking into account the nature and circumstances of the case and the personal characteristics of the victim (Criminal Evidence Act 1992, s 14AA).

Persons with 'mental handicap' [sic] may also give evidence other than on oath or affirmation if the court is satisfied that they can give an intelligible account of events that is relevant to the proceedings (s 27(3)). This applies in all criminal proceedings. However, there has to be an enquiry (*O'Sullivan v Hamill* [1999] 3 IR 9) and this may require medical evidence. It might be noted that, unlike in other updated provisions of this act, 'mental handicap' has not otherwise been defined.

The Absent Witness

The CJA 2003, s 116(1) provides that if witnesses are unable to give evidence, their statement may be read to the court if they are 'unfit to be a witness' by reason of a 'bodily or mental condition'. A report in such a case should not only identify the witness's mental condition, but also explain clearly how it makes the person unfit to give oral evidence.

Credibility

It is not for the expert to tell the court whether a witness (or indeed an accused) is credible or honest. This is for the court to decide. However, a psychiatrist may be asked to give an opinion as to whether a witness 'is or was suffering from some recognised mental illness, disability or abnormality . . . that undermines his credibility' and it 'must be allowable to call medical evidence of mental illness which makes a witness incapable of giving reliable evidence, whether through the existence of delusions or otherwise' (*Toohey v Metropolitan Police Commissioner* [1965] AC 595) or about a mental or physical condition which would 'substantially affect the witness's capacity to give reliable evidence' (*R v MacKenney* (1983) 76 Cr App R 271).

In Scotland, the CP(S)A, s 275C permits the admission of expert psychological or psychiatric evidence to explain the behaviour of the complainer or to rebut any inference that might be adverse to the credibility or reliability of the complainer which might otherwise be drawn from that behaviour.

In *R v S* [2006] EWCA Crim 2389, it was held that the court properly admitted the evidence of an expert witness that a complainant with autism would not have been capable of inventing the evidence that she had given. In *R v H* [2005] EWCA Crim 1828, expert evidence was admitted as to the potential unreliability of a childhood memory described in unrealistic detail and the conviction was quashed on appeal. However, normally a witness's memory would be within the knowledge of a jury. Nevertheless, in *The People (DPP) v Kavanagh* [2008] IECCA 100, the Irish Court of Criminal Appeal found that the proposed evidence of a psychologist, which was sought to be admitted to support the credibility of evidence given by the accused that she was subject to panic attacks and would not have reacted as a normal person would to a particular situation, would not have been relevant to her guilt or innocence. The purpose was to explain why she would have found it difficult to refuse to obey the instructions of the co-accused. The court pointed out that the evidence did not raise a question of mental illness; in any event, the appellant's evidence had not been that her will had been overborne, but that she had been unaware of either the plan to commit the offence or that it had been committed.

Albeit in two family cases, but illustrative of the judicial approach, it was made clear that psychometric testing has no place where the credibility of an adult witness is an issue (*Re S (Care: Parenting Skills: Personality Tests)* [2004] EWCA Civ 1029; *Re L (Children)* [2006] EWCA Civ 1282).

Reliability

Most commonly, the issue of reliability, or accuracy, arises in cases of adults alleging sexual abuse in childhood and in which case it is common to be asked to address the issue of 'false memory syndrome'. This is a highly specialised area and one where, in any event, it is usually best to work collaboratively with a psychologist, especially if issues arise as to the genuineness of reported childhood memories. Where the evidence of a complainant is based on 'recovered memories', the psychiatrist should be familiar with the literature on this subject.

False memory syndrome and the reliability of the account of a complainant as to sexual assaults in childhood were the issue in *R v H* [2014] EWCA Crim 1555, where the trial judge excluded a psychiatrist's evidence on the grounds that her reports:

> ... were littered with wholly inappropriate, adverse comments on the credibility and reliability of X. He believed that [she] had also advanced her opinion in a wholly inappropriate way for an expert witness, and had assumed the role of the advocate arguing the case for the defence forcefully carrying out what amounted to a deconstruction, if not demolition, of the reliability of this 16 year old girl. The judge noted that [defence counsel] conceded that much of the expert's evidence insofar as it amounted to no more than a comment on the complainant's credibility and reliability would be inadmissible.

Having reviewed the authorities, the judge concluded that the principles which emerged were:

[1] The defence were not permitted to call an expert to examine the detail of a complainant's statement/evidence, and other relevant evidence such as medical or counselling notes, and then pass judgement or adverse comment on whether the witness was a credible or reliable witness. To do so would be to usurp the jury's function.
[2] The defence were entitled, in an appropriate case, to call expert evidence on a specific subject which would be outside the knowledge and experience of the jury and which might assist them in their task of assessing the credibility and reliability of allegations of historic sexual abuse.
[3] False Memory Syndrome, or Recovered Memory Syndrome, was just such a subject where defence expert evidence was potentially admissible.
[4] There had to be a sound factual foundation for such expert opinion which had to be established in evidence prior to such expert evidence becoming admissible. It was for the trial judge to decide whether such foundation had been laid.

Just because someone suffers from a mental disorder, it does not follow that they are any more unreliable on matters unaffected by the mental disorder than any other witness: 'The fact of mental ill health, however, does not mean that the witness . . . cannot accurately be describing what has happened to her or that it would prevent her from (or make her incapable of) being reliable in her account.' In *The People (DPP) v Gillane* (Irish Court of Criminal Appeal, unreported, 14 December 1998), the appellant had been convicted of soliciting two men to murder his wife. Under cross-examination, one of the men volunteered that he had had a microchip inserted in his head in the course of a hospital operation, that it was connected to his mouth and that people could read his mind. The Irish Court of Criminal Appeal held that the fact that the witness had such 'very strange ideas' did not mean that he was incapable of giving evidence; he had been a positive, clear and forceful witness in relation to the events concerning the appellant. His testimony had to be given the same attention and respect as the testimony 'of the more comfortably circumstanced'. In *R v Barratt* [1996] Crim LR 495, a witness had what had been described as 'fixed belief paranoia' and she had various bizarre beliefs about her personal life, but the court could see no reason not to rely on her evidence on matters unaffected by her mental condition. Likewise, in *R v H* [2005] EWCA Crim 1828, the judge also held that the fact of mental ill health did not mean that X could not accurately be describing what had happened to her or that it would prevent her from (or make her incapable of) being reliable in her account. He held that these issues of fact were not for resolution by doctors, but for determination by the jury. What he did accept was that, as it was put in *R v Bernard V* [2003] EWCA Crim 3917, evidence is admissible when it is necessary 'to inform the jury of experience of a scientific and medical kind of which they might be unaware, which they ought to take into account when they assess the evidence in the case in order to decide whether they can be sure about the reliability of a particular witness'.

In Ireland, the much more limited admissibility of such expert evidence is illustrated by *The People (DPP) v Campion* [2015] IECA 190, and upheld in *The People (DPP) v Campion* [2018] IESC 35, where the reliability of a witness (whose evidence was central to the murder conviction that followed) may have been impaired by reason of mental illness: 'The scope for expert professional evidence on whether a witness is reliable or indeed capable of telling the truth will be very limited. The decision making process will normally not be enhanced by the prospect of professional witnesses intervening and offering conflicting and competing opinions on a matter that is so quintessentially one for a jury.' However, the court declined to attempt to resolve the question of the parameters of the admissibility of expert psychiatric evidence bearing upon the mental condition of the witness insofar as it affected his reliability and so whether developments in England and Wales (*MacKenney*) will be followed in Ireland must abide a case in which the issue properly arises.

Where there is evidence of a form of personality disorder that manifests in dishonesty or exaggeration, medical (and particularly psychiatric) records should be carefully studied for examples of dishonesty or exaggeration. However, it does not follow that everyone with a particular personality disorder lies or exaggerates.

Even if there is expert psychiatric evidence that calls into question a witness's or complainant's credibility or reliability, it is important not to suggest that the person has not given or is not capable of giving credible or reliable evidence. This is for the court to decide: 'Evidence given by experts which tends to convey to the jury the expert's opinion of the truth or otherwise of the complaint is clearly inadmissible. The truth and reliability of the evidence was a matter for the jury not for the expert' (*R v WC* [2012] EWCA Crim 1478).

This has been confirmed in *Pora* (see Chapter 6, 'Treading on the Judge's Toes'). The evidence of a forensic psychologist, who was asked to consider the appellant's reliability and who could not be faulted by the court for any lack of thoroughness in his approach, which involved a review of the evidence in painstaking detail, was ruled inadmissible on the basis that, in trenchantly asserting that the appellant's confessions were unreliable, he was supplanting the court's role as the ultimate decision-maker on a matter that was central to the outcome of the case. The court observed that the expert:

> . . . could have expressed an opinion as to how the difficulties that Pora faced might have led him to make false confessions. This would have allowed the fact finder to make its own determination to whether the admissions could be relied upon as a basis for a finding of guilt, unencumbered by a forthright assertion from the expert that the confessions were unreliable.

By contrast, the evidence of another forensic psychologist about Pora's foetal alcohol syndrome disorder as providing 'a possible explanation for his having admitted to something that he did not do' was accepted as evidence which was relevant and, at least potentially, extremely helpful in determining the reliability of Pora's confessions.

If a person with mental disorder gives evidence as a witness, the jury will decide what weight to attach to the evidence because if the witness's evidence is so 'tainted with insanity as to be unworthy of credit', it is the proper function of the jury to disregard it and not act on it (*R v Hill* (1851) 2 Den CC 254).

R v Brown [2004] EWCA Crim 50 illustrates the potential admissibility of evidence by a neuropsychiatrist specialising in sleep disorder as to the reliance that can be placed on the recollection of someone being woken from sleep. This was an issue because the rape conviction depended in part on what a witness heard when she may have been woken by sounds from the next-door property. It was the expert's evidence that 'there must be doubt not as to the integrity but as to the reliability of the evidence', but the court found that it was 'not necessary or expedient in the interests of justice for that evidence to be received'. However, a successful application was made to admit the same expert's evidence which cast doubt on the reliability of the complainant in a sexual assault case who said that she woke to find the accused licking her clitoris (*R v JLW* [2000] 5 WLUK 391).

Sexual Offences against Persons with a Mental Disorder Impeding Choice and Protected Persons

In England and Wales, the SOA has created 'Offences against persons with a mental disorder impeding choice'. Under s 30(1), a person (A) commits an offence if A touches sexually a person (B) who is 'unable to refuse because of or for a reason related to a mental disorder' and 'A knows or could reasonably be expected to know that B has a mental disorder and that because of it or for a reason related to it B is unlikely to be able to refuse'. Section 1(2) sets out a capacity test for refusal in the following terms: 'he lacks the capacity to choose whether to agree to the touching (whether because he lacks sufficient understanding of the nature or reasonably foreseeable consequences of what is being done, or for any other reason), or he is unable to communicate such a choice to A'. Sections 31 to 37 create further similar offences.

In *Hulme v Director of Public Prosecutions* [2006] EWHC 1347 (Admin), a woman with what would appear to have been an intellectual disability was found to have been unable effectively to communicate her choice when a man she met in her parents' public house touched her vagina over her clothing and put his hand on his flaccid, exposed penis. Whereas many people, even those with dementia or an intellectual disability, would probably be able to say 'no' to an unfamiliar person requesting sexual intercourse, they are still very vulnerable to being surreptitiously 'groomed' by others with the intention of performing inappropriate sexual activity (Curtice and Kelson 2011).

In Ireland, it is an offence to engage in a sexual act where it is known, or one is reckless as to whether, the other person is a 'protected person'. It is also an offence to invite, induce, counsel or incite a protected person to engage in a sexual act knowing or being reckless as to whether the person is a protected person. A 'protected person' is one who lacks the capacity to consent to a sexual act by reason of a mental or intellectual disability or a mental illness that renders them incapable of understanding the nature, or the reasonably foreseeable consequences, of the act, evaluating relevant information for the purposes of deciding whether or not to engage in the act or communicating consent by speech, sign language or otherwise. In relevant criminal proceedings, it is presumed, unless the contrary is shown, that the defendant knew or was reckless as to whether the person against whom the offence is alleged to have been committed was a protected person (Criminal Justice (Sexual Offences) Act 2017, s 21). Thus, the ingredients of the offences are (1) knowledge or (2) recklessness in respect of the disability and incapacity, with a rebuttable presumption in respect of each against the accused. Second, the incapacity is not pegged to a mental disorder within the meaning of the MHA 2001, but is functionally related to mental disability, intellectual disability or mental illness, however classified or however occurring.

Box 7.30 sets out the issues to be addressed in a report on a complainant in a case of this nature. Capacity to consent to sexual relations and the case of *R v C* [2009] UKHL 42 are considered in more detail in Chapter 10.

Causing or Allowing the Death of a Vulnerable Adult

Under the DVCVA, s 5, it is an offence to cause or allow the death of a vulnerable adult. Section 5(6) defines a vulnerable adult as 'a person aged 16 or over whose ability to protect himself from violence, abuse or neglect is significantly impaired through physical or mental disability, through old age or otherwise'. The words 'or otherwise' were given meaning in *R v Uddin* [2017] EWCA Crim 1072: 'A victim of sexual or domestic abuse or modern slavery,

Box 7.30 Issues to Be Addressed in Reporting on a Complainant in a Case of Sexual Activity with a Person with a Mental Disorder Impeding Choice or with a Protected Person

- Does the complainant have a mental disorder?
- Does the complainant have the capacity to consent to sexual activity?
- Is any incapacity to consent to sexual activity due to the mental disorder?
- Does the complainant have any external distinguishing features that might indicate the presence of mental disorder and, if so, make it evident that the complainant was unable to consent?
- Could the complainant communicate a decision about sexual activity to the accused?

for instance, might find himself in a vulnerable position, having suffered long term physical and mental abuse leaving them scared, cowed and with a significantly impaired ability to protect themselves.' There is a similar offence under s 6A of allowing a vulnerable adult to suffer serious physical harm.

Psychiatric Harm

In England and Wales, the courts have recognised that psychiatric illness or injury, including hysterical or nervous shock (*R v Morris* [1997] 10 WLUK 404), can constitute harm that may form the basis of a charge of causing really serious harm amounting to grievous bodily harm (*R v Ireland* [1998] AC 147; *R v D* [2006] EWCA Crim 1139) or harm amounting to actual bodily harm (*R v Chan-Fook* [1994] 1 WLR 689) under the OAPA. In order to prove such harm, the prosecution needs psychiatric evidence as to cause and effect, whether the accused's conduct resulted in the injury. Distress, grief, anxiety or other psychological harm that does not amount to a recognisable psychiatric illness is not bodily harm for the purposes of the OAPA (*R v D*). *In Ireland*, in the NFOAPA, s 1(1), harm is defined as meaning 'harm to body or mind and includes pain and unconsciousness'. At the level of principle, psychiatric harm seems sufficient.

Extradition

A person's mental condition may be grounds for adjourning extradition proceedings and be a bar to extradition if it makes it unjust or oppressive to extradite them (Extradition Act 2003, ss 25 and 91) and the *Framework decision on the European arrest warrant and the surrender procedures between Member States*, art 23.4 provides for temporary postponement 'for serious humanitarian reasons, for example if there are substantial grounds for believing that it would manifestly endanger the requested person's life or health'. However, '[a] high threshold has to be reached' and, where the mental condition is linked to a risk of a suicide attempt if the extradition order were made, there has to be a 'substantial risk that the [requested person] will commit suicide' (*Turner v Government of the USA* [2012] EWHC 2426 (Admin)). Furthermore, so far as suicide risk is concerned, '[t]he mental condition of the person must be such that it removes his capacity to resist the impulse to commit suicide, otherwise it will not be his mental condition but his own voluntary act which puts him at risk of dying and if that is the case there is no oppression in ordering extradition' (*Turner*).

In these proceedings, 'oppression' refers to hardship to the requested person from changes in his circumstances, but the bar is set high because it is recognised that extradition is ordinarily likely to cause stress and hardship.

In such cases, adequate medical evidence must be provided. Relevant considerations are suicide risk and what might happen to the requested person following extradition. For example, if suicide risk is to be managed by 'suicide watch' or 'segregation' or if the person's mental illness is likely to result in them being put in solitary confinement, such arrangements may in themselves be oppressive because, as in *Love v Government of the USA* [2018] EWHC 172 (Admin), where the requested person had a unique combination of depression, Asperger syndrome and eczema, it was held that 'those measures would themselves be likely to have a seriously adverse effect on his very vulnerable and unstable mental and physical wellbeing'. Here, assessment involved taking a holistic view that encompassed the relationship between physical and mental conditions. Other considerations are the impact of a custodial environment on a requested person and their removal from family networks, as well as the impact that previous torture and mistreatment has on someone being extradited.

Oppression can also encompass a loss of dignity. In *Magiera v District Court of Krakow, Poland* [2017] EWHC 2757 (Admin), the requested person had a stoma, following surgery for bowel cancer. It was held that being:

> ... unable to care for himself in a hygienic and dignified way for any length of time would unquestionably be oppressive ... and would also be a disproportionate interference with his right to a private and family life. It constitutes the sort of particular, distinct and severe hardship which is necessary to reach the necessary thresholds for these provisions.

In *Jansons v Latvia* [2009] EWHC 1845 (Admin), the appellant successfully appealed against an order for extradition to Latvia in what the courts recognised as a most unusual but also exceptional case: the appellant had hanged himself in his cell, he was cut down at the last possible moment, his life was saved by lengthy and skilled medical treatment, he spent ten days in intensive care and did not recover consciousness until day nine. There was uncontested medical evidence that the appellant was going to kill himself if returned to Latvia.

By contrast, in *Howes v Her Majesty's Advocate* [2010] HCJAC 123, the appellant unsuccessfully opposed extradition; the suicide risk was not sufficiently high. In *R (Prosser) v Secretary of State for the Home Department* [2010] EWHC 845 (Admin), dismissal of the appellant's appeal against an order for extradition to the USA took into account the fact that 'proper medical care would substantially reduce the risk of suicide', but the court recognised that a 'very high risk would doubtless be capable of achieving the art 3 (prohibition on torture) threshold'. Likewise, in *S v The Court of Bologna* [2010] EWHC 1184 (Admin), where an appeal against an extradition order on the grounds of suicide risk was unsuccessful, the court highlighted 'the need for circumspection in evaluating the evidence when such an issue is raised in case there is a perception that raising the issue is an easy way of avoiding extradition'.

In *Rot v Poland* [2010] EWHC 1820 (Admin), a similarly unsuccessful case, the court nevertheless expressed misgivings about *Jansons*:

> Until and unless the reasoning in *Jansons* is disproved, the risk of suicide must be accepted to be a relevant risk for the purpose of section 25. The question must therefore be addressed

> and answered in such a case: would the mental condition of the person to be extradited make it oppressive to extradite him? Logically, the answer to that question in a suicide risk case must be no unless the mental condition of the person is such as to remove his capacity to resist the impulse to commit suicide, otherwise it will not be his mental condition but his own voluntary act which puts him at risk of dying, and therefore may make it oppressive to extradite him. Untidy though it may be, and while *Jansons* remains good authority, the question must be approached in a somewhat less logical manner. When, as in *Jansons*, there is uncontradicted evidence that an individual who has made a serious attempt to kill himself will kill himself if extradited, it may be right to hold that it would be oppressive to extradite him. Anything less will not do.

In *Wrobel v Poland* [2011] EWHC 374 (Admin), the court quashed an extradition order on the grounds that there was a very high risk of the appellant committing suicide if extradition proceeded. The court rejected the argument that the appellant had to establish a certainty that he would kill himself if extradited; the test had been put too high in *Rot*. It found that it was sufficient if the appellant could establish a very high risk of suicide.

In *Mazurkiewicz v Rezeszow Circuit Court* [2011] EWHC 659 (Admin), although the court applied the test in *Wrobel* and found that undoubtedly it was a case where there was a suicide risk, it found that it was not so high that the appellant's rights under ECHR arts 2 (right to life), 3 (prohibition on torture) or 8 (right to respect for private and family life) were infringed, or that extradition would be 'unjust or oppressive' under the Extradition Act 2003, s 25. However, the court shared the misgivings expressed in *Rot*:

> A person who is otherwise fit to serve a sentence of imprisonment does not escape such a sentence in this country simply by pointing to a high risk that he will commit suicide. Obviously mistakes are sometimes made, but the prison service has systems in place to protect vulnerable prisoners against self harm. Our criminal justice system operates on that basis.

Wolkowicz v Polish Judicial Authority [2013] EWHC 102 (Admin), where the court rejected three appellants' appeals against extradition, sets out the general approach in such cases, relying heavily on *Turner*, but points out that such cases are highly fact-sensitive. In the case of Mariusz Wolkowicz, the court found that, even if it accepted that he was at high risk of suicide, and as an attempted suicide in prison in England had been prevented, there was nothing to suggest that effective steps could not be taken to mitigate the risk whilst in custody in the UK and during removal to Poland; furthermore, there was no evidence to impugn the ability of the Polish authorities to take similar steps. Likewise, in the case of Wojciech Biskup, although it was accepted that he had a serious mental illness, there was no doubt that his condition and the risks had been properly managed by the UK authorities and there was no evidence for contending that his condition could not be properly managed when being transferred to, and in custody in, Poland. And in the case of Vilma Rizleriene, who clearly had a mental illness associated with a significant risk of self-harm and suicide, and where there was evidence from a UK psychiatrist who believed that the quality of treatment in Lithuania would not be as good as in the UK and that she should not be in prison anywhere, the court was provided with information by the Ministry of Justice of Lithuania that was sufficient to establish that in Lithuania there was provision for prisoners with recognised mental illnesses.

The issue of what might happen to a requested person who is extradited was considered in *South Africa v Dewani* [2014] EWHC 153 (Admin). There was disputed medical evidence as to Dewani's FTP. Although it was held that it was for the requesting state to determine this as part of the trial process, it was recognised that the English court could consider whether in a particular case this would result in unjustness or oppression – for example, if the person might remain permanently unfit. If there was such a prospect, it was open to the English court to require an undertaking to allow the person's return if, following treatment over a reasonable time, he was still likely to remain unfit.

FTP was also an issue for Wojciech Biskup in *Wolkowicz*. There was psychiatric evidence as to his ability to participate properly in any trial process in Poland, specifically evidence that under stress he tended to regress and become anxious and agitated, would try to avoid being confronted with reality and passively refuse to engage with his legal team, and avoid reading letters and require assistance of people he knew in meetings with his legal representatives. However, the court found that this evidence as to his ability to instruct lawyers came nowhere near raising an issue of FTP; his appeal was dismissed.

As not all jurisdictions have effective mental health provision within the custodial environment, cases may turn on whether a particular country is able to provide adequate custodial mental healthcare.

Other cases where PTSD or effects of abuse and torture are such that someone should not be extradited cut across the issues for lawyers, as this is a specific issue that the courts must determine. In *LMN v Government of Turkey* [2018] EWHC 210 (Admin), there was expert psychiatric evidence that the appellant, who faced extradition to Turkey, had a severe depressive episode with some features of PTSD and would be at high risk of suicide if extradited. It was held that taking into account the risk of suicide, a failure to meet his mental healthcare needs would attain the minimum standard of severity necessary to breach his art 3 right to prohibition on torture. However, it is important that expert psychiatric witnesses should not give evidence as to mental health provision in other countries unless they have knowledge of such. As in the case of Vilma Rizleriene, a view as to the adequacy of medical treatment in another country may be challenged by evidence from that country.

In *Attorney General v Davis* [2018] IESC 27, there was a question of suicide risk on the extradition to the USA of a man with Asperger syndrome who, it was alleged, was an administrator of the 'Silk Road'. His essential ground of objection was that there was a real risk, given the severity of his mental disorder and the state of his psychological health, that pre-trial and/or post-conviction incarceration in the USA would cause his condition to deteriorate and could foreseeably put his life at risk. The court was satisfied of the state's obligation to protect vulnerable persons suffering from mental illness within the context of an extradition application, but rejected the application because he failed to establish by evidence that there were substantial grounds for believing that if he were extradited to the requesting country, he would be exposed to a real risk of being subjected to treatment contrary to ECHR, art 3 or equivalent fundamental rights under the Irish Constitution.

Appeals

A person convicted can appeal on the basis that the conviction was unsafe or on the basis that the sentence was too severe.

In England and Wales, under the Criminal Appeal Act 1968, the court must give 'leave to appeal' or what is now known under CrPR as 'permission to appeal'. Someone who has served a notice to appeal but has not been granted permission to appeal is an 'applicant' and a person who has been granted permission is an 'appellant'. An application to appeal should only be made where there are grounds that indicate a real prospect of success. *In the Isle of Man*, leave is not required to appeal conviction.

Where the appeal depends on the admission of fresh evidence, there has to be a reasonable explanation for the failure to adduce the evidence at trial. In *R v Gilbert* [2003] EWCA Crim 2385, the court allowed the application to adduce evidence on the basis that there was a chance that the appellant did not advance the true facts because he was ill. *Moyle*, who was convicted of murder, is a similar case. He had refused to see a psychiatrist because he felt that he was part of a conspiracy to have him hung, drawn and quartered. He felt that if he had disclosed his symptoms at the time, he would have been convicted of witchcraft. The court accepted that the appellant's decisions at the time of his trial were affected by the illness itself, quashed the conviction and substituted a conviction for manslaughter on the grounds of diminished responsibility. Thus, in appeal cases, it is important to consider the effects of the appellant's illness on his thinking and behaviour at the time of the trial.

The evidence of a further expert to the same effect as that of an expert at the trial is not likely to be regarded as fresh evidence. It is regarded as a potential subversion of the trial process to allow at appeal another and supposedly more persuasive expert to give the same opinion evidence that was unsuccessfully given at the trial or to present an alternative expert opinion based on the same factual evidence that was available at the trial (*R v Meachen* [2009] EWCA Crim 1701). Retrospective medical evidence will generally be viewed with scepticism (*R v Andrews* [2003] EWCA Crim 2750). Although the expert may be provided with transcripts of parts of the trial, in *R v Cleobury* [2012] EWCA Crim 17, there is a warning that the expert should remain within their area of expertise and not provide an advocate's critique either of what happened at the trial or the judge's summing-up.

In Ireland, the provision whereby leave to appeal had to be obtained first has been abolished. New or additional evidence may be heard on an appeal, but leave must be obtained to adduce new evidence. In an application to introduce new or fresh evidence:

> ... exceptional circumstances must be established before the court should allow further evidence to be called. That onus is particularly heavy in the case of expert testimony, having regard to the availability generally of expertise from multiple sources ... the evidence must not have been known at the time of the trial and must be such that it could not reasonably have been known or acquired at the time of the trial [and] [i]t must be evidence which is credible and which might have a material and important influence on the result of the case. (*The People (DPP) v Buck* [2010] IECCA 88)

Where a new, or newly discovered, fact shows that there has been a miscarriage of justice in relation to a conviction or that the sentence imposed is excessive, a person may apply to the court for an order quashing the conviction or reviewing the sentence. Reference to a newly discovered fact is to a fact discovered by, or coming to the notice of, the convicted person after the relevant appeal proceedings have been finally determined or a fact the significance of which was not appreciated by the convicted person or his advisors during the trial or appeal proceedings (Criminal Procedure Act 1993, s 2).

Appeals relating to FTP and diminished responsibility have since received particular attention from the Court of Appeal. The bar is high. In *R v Erskine* [2009] EWCA Crim 1425, the court said that:

> ... it will be very rare indeed for a later reconstruction, even by distinguished psychiatrists who did not examine the appellant at the time of trial, to persuade the court that

> notwithstanding the earlier trial process and the safeguards built into it that the appellant was unfit to plead, or close to being unfit or that his decision to deny the offence and not advance diminished responsibility can properly be explained on this basis. The situation is, of course, different if . . . serious questions about his fitness to plead were raised in writing or expressly before the judge at the trial.

However, *R v Shulman* [2010] EWCA Crim 1034 (Wood and Rix 2016) is an example of a case in which study of the transcripts of the defendant's evidence and his interruptions of court proceedings, along with notes of his conferences with counsel, revealed evidence of his schizophrenic thought disorder and this, along with evidence of his delusions about the female complainant, who alleged rape, false imprisonment and assault, persuaded the Court of Appeal to quash his convictions and make a finding of unfitness to plead and stand trial. In *Williams*, a psychiatrist prepared a report which did not support a plea of diminished responsibility and the defendant was convicted of murder. However, on appeal, the psychiatrist was criticised for not having considered the general practice records and CT scans of the brain made shortly before the killing and the court found that the psychiatrist had misunderstood the law of diminished responsibility. Fresh psychiatric evidence was successfully admitted to the effect that, as a result of long-standing alcohol dependence, the defendant had suffered brain damage which caused serious and significant impairment of his judgement and his ability to control his impulses.

Reports for the Parole Board and Discretionary Lifers Panel

The word 'parole' derives from the French expression for 'word of honour', so the implication is that, if released, the offender is honour-bound not to commit further offences. Parole Boards are courts for the purposes of reviewing detention in relation to the right to liberty under ECHR, art 5.

The Parole Board makes decisions on the applications for parole of prisoners serving sentences of between four and seven years and in the case of prisoners serving seven or more years it makes a recommendation to the Home Secretary. It reviews the cases of prisoners serving a mandatory life sentence and the first review is usually about three years before the expiry of their tariff, which is the minimum period they are ordered to serve before becoming eligible for parole, and it reviews, as a 'Discretionary Lifer Panel', the cases of prisoners serving a discretionary life sentence as soon as they have served their tariff. The primary concern is the risk to the public of a further offence being committed when the prisoner would otherwise be in prison. It can recommend a transfer to open conditions.

The Parole Board also makes decisions about those who were aged under 17 years on the date of the commission of the offence and who have been detained during Her Majesty's Pleasure. This is known as an HMP Panel.

Parole Board members are advised to take into account 'medical or psychiatric considerations' and so an up-to-date psychiatric report is likely to be requested. It should deal with any psychiatric history, including responsiveness to treatment and the relationship between the psychiatric disorder and offending, any requirement as to psychiatric treatment that might be made a condition of release and the likelihood of cooperation with and a response to such treatment. Insofar as they fall within the expertise of the psychiatrist, which will depend on the nature of the case, the report should address any risk to the victim or other persons, attitude and behaviour in custody, remorse, insight into offending behaviour, steps taken to achieve any treatment objectives and the likelihood of cooperation with supervision in the community. The report should be based on study of the parole dossier and it should pay particular attention to the psychology reports.

The report will form part of the final parole dossier and will be made available to the prisoner in advance of the hearing. However, exceptionally, the report could be withheld if, on psychiatric grounds, it is felt necessary to do so where the mental and/or physical health of the prisoner could be impaired by disclosure. Alternatively, parts of the report could be redacted and the prisoner provided with the redacted version. It is the governor who decides on withholding and redaction.

Provide a psychiatric analysis of the prisoner's case, not a mere recitation of their history, consider the risk to others and give the reasons for the particular statement as to risk if possible by reference to a structured professional judgement risk assessment. If the prisoner is going to need psychiatric supervision in the community, set this out in as much detail as possible, even though the area to which the prisoner may be released is uncertain. This may require liaison with the health and probation services in the relevant area.

If called to give evidence, remember that although the Criminal Justice Act 1991, s 32(3) adds an inquisitorial quality to Parole Board proceedings, the judges who chair them come from an adversarial tradition and will often conduct hearings as if they are adversarial.

The Parole Commission *in Northern Ireland* and the Parole Committee *in the Isle of Man* fulfil a similar role. *In Ireland*, the Parole Board has a similar function and when the Parole Act 2019 is implemented it will have the power to direct expert reports and, specifically, from psychiatrists, whether inside or outside Ireland.

Further Reading

Gledhill, K. (2012) *Defending Mentally Disordered Offenders* (Legal Action Group).

Hallett, N., Smit, N. and Rix, K. (2019) 'Miscarriages of justice and expert psychiatric evidence: lessons from criminal appeals in England and Wales', *BJPsych Advances*, 25, 251–64.

Ormerod, D. and Perry, D. (gen. eds) (2020) *Blackstone's Criminal Practice* (Oxford University Press).

Taylor, C. and Krish, J. (2010) *Advising Mentally Disordered Offenders: A Practical Guide* (The Law Society).

Reports in Personal Injury Cases

Laurence Mynors-Wallis and Keith Rix

I cannot leave this case without expressing my profound gratitude to counsel on both sides ... for the deep humanity with which they have conducted this tragic case.
Hirst J in *Aboul-Hosn v Trustees of the Italian Hospital* [1993] 1 WLUK 646

Psychiatric reports in personal injury cases are requested in the following circumstances:

- road traffic and industrial accidents involving physical injury;
- clinical negligence cases:
  - medical negligence resulting in psychiatric injury;
  - negligence in mental healthcare;
- employment stress;
- historical child abuse (HCA);
- 'nervous shock';
- mere mental or emotional distress.

Related issues are limitation and malingering.

Limitation

In England and Wales, there is a three-year limitation period in most personal injury actions. In some HCA cases, and in professional negligence cases, it is six years. This is the period during which the claim must be brought. It begins in theory when the cause of action (i.e. the index incident) occurred. In HCA and clinical negligence cases, it begins when the claimant has the relevant 'knowledge': (1) that the injury was significant (whether a reasonable person with the claimant's knowledge would have considered the injury sufficiently serious to justify suing a defendant who did not deny liability and had the means to pay, an objective test for which the impact of the claimant's injuries on his ability to issue proceedings is not a relevant consideration (*A v Hoare* [2008] UKHL 6); (2) that the injury is attributable in whole or part to the act or omission which constitutes the alleged negligence or breach of duty; and (3) the identity of the defendant. 'Attributable' means 'capable of being attributed to' or 'a real possibility' (*Spargo v North Essex Health Authority* [1997] 3 WLUK 252).

This leads to questions such as when actual knowledge was acquired and whether the claimant had constructive knowledge at an earlier date. In a negligence case, a claimant may not acquire actual knowledge until their solicitors receive a report from an expert who attributes significant injuries to a breach of duty. In an HCA case, the claimant may not acquire actual knowledge until receipt of a report that attributes significant psychiatric damage to the alleged abuse.

What constitutes 'actual knowledge' partly depends on the 'particular patient':

> Whether or not a state of mind ... is properly to be treated ... as knowledge seems ... to depend, in the first place, upon the nature of the information which the claimant has received, the extent to which he pays attention to the information as affecting him, and his capacity to understand it. There is a second stage at which the information, when received and understood, is evaluated. It may be rejected as unbelievable. It may be regarded as unreliable or uncertain. The court must assess the intelligence of the claimant; consider and assess his assertions as to how he regarded such information as he had; and determine whether he had knowledge of the facts by reason of his understanding of the information. (*Nash v Eli Lilly & Co.* [1993] 1 WLR 782)

'Constructive knowledge' refers to how a claimant would have had 'actual knowledge' if they had asked the right questions or sought the right advice earlier. The Limitation Act 1980, s 14(3) refers to 'knowledge which he might reasonably have been expected to acquire ... from facts observable or ascertainable by him', including 'facts ascertainable with the help of medical or other appropriate expert advice which it is reasonable for him to seek'. Although the words 'reasonable' and 'reasonably' represent an objective test, personal or individual characteristics can be taken into account. Psychiatric evidence may be needed as to their nature and potential effects.

What amount to relevant characteristics can be problematic. In *Adams v Bracknell Forest Borough Council* [2004] UKHL 29, an intelligent man with severe dyslexia had not sought any advice about his literary difficulties because he did not want to talk about them. However, even though he had a social phobia, which arguably could have accounted for, or been connected with, his shyness and embarrassment, the court, on the basis that others with a similar dyslexia would not be so inhibited from asking the right questions or seeking expert help, ruled that his shyness and embarrassment should be disregarded; these characteristics were not relevant as they were strictly personal characteristics. There are likely to be further cases that require judicial decisions on the eligibility of characteristics. In such a case, you should do the following. Ensure that characteristics are specified with clarity. Refer to the evidence for their existence. Make clear whether they are a feature of a recognised mental disorder, thus allowing a distinction to be made between, for example, shyness as an ordinary personality characteristic and shyness as a feature of Asperger syndrome. Explain how the characteristic affects such processes as the abilities to pay attention to, understand and evaluate personally relevant information and make reasonable enquiries.

In England and Wales, the limitation period does not begin to run if the person was 'under a disability': 'the action may be brought before the expiration of three years from the date when he ceased to be under a disability or died, whichever first occurred, notwithstanding that the limitation period has expired' (Limitation Act 1980, s 28(1)). Section 38(2) defines 'disability' as a person who is 'an infant or of unsound mind' – the latter meaning 'lacks capacity (within the meaning of the Mental Capacity Act 2005) to conduct legal proceedings'.

The Limitation Act 1980, s 33 provides the court with a discretion to allow a case to proceed 'out of time'. This is the fall-back position for claimants in HCA cases who fail the objective test as to their date of knowledge because the impact of their injuries on their ability to issue proceedings is regarded as a relevant consideration for the court in deciding whether to exercise discretion.

A psychiatric report addressing limitation issues should have regard to some of the circumstances to which the court is particularly directed: factors which have influenced the claimant's decision to come forward at the stage at which he did and the corollary, which is: reasons for delay on the part of the claimant; the duration of any disability of the claimant arising after the date of accrual of the cause of action; the extent to which the claimant acted promptly and reasonably once he knew whether the act or omission of the defendant, to which the injury was attributable, might amount to a cause of action; the steps, if any, taken by the claimant to obtain medical advice and the nature of such advice as he may have received; and the effect of his psychiatric injuries on his ability to issue proceedings. An impairment of health that falls short of a 'disability' may be relevant (*Davis v Jacobs* [1999] 3 WLUK 90).

In Ireland, the limitation period for most personal injury actions is two years from the date of accrual of the cause of action or the date of knowledge (if later). As an authorisation from the Injuries Board is a condition precedent to the issuing of any proceedings claiming damages for personal injuries (other than clinical negligence claims), in reckoning any period of time for limitation purposes, the period beginning on the making of an application to the Board and ending six months from the date of authorisation is disregarded, so in effect the limitation clock stops. There is a proposal to increase the limitation period to three years in clinical negligence cases only.

The 'date of knowledge' requirements and the tests are similar to those in England and Wales. However, there is no provision for the discretionary judicial extension of the limitation period other than in 'exceptional circumstances' in cases brought under the Residential Institutions Redress Act 2002, which provides for financial awards to adults who have, or had, injuries received in residential care, and the Hepatitis C Compensation Tribunal Acts 1997–2006. Such exceptional circumstances could include the effect or impact of mental or physical health problems or conditions on the plaintiff. A person is under a disability if of 'unsound mind', which is not defined in the Statute of Limitations 1957. There is a conclusive presumption of such under the Lunacy Regulation (Ireland) Act 1871, s 48(2) for any person detained pursuant to any enactment authorising 'the detention of persons of unsound mind or criminal lunatics'. This means persons detained under the MHA 2001 or because of unfitness to plead or following the special verdict of NGRI. Additionally, in cases of historical sexual abuse, under the Statute of Limitations (Amendment) Act 2000, s 2, a plaintiff is under a disability while suffering from any psychological injury caused by the perpetrator of the abuse and of such significance that their will, or ability to make a reasoned decision, to bring such an action is substantially impaired.

In Scotland, there is a 'prescription period' of three years in personal injury actions. It can be extended to account for any period when the claimant was not aware, and could not with reasonable diligence have been aware, of the claimed loss. However, the Limitation (Child Abuse) (Scotland) Act 2017 has removed the limitation period in child abuse personal injury claims.

Road Traffic and Industrial Accidents and the Effects of Allegedly Negligent Medical Care

In accident and medical negligence cases, the questions asked are often in the form:

> To provide a medical report detailing relevant pre-accident/incident medical history, the injuries sustained, treatment received and present condition dealing in particular with the capacity for work and giving a prognosis. To specifically comment on any areas of

continuing complaint, disability or impact on daily living and, if there is such continuing disability, the level of suffering or inconvenience caused and when, or if, the complaint or disability is likely to resolve.

The facts or assumed facts that you should set out include:

- an account of the accident or alleged medical negligence (the index event);
- a summary of the physical injuries sustained, if any, by the claimant – you are not an expert on physical injury, but this can help in understanding the psychological injuries;
- the social consequences of the index event (e.g. mobility, employment, self-care, leisure activities);
- psychological symptoms subsequent to the index event, often as described by the claimant, but ideally including information from any informants;
- relevant medical history, derived both from the claimant and also medical records, including all psychiatric symptoms documented both pre and post the index event;
- mental state examination.

In the Opinion, set out:

- any relevant medical history;
- any psychiatric diagnosis;
- causation, considering predisposing, precipitating and maintaining factors;
- treatment given and recommended;
- present condition;
- prognosis, including employment and life expectancy.

Any Relevant Medical History

A history of psychiatric disorder may indicate a predisposition, or what the law recognises as a vulnerability, to psychiatric disorder. This does not weaken or invalidate the claim. According to the 'egg-shell skull' doctrine, the defendant must take the victim as they find him. If as a result of unforeseen vulnerability, the injury is more severe, the defendant may nevertheless be liable for the injury in full. There may also be the issue of whether a psychiatric disorder was present at the time of the index event or would have occurred in any event.

Where previous physical ill-health has been complicated by psychiatric symptomatology, and especially if, with recurrence, chronicity or deterioration, the psychiatric symptoms have become more frequent or more severe, there will be the question of whether psychiatric symptomatology subsequent to the index event is related to the pre-existing and ongoing physical ill-health.

Diagnosis

Set out any psychiatric diagnosis or diagnoses. In straightforward cases, a paragraph on each diagnosis may suffice. It has become common convention to use ICD or DSM diagnoses. This is unnecessary unless you are asked to use them, but it can facilitate comparison of the opinions of two or more experts. If you rely on them, be aware of, and consider referring to, the cautions about their medicolegal application.

ICD-10 does not include any caution as to medicolegal application, although it makes it clear that it provides 'general diagnostic guidelines' and (p. x):

> These descriptions and guidelines carry no theoretical implications, and they do not pretend to be comprehensive statements about the current knowledge of the disorders. They are simply a set of symptoms and comments that have been agreed, by a large number of advisors and consultants in many different countries, to be a reasonable basis for defining the limits of categories in the classification of mental disorders.

Similarly, DSM5 (p. 21) states: 'Diagnostic criteria are offered as guidelines for making diagnoses, and their use should be informed by clinical judgment.'

DSM5 (p. 25) is also more explicit and specific, referring to how it was not developed:

> . . . to meet . . . all of the technical needs of the courts and legal professionals . . . the use of DSM-5 should be informed by an awareness of the risks and limitations of its use in forensic settings. When . . . employed for forensic purposes, there is a risk that diagnostic information will be misused or misunderstood . . . because of the imperfect fit between the questions of ultimate concern to the law and the information contained in a clinical diagnosis. In most situations, the clinical diagnosis of a DSM-5 disorder . . . does not imply that an individual with such a condition meets legal criteria for the presence of a mental disorder or a specific legal standard.

ICD and DSM are the product of committees. The ICD provides broader criteria, allowing more people to be diagnosed; the DSM is more restrictive, so a smaller number of people meet the diagnostic criteria. Their diagnoses are not based on research to establish their validity or on any objective laboratory test, but it is not unusual at an experts' meeting to find a psychiatrist ruling out a diagnosis because the claimant is one short of the required number of symptoms required by DSM. In *R (B) v S (Responsible Medical Officer, Broadmoor Hospital)* [2005] EWHC 1936, the court held that it was 'a fair criticism of Professor H's reports that . . . he adopted an over-rigid application of the DSM and ICD criteria'. One of the court's findings was that 'the setting of four days [for the duration of symptoms] is an arbitrary minimum'. This is entirely consistent with the Introduction to ICD-10 (p. x): 'Statements about the duration of symptoms are also intended as general guidelines rather than strict requirements; clinicians should use their own judgement about the appropriateness of choosing diagnoses when the duration of particular symptoms is slightly longer or shorter than that specified.'

Whether relying on DSM or ICD, be familiar with the potential legal challenges to diagnostic testimony (Hagan and Guilmette 2015). Notwithstanding such challenges, their use is encouraged by lawyers. In *Litigating Psychiatric Injury Claims*, Marshall, Kennedy and Azib advocate the use of ICD or DSM as 'a framework to "fit" an illness to and therefore justify it as recognisable . . . [because] without a label that is recognisable, a claimant is likely to have an uphill struggle to achieve compensation without a psychiatric condition that will fit one, or more, of the diagnostic descriptions'.

In *Hussain v The Chief Constable of West Mercia Constabulary* [2008] EWCA Civ 1205, we are told that: 'A recognised psychiatric illness is one which has been recognised by the psychiatric profession. In general, they are illnesses that are within the ICD . . .', and for ICD also read DSM.

That was unfortunate for the pursuer in *Rorrison v West Lothian College* (1999) Rep LR 102. A psychologist's evidence that her 'emotional symptoms constituted psychological damage' was accepted, but the court found that she 'had not pleaded any disorder that was recognised in DSM-IV . . . There is no evidence that she has ever been diagnosed by a psychiatrist as suffering from a recognised psychiatric disorder . . . The action accordingly falls to be dismissed.'

Not all judges are taken with ICD and DSM. His Honour John Cockroft said that between one case and another he forgot what the acronyms stood for. He also commented that there is too much emphasis on attaching a label to the claimant's condition; it is the contents of the jar, not the label, that matters. He recalled psychiatrists agreeing everything relevant to the claim, but vehemently disagreeing as to diagnosis. His approach concurs with that taken in *Noble*: '[T]he precise characterisation of Mr. Noble's psychiatric disorder does not signify. What matters are the symptoms of Mr. Noble's condition and the prognosis.' This echoes Gunn and Taylor (1993, pp. 102–103):

> The doctor thus must attempt to determine the existence of any psychiatric disorder and its relation to the incident. The court is more concerned with the existence of disorder in itself, its attribution, and its consequences than with niceties of diagnosis and classification. Diagnostic terms should be used simply and conventionally, but it is unnecessary to follow slavishly definitions from textbooks and glossaries such as DSM III or ICD.

Justify the diagnosis by reference to the psychopathology. Indicate the extent to which the evidence from the medical records and any other corroborative evidence supports the diagnosis. Make clear if the diagnosis is based entirely on self-report. If diagnoses made by other experts are not supported, indicate this and say why. Where there is a range of reasonable opinion, state what other diagnoses may reasonably be made and indicate why yours is to be preferred.

Causation

Identify the conditions or disorders that would not have occurred 'but for' the index event (see Chapter 2, 'The Liability (Breach of Duty and Causation) Report'). Identify those which would have occurred in any event. If there are multiple causes, distinguish them and distinguish between tortious and non-tortious causes. The doctrine of material contribution, which does not apply in Ireland, acknowledges that injury may have several causes which are not divisible. If the injury is indivisible, make this clear.

Beware of percentage apportionments between predisposing factors, the index event and independent precipitating or maintaining factors. It is common to see an apportionment along the lines: 20 per cent genetic predisposition, 20 per cent vulnerability from earlier life experiences, 40 per cent the index event and 20 per cent subsequent independent life experiences. This does not assist. It does not explain what difference the index event has made – 'but for . . . ?' Instead, have one paragraph beginning 'As a result of the accident . . .', then a paragraph beginning 'In the absence of the accident . . .'.

Beware relying on epidemiological evidence to prove causation: 'by its very nature, the statistical evidence does not deal with the individual case' (*Sienkiewicz v Greif (UK) Ltd* [2011] UKSC 10). If you rely on epidemiological evidence, be able to assist as to 'how reliable the evidence is – whether, for example, the study has been properly constructed and, in particular, what the confidence intervals are' because '[w]hat significance a court may attach to (epidemiological evidence) must depend on the nature of the epidemiological evidence'.

Treatment Received and Recommended

This section can often be brief. Set out the form or forms of drug or psychological therapy that have been employed. Make clear if treatment has been insufficient, such as an inadequate antidepressant dosage or too little cognitive behavioural therapy (CBT). Make clear if there is treatment that ought to have been given that has not been given.

If the claimant has not complied with treatment, explain why. So, ask about failure to attend appointments, discontinuation of medication or a frequency of repeat prescriptions which suggests that medication has been missed. This is because a claimant is under a duty to mitigate her loss. A distinction has to be made, by the parties or the court, between the claimant who is simply uncooperative with treatment and one whose failure to comply with treatment is understandable – misunderstandings, appointments at genuinely inconvenient times or places, intolerable drug side effects, difficulty in engaging with the therapist, etc.

If there are outstanding requirements as to treatment, these have to be set out with sufficient detail for the treatment to be costed, as it may need to be obtained independently, and for it to be arranged.

Present Condition

'Present condition' means the severity of the injury in terms of the degree of suffering and impairment of functioning or functional deficit. Although the categories of damage in the Judicial College Guidelines mix up condition and prognosis, it is usually helpful to consult them and ensure that here information is provided as to matters taken into account in deciding the severity of the injury (Box 8.1).

It is then possible to grade the claimant's condition by reference to the categories of severity in the Judicial College Guidelines, but this is not essential and it can be argued that this is for the parties or the court having regard to their evaluation of all of the evidence. Experts have been criticised for not using the classification, and experts have been criticised for doing so! Criticism may be avoided by using the classification and adding your acknowledgement that this is an ultimate issue 'for the parties to agree or for the court to decide' (an often helpful phrase in any report). The categories of psychiatric damage generally and specifically for PTSD are 'severe', 'moderately severe', 'moderate' and 'minor', but the criteria differ slightly.

Box 8.1 Matters Taken into Account by Lawyers and the Courts in Deciding the Severity of the Damage Sustained under the Judicial College Guidelines

(i) the injured person's ability to cope with life and work;
(ii) the effect on the injured person's relationships with family, friends and those with whom he or she comes into contact;
(iii) the extent to which treatment would be successful;
(iv) future vulnerability;
(v) prognosis;
(vi) whether medical help has been sought;
(vii) claims relating to sexual and physical abuse usually include a significant aspect of psychiatric or psychological damage . . . Others have an element of false imprisonment. The fact of an abuse of trust is relevant . . . A further feature, which distinguishes these cases from most involving psychiatric damage, is that there may have been a long period during which the effects of the abuse were undiagnosed, untreated, unrecognized, or even denied. Awards should take into account not only the psychiatric effects of the abuse on the injured party but also the immediate effects of the abuse at the time that it was perpetrated, including feelings of degradation.

Box 8.2 Questions to Guide the Assessment of the Severity of a Given Injury in Ireland

(i) Was the incident which caused the injury traumatic, and if so, how much distress did it cause?
(ii) Did the plaintiff require hospitalisation, and if so, for how long?
(iii) What did the plaintiff suffer in terms of pain and discomfort or lack of dignity during that period?
(iv) What type and number of surgical interventions or other treatments did they require during the period of hospitalisation?
(v) Did the plaintiff need to attend a rehabilitation facility at any stage, and if so, for how long?
(vi) While recovering in their home, was the plaintiff capable of independent living? Were they, for example, able to dress, toilet themselves and otherwise cater to all of their personal needs or were they dependent in all or some respects, and if so, for how long?
(vii) If the plaintiff was dependent, why was this so? Were they, for example, wheelchair-bound, on crutches or did they have their arm in a sling? In respect of what activities were they so dependent?
(viii) What limitations had been imposed on their activities such as leisure or sporting pursuits?
(ix) For how long was the plaintiff out of work?
(x) To what extent was their relationship with their family interfered with?
(xi) Finally, what was the nature and extent of any treatment, therapy or medication required?

Shannon v O'Sullivan [2016] IECA 93

In Ireland, questions to guide the assessment of the severity of an injury were set out in *Shannon v O'Sullivan* [2016] IECA 93 (Box 8.2). The standard form assessment report used by the Injuries Board asks the examining clinician to indicate the degree, if any, to which the claimant's condition is currently affecting their ability in a range of activities, whether normal, mildly, moderately, severely or profoundly impaired. It also asks for the ICD classification of the claimant's disease, and for the reporting clinician to indicate the degree (in 25 per cent quanta) to which they feel the claimant's symptoms/disability have been caused by the index event.

The effect on capacity for work or 'earning capacity' is usually of importance because often the loss of earnings claim is a major, and sometimes the only contentious, element of the sum of compensation claimed. So, state whether the claimant is under a disadvantage on the labour market and whether they are under a disability, as this affects the way in which their future loss of earnings is calculated. To be classified as disabled, three conditions have to be met:

- the claimant has had an illness or disability which has lasted or is expected to last for over a year or is a progressive illness;
- the claimant satisfies the Equality Act 2010 definition that their disability substantially limits their ability to carry out normal day-to-day activities (see Chapter 13, 'Normal Day-to-Day Activities'); and
- the condition affects either the kind or amount of paid work they can do.

The claimant may take longer to find work and they may be unable to do the same work as previously.

Prognosis

Cases cannot go on forever, but if you have not been paid for your report it may seem like it. Cases have to be settled by the parties or decided by the court on the basis of a prediction as to the course and outcome of the claimant's condition, including the award of damages for what might happen in the future. This is often one of the most difficult parts of a condition and prognosis report. It is difficult enough to predict the course and outcome of a psychiatric disorder in clinical practice; it is more so where people know that the level of damages will take into account the duration and outcome of their condition. Here, the test *in England and Wales* is the 'real' likelihood of future events occurring or not occurring.

A further matter that sometimes has to be addressed is the risk of deterioration because in some jurisdictions a judge can award 'provisional damages' where the evidence persuades her that, although the chances of deterioration are less than 50 per cent, there is nevertheless a real risk that a substantial deterioration may occur in the future. Here, lawyers can and do expect percentages, set out for example as a 20 to 30 per cent risk, and accompanied by an estimate of how long the deterioration would last and with what effect on activities of daily living and employment. *In Ireland*, there is no provision at common law for 'provisional awards' and it is not provided for by statute other than in the context of awards made by the Hepatitis C Compensation Tribunal. The possibility of further adverse effects falls to be provided for, insofar as intuitively possible, by the making of a one-off award of damages, based on the probabilities, but noting the non-probable possibilities.

Also indicate whether or not the claimant has been rendered more vulnerable to psychiatric disorder in the future.

When the issue is life expectancy, psychiatrists are likely to identify with the neuropsychiatrist in *Arden v Malcolm* [2007] EWHC 404 (QB) who sought to defer to a medical statistician, declaring that he was 'no expert on matters of life expectancy, although like anybody else in the field I am familiar with the literature, but I am not an epidemiologist, and the mathematics of calculating reduced life expectancy . . . is complicated'. However, the court followed *Royal & Sun Alliance Insurance v T&N Ltd* [2002] EWCA Civ 1964, holding that clinician experts should be the normal and primary route through which statistical evidence should be put before the court. Not least with *Meadow* in mind, psychiatrists ought to decline to give such statistical evidence. Fortunately, *Mays v Drive Force (UK) Ltd* [2019] EWHC 5 (QB) is supportive of such a position, it being held that statistical evidence is admissible in appropriate cases alongside the evidence of clinicians. Appropriate cases were identified as ones in which a number of potential co-morbid factors are in issue. So, in cases where the claimant smokes, is obese or has co-morbid physical diseases, recommend the instruction of a medical statistician.

Clinical Negligence in Mental Healthcare

In a case of allegedly negligent psychiatric care, you are likely to have your attention drawn to what appear to the instructing solicitors to be failings which have resulted in harm to or even death of the patient or others. But consider the case in the round; there may be other unrecognised failures. Begin with a chronology (see Chapter 2, 'The Liability (Breach of Duty and Causation) Report'). Some of the potential issues are set out below.

Standard of Care

Do not set the standard of care too high; it is the standard of the ordinary competent practitioner (*Chin Keow v Government of Malaysia* [1967] 1 WLR 813). Remind yourself of the legal tests for negligence (see Chapter 2, 'The Liability (Breach of Duty and Causation) Report'). Where you identify care which falls below the expected standard, ask if a reasoned case could be made for doing what was done. Anticipate the defence. Try to find a published authority to justify your criticism. Although often asked to cite passages from textbooks, in psychiatry it is the published guidelines and protocols of national bodies and organisations that are most likely to assist, such as Maudsley Prescribing Guidelines, Department of Health publications, Royal College of Psychiatrists guidance and NICE guidelines. Make sure that the guidance existed at the relevant time. Make allowances for how long it takes for new or changed guidance to be implemented. It is also helpful if your criticisms are evidence-based, but beware reliance on NICE quality standards; they are markers of high quality care. Beware guidance that sets out best or even prudent practice; they too set the standard too high. Furthermore, be prepared for cross-examination which 'may extend to the scope of the guidelines, their development, whether they are mandatory or not, known exceptions to their application, and whether any responsible body of medical thought recommends a different approach' (Ellis).

Diagnostic Error

A wrong diagnosis does not necessarily amount to negligence. It may assist the defence in such a case if the correct diagnosis was included in the differential diagnosis and it can be demonstrated why a reasonable, responsible body of psychiatrists would not have made this the preferred diagnosis. Be prepared to explain to the court that establishing a diagnosis in psychiatry is not an exact science and that there can be an overlap between different diagnoses.

The court may need to understand that once a psychiatric diagnosis is made, it is not set in stone, but reviewed regularly and may change if and when new information becomes available. The test is not whether the doctor has made a fully accurate diagnosis, but whether the diagnosis would likely have been made by a body of colleagues and is logical on the information available.

The error may be the misdiagnosis of a physical disease as a psychiatric disorder, delayed diagnosis of a physical disease or failure to diagnose a physical disease. But if the association between the physical disease and the presenting psychiatric symptomatology is little known, this may afford a defence.

The Challenge of Multi-Professional Care

Patients have a right to receive care from someone with suitable skills and knowledge. If an assessment has been done by a trainee, the questions are about the doctor's training and experience and their supervision. Psychiatrists specialise in different areas and there is considerable overlap in training and experience, but all psychiatrists should be competent in their area of practice. If working outside their specialism, they may be required to demonstrate their competency.

Where care is given by someone other than a doctor, having regard to the health professional's training and experience, you may identify shortcomings which it will be advised that an expert from the appropriate profession will need to confirm. In the event that they should have referred the patient to a doctor, your role will be to describe the assessment a psychiatrist would have carried out and indicate what its outcome would have been. Would the outcome have been any different?

The Assessment and Management of Risk

In considering the standard of risk assessment, which often determines not only the pathway into psychiatric care, but decisions as to observation levels, leave and discharge, bear in mind that risk cannot be eliminated. Taking risks is often necessary in order to avoid putting the patient into a therapeutic strait-jacket. This was recognised in *G v Central and North West London Mental Health NHS Trust* [2007] EWHC 3086 (QB):

> Psychiatry – perhaps more than any other branch of medicine – is not an exact science. A doctor practising in this field has to make difficult decisions about the management and treatment of patients suffering from a range of mental illnesses and distress. Many of these decisions inevitably involve the assessment of risk, together with the balancing of any risk which may be present against the benefits of making progress with the patient's rehabilitation.

In this case, the patient was informal and made her way to a railway line where she was hit by a train. The issues included being permitted by medical staff to have periods of unescorted leave from the psychiatric unit provided that she remained on hospital premises and whether the staff's encouragement of her to control herself and to take responsibility for her actions was an appropriate way of managing her very difficult behaviour. In finding in favour of the defendant hospital, the judge made a number of observations which illustrate factors that need to be considered when assessing the quality of risk assessments:

> It is clear from the records that [Dr G] carried out regular reviews of the Claimant's condition and that those reviews included discussions (often quite lengthy discussions) with the Claimant and her husband, as well as with other members of her team. Her reviews were supplemented by reviews made at other times by junior doctors. During the period of the Claimant's admission, Dr G made a number of adjustments to her medication in response to problems that were reported to her. These adjustments continued to be made right up to the time of the Ward Round immediately preceding the Claimant's suicide attempt. She was, in my judgment, making every effort to respond to the Claimant's needs throughout the period of her admission.
>
> There is no doubt that Dr G had the risks associated with leave in mind and that she discussed them with the Claimant and her husband. The medical records make this clear. I accept her evidence that she was seeking to balance those risks against the benefits to the Claimant that a greater degree of freedom would bring.

So, the questions include these. Was the patient's condition kept under regular review by the consultant? Were family members involved in the reviews? Were the views of other team members considered? Was there a junior doctor also reviewing the patient? Was the treatment itself being reviewed with sufficient frequency and in the light of which that treatment was being adjusted? Do the records show evidence of discussion of the balancing of risks and benefits?

It is not simply a matter of using a risk assessment instrument. It is possible adequately to assess risk without using a risk assessment tool or scale. When used, they are not a substitute for common clinical sense and judgement. They are not predictive of suicide or repetition of self-harm. Where an instrument has been used, pay attention to the following. Is the assessment based on all of the information which was, or reasonably should have been, known to those carrying it out? Comparison of the information taken into account with that documented in records which were, or should have been, considered may reveal that risk factors have been overlooked. Has the assessment been updated to take into account new information or changed circumstances? With computerisation of medical records, it is easy to bring forward an assessment giving the impression that it is up to date when in fact it is out of date.

It matters how risk is described. It is insufficient to state that the risk is, for example, 'low' or 'moderate'. A comprehensive risk assessment addresses what might happen, how likely it is to happen, how serious the harm might be, how imminently it might happen, and what makes it more or less likely that the event might occur. This means considering factors that may increase risk and factors that may mitigate against risk and how they can be modified. Where the records reveal that such matters have been carefully considered, it may be possible to defend the risk assessment and management processes as *Bolitho*-defensible because the risk assessment is logically based and the risk management plan is one which it was responsible and reasonable to follow.

To Admit or Not to Admit

In-patient psychiatric care has decreased significantly, as has duration of admissions. This reflects the increasing use of crisis response and home treatment teams which provide intensive support to patients at home as an alternative to admission. Hospital admission is now reserved for the most ill patients who cannot be safely managed at home. If a patient harms themselves or others following an assessment which has not led to a hospital admission, relatives will rightly question whether admission would have prevented this. To answer this question, the quality of the assessment and whether the judgement following that assessment can be justified will be scrutinised.

It is likely to be difficult to prove that a decision not to admit to hospital was negligent due to:

- the expectation that patients will be treated at home where possible;
- the expectation that in considering whether to use mental health legislation the least restrictive options are to be used;
- the recognition that in-patient care rarely offers specific interventions that cannot be delivered in the community.

If a patient is known to be at significant risk to themselves or others and the decision is taken not to admit or to use powers under mental health law, what matters is whether the reasons are set out in the clinical record and whether the decision not to admit was a logical and reasonable decision or one which no clinician acting responsibly would make. It is not acceptable to record that the reason for not admitting a patient was the unavailability of beds or to use risk assessment tools and scales to decide on admission. If the treatment plan fails adequately to address the risks identified, the decision not to admit will be questionable.

Observations

A key decision following and throughout in-patient admission is observation level. All in-patient units will have an observation policy and it is usually helpful to see it. A case may be easier to defend if there has been adherence to the policy, but harder to defend if there has been a failure to adhere to it.

Observation levels vary from general observations through timed observations to constant observations, where patients are within line of sight at all times, and then special observations, where patients are within arm's length. Timed observations are controversial, although they continue to be widely used. Bowers, Gournay and Duffy (2000) offer a useful description of general and constant observation:

> General observation can be thought of as the observation and monitoring of the physical geography of the ward and as a component of constant review of safety in the light of opportunities the ward and its contents provide for harm to come to patients. The general observation should be an established part of ward routine and followed rigorously and regularly by nurses as part of their everyday practice to maintain the safety of patients. Constant observation should be used for patients who are considered to present a significant risk to self or others. An allocated member of staff should be constantly aware at all times of the precise whereabouts of the patient through visual observation or hearing.

The only observations that can prevent suicide are keeping patients in line of sight, but suicide can occur even under such a high level of observation. At all other times, clinicians have to take a risk because there will be times when the patient is not in direct observation of nursing staff. A balance needs to be struck between keeping the patient safe by watching them and the often intrusive and unpleasant nature of being kept under close scrutiny, which can be counter-therapeutic. Current nursing practice is to limit the use of timed observations in favour of using skilled nursing time to engage with the patient and build up a rapport and a relationship in order that the patient will let staff know how they are feeling and if they have suicidal thoughts.

Where the level of observation is an issue, it may be necessary to see not only the observation record, but also take into account the number of staff on the ward, their allocated duties, the number of patients, their observation levels and the timing of sightings of the patient in between scheduled observation times. In some cases, it is possible to show that it was impossible for the staff to have carried out the observations as they claim to have done in their witness statements and as charted. It is sadly not an infrequent finding that observation charts, usually at night, record 'observations' of the patient for a while, sometimes hours, after the time at which the patient has been found hanging or is known to have absconded.

Care in Hospital

Most providers of in-patient care will have standards and protocols which staff are expected to follow and these should be obtained. Central to care delivery in hospital is the care plan. Increasingly, these are not nursing, but multi-professional, care plans. With computerised records, the easy creation of templates and ease of 'copying and pasting', there has been an unfortunate tendency to have standardised care plans, with the result that all patients have the same care plans instead of individualised, holistic care plans, or for patients to have care plans copied and pasted from one review to the next without reflecting the outcome of interventions or changes in their condition or without incorporating changes agreed in the meeting. However, it is one thing to identify such failings and another to prove that they were causative of harm.

Pay attention to family involvement. Families are sometimes not involved at all. Sometimes they are involved, but either insufficient time is allowed for their input or what they have to say is ignored.

Sometimes, communication failures can be identified. Night staff are handed a patient's suicide notes, they are filed away and nothing is communicated at handover to the morning staff. A patient communicates suicidal thoughts to a member of staff, such as an occupational therapist or psychologist, who keeps records separate from the main written or computerised record and fails to report this to the nursing staff or, if it is reported, it is not recorded or mentioned at handover.

Medication errors can give rise to clinical negligence allegations. So, consider choice of medication, dose, combinations used and monitoring, in particular for common side effects. The drug administration chart may reveal that medication has been repeatedly refused, but this has not been reported to the clinical team. Assessment of capacity to consent to take prescribed medication may be in issue.

Leave and Discharge from Hospital

Leave, either accompanied or unaccompanied, is a time of increased risk. Were leave decisions made by a multidisciplinary team involving senior clinicians? It is usual for there to be an assessment of the patient prior to going on leave and on return to ensure no new risk issues have emerged. Decisions about discharge should be made on a similar basis. Did the decision involve patients and their immediate family, where appropriate, and community staff who were going to be responsible for the patient's care following discharge? There may be evidence of a breakdown of communication on discharge. A discharge care plan that reads 'care coordinator', followed by a failure to appoint a care coordinator, is anything but a care plan.

As the greatest risk of suicide following discharge from hospital is in the first two weeks, there is an expectation that all patients discharged from hospital are followed up within seven days and for those at high risk within forty-eight hours. Check that this is not simply a tick-box exercise, but a planned meeting at which the patient is able to talk about their experience since discharge and how they are feeling, and a thorough and professional assessment is made of current suicidal intent.

Care in the Community

Whether or not formally registered under the 'Care Programme Approach', look for evidence that its principles have been applied: an identified care coordinator or key worker whose identity and contact details were known to the patient and family or carers, who saw the patient sufficiently often; a plan of care tailored to the patient's needs, sufficiently frequently reviewed and amended; and a crisis plan, including relapse indicators, known to the patient, family or carers and those expected to deliver the care.

Employment Stress

Walker v Northumberland County Council [1995] 1 All ER 737 established that an employer could be held liable in damages for psychiatric injury caused by employment stress. Cases

Box 8.3 Likely Issues in an Employment Stress Case

- Has the claimant suffered an injury to health (as distinct from occupational stress)?
- Is the psychiatric injury attributable to stress at work as distinct from other causes?
- If there are other causes for the employee's psychiatric injury, can it be obviously inferred that the employer's breach(es) of duty made more than a minimal contribution to the psychiatric injury?
- Is there evidence that the employer knew of some particular problem or vulnerability such that he was not entitled to assume that the employee could withstand the normal pressures of the job? Because of the nature of mental disorder, it may be easier to foresee in a known individual than in the population at large.
- Is the workload much more than is normal for the particular job?
- Is the work particularly intellectually or emotionally demanding for the employee?
- Are the demands being made of the employee unreasonable when compared with the demands made of others in the same or comparable jobs?
- Has the employee already suffered from illness attributable to stress at work?
- Have there recently been frequent or prolonged absences which are uncharacteristic of the employee, or something such as a request for a sabbatical, and, if so, is there reason to think that these are attributable to stress at work – for example, because of complaints or warnings from him to others?
- Having regard to any pre-existing disorder or vulnerability, would the employee have succumbed to a stress-related disorder in any event?

Based on *Hatton* and *Dickins*

such as *Hartman v South Essex Mental Health and Community Care NHS Trust* [2005] EWCA Civ 6 established that liability for psychiatric injury caused by stress at work is in general no different in principle from liability for physical injury.

Box 8.3 sets out the issues that usually have to be addressed in employment stress cases based on the relevant guidelines of Hale LJ in *Hatton v Sutherland* [2002] EWCA Civ 76 and as modified by *Dickins v O2* [2008] EWCA Civ 1144. Note the following. The test is the same whatever the nature of the employment, as no occupations should be regarded as intrinsically dangerous to mental health. It is necessary to take into account the nature and the extent of the work done by the employee – for example, whether the workload is more than is normal for that particular job, whether the work is particularly intellectually or emotionally demanding, or demands are being made of the employee that are unreasonable compared to the demands made of others in the same or comparable jobs. An aetiological formulation will be necessary, but the psychiatrist will avoid difficult questions of apportionment of causes on a fractional or percentage basis.

At common law, in contrast to the position under the Protection from Harassment Act 1997 (PHA) and the Equality Act 2010 (see Chapter 13, 'Statutory Law'), the claimant must prove that the defendant reasonably foresaw psychiatric damage: 'The defendant will be deemed liable for those consequences . . . only if they were caused by his failure to take precautions against a foreseen or foreseeable and legally relevant danger' (*Pratley v Surrey County Council* [2003] EWCA Civ 1067) and foreseeability depends on what the employer knew or ought to have known about the individual employee (*Hatton*). It is foreseeable injury flowing from the employer's breach of duty that gives rise to the liability. It does not follow that because a claimant suffers stress at work and that the employer is in some way in breach of duty in allowing that to occur that the claimant is able to establish a claim in negligence. It is not enough to show that occupational stress has caused the harm:

> Many, alas, suffer breakdowns and depressive illnesses and a significant proportion could doubtless ascribe some at least of their problems to the strains and stresses of their work situation: be it simply overworking, the tension of difficult relationships, career prospect worries, fears or feelings of discrimination or harassment, to take just some examples. Unless, however, there was a real risk of breakdown which the claimant's employers ought reasonably to have foreseen and they ought properly to have averted there can be no liability. (*Garrett v Camden LBC* [2001] EWCA Civ 395)

Where reasonable foreseeability is required, you may have to address the issues of vulnerability or predisposition to psychiatric injury. If the employer knew or ought to have known of an employee's vulnerability to stress, he owes a greater duty of care to his employee (*Walker*); if he was not made aware of it, he is entitled to assume that the employee can cope with the normal stresses and strains of working life. The employer is generally entitled to take what he is told by his employee at face value, unless he has good reason to think to the contrary. He does not generally have to make searching enquiries of the employee or seek permission to make further enquiries of his medical advisors.

An employer cannot be said to have been in a position to foresee psychiatric injury where an employee had disclosed information about their mental condition in confidence to the occupational health department as no other employee had a right of access to that information without the employee's consent (*Hartman*).

The employer is only in breach of duty if he has failed to take the steps, which are reasonable in the circumstances, to prevent injury to the employee. In all cases, it is necessary to identify the steps which the employer both could and should have taken before finding him in breach of his duty of care and the court is likely to need expert evidence on these matters. But an employer who offers a confidential advice service, with referral to appropriate counselling or treatment services, is unlikely to be found in breach of duty.

Historical Child Abuse

In cases of HCA, three issues are particularly likely to engage the expert: limitation (see also above, 'Limitation'), consent and causation.

Limitation

As was recognised in *Hoare*: 'These perpetrators have many ways, some subtle and some not so subtle, of making their victims keep quiet about what they have suffered. The abuse itself is the reason why so many victims do not come forward until years after the event.'

The expert may be able to help the court understand how a perpetrator can continue to exert an influence over the victim. This is especially likely in male-on-male abuse where the victim is a teenager. There may be a power imbalance which leads to the claimant's silence, such as where the abuse is perpetrated by someone in a position of authority or dominance. The claimant may have been so well-groomed that they do not appreciate that what was done was wrong. The expert can explain how the effects of the abuse may have prevented the complainant from taking steps to bring their claim – for example, by making it difficult or impossible to explain what happened, perhaps through shame or embarrassment. Alcohol and drug misuse may not only be a consequence of the abuse – they may also be used to repress memories. Mental ill health can contribute to an inability to address past trauma.

It is often the case that a complaint has been made about the abuse to the police or other authority figures and no appropriate action has been taken. This can explain unwillingness or reluctance to bring forward a claim. The potential claimant may fear that again they will not be believed. They may want to avoid the distress or worsening of their mental condition that will result.

So, often, children who have been abused grow into adulthood using alcohol or drugs or both to cope with the consequences of the abuse. But alcohol and substance misuse or dependence and other mental disorders can make it difficult for them to bring claims.

Care is needed in exploring such a history. In *Wilde v Coventry City Council* [2017] 3 WLUK 750, when it was submitted on behalf of the claimant that past experiences of repeatedly complaining and no action being taken was the main or principal reason for not bringing forward a claim earlier in her adult life and there was no evidence of this until the preparation of a psychiatric report, it was submitted on behalf of the defendant that she got the idea from the psychiatrist and not the other way round.

This case also illustrates the need to take into account the content of the medical records. The judge held that even though she may have been disbelieved as a young girl, in her 20s and 30s, her medical records revealed no difficulty discussing the general topic of sexual abuse and some details with her medical advisors, thus indicating that she was able to make complaints and discuss the abuse when she needed to do so. Nevertheless, she was allowed to bring her claim out of time on the grounds that there was an understandable delay in that effectively she was unaware of the possibility of bringing a civil claim. In another case, where a claimant told the psychiatrist it was embarrassment and shame which explained the delay in bringing her case, this was called somewhat into question, as her medical records documented that she did not feel guilty about what had happened.

Where the claimant has sought and received treatment of a psychological or psychotherapeutic nature that has involved making a connection between early life experiences and difficulties in adult life, the psychiatric expert may need to assist in the interpretation of records that may shed light on when the claimant became aware of a psychiatric injury attributable in whole or in part to the abuse or when they should have asked their therapist or another suitable person whether they had suffered psychiatric damage as a result of the abuse. Where the claimant has suffered a multitude of adverse events and circumstances and where the therapy is not for what has been diagnosed at the outset as a specific psychiatric disorder, it cannot be assumed that seeking therapy in itself is proof of 'actual knowledge' or receipt of therapy that 'makes the links' is proof of 'constructive knowledge'.

Consent

It is a potential obstacle in an HCA case that, in the civil courts, claimants can be deemed to have consented in fact, even if they are below the age of criminal consent at the time of the abuse. Psychiatric evidence may be necessary to the effect that a consequence of grooming can be for a child to continue to engage in sexual acts with their abuser beyond the age of criminal consent and well into adulthood. However, *in Ireland*, the 'consent' of a minor below the age prescribed by the criminal law is irrelevant.

Causation

Causation is often a crucial problem in HCA cases. In many HCA cases where the abuse has occurred to a claimant in care and the case is against those providing that care, the fact that the claimant was taken into care as a result of abandonment, neglect, violence or sexual abuse and arrives in a highly disturbed state requires consideration to be given to the relative effects of what necessitated the claimant going into care and the abuse suffered in care. There is the further complication of the claimant leaving care and deteriorating into alcohol and drug misuse and crime.

In such cases, some experts suggest a percentage apportionment. An expert in *B v Nugent Care Society* [2009] EWCA Civ 827 estimated that 'the attribution can be divided 60% pre-care, 20% alleged abuse in care and 20% the process of being in care generally', but this seemed to the court to be 'a throwaway and clearly very approximate conclusion'. What the court concluded was that:

> There can be no doubt that these are extremely difficult waters. The debate as to the proper degree of emphasis to place on genetic inheritance, the effect of early childhood and personality development in the childhood environment, the contribution of rather later adverse experiences of an extreme kind, undergone whilst yet in early life, are questions which can never be solved in a case such as this. In my judgment, one is on surer ground in concluding that all of these components may have a major effect; that the effect may vary greatly from individual to individual and that it is difficult to draw any precise conclusions from the scientific literature.

The interplay of causal factors was also addressed in *Irvine v Sisters of Nazareth* [2015] NIQB 94. The court found that it was 'not a case where the Plaintiff can establish that as a result of tortious acts by the defendant she has suffered an actual psychiatric injury. At best she has been rendered vulnerable to psychiatric injury and that injury has materialised because of other stressors in her life.' But a vulnerability may still sound in damages.

Nervous Shock

The Law

There is a form of psychiatric injury which the law calls 'nervous shock'. Two leading cases provide definitions (Box 8.4). Both make it clear that there has to be a psychiatric illness or what was described in *McLoughlin v O'Brian* [1983] 1 AC 410 as 'not merely grief, distress or any other normal emotion, but a positive psychiatric illness'. Shock, on its own, and in the lay sense, anxiety or depression as symptoms but not amounting to psychiatric illness, disappointment or grief, unless pathological, do not amount to 'nervous shock' as defined. There has to be something more than what are regarded as normal or ordinary emotional responses to events:

> In English law no damages are awarded for grief and sorrow caused by a person's death. No damages are to be given for worry about the children, or for the financial strain or stress, or the difficulties of adjusting to a new life. Damages are however recoverable for nervous shock, or to put it in medical terms, for any recognisable psychiatric illness caused by the breach of duty of the defendant. (*Hinz v Berry* [1970] 2 QB 40)

Box 8.4 'Nervous Shock'

> I understand 'shock' in this context to mean the sudden sensory perception – that is, by seeing, hearing or touching – of a person, thing or event, which is so distressing that the perception of the phenomenon affronts or insults the claimant's mind and causes a recognizable psychiatric illness.
>
> Brennan J in *Jaensch v Coffey* (1984) 155 CLR 549

> 'Shock' in the context of this cause of action, involves the sudden appreciation by sight or sound of a horrifying event, which violently agitates the mind. It has yet to include psychiatric illness caused by the accumulation over a period of time or more gradual assaults on the nervous system.
>
> Lord Ackner in *Alcock v Chief Constable of South Yorkshire* [1992] 1 AC 310

As Lord Oliver put it in *Alcock v Chief Constable of South Yorkshire Police* [1992] 1 AC 310: 'grief, sorrow, deprivation and the necessity for caring for loved ones who have suffered injury or misfortune must, I think, be considered as ordinary and inevitable incidents of life which, regardless of individual susceptibilities, must be sustained without compensation'. It follows that '[o]nly recognisable psychiatric harm ranks for consideration. Where the line is to be drawn is a matter for expert psychiatric evidence' (*White v Chief Constable of South Yorkshire* [1998] 3 WLR 1509).

Policy decisions of the courts limit the extent to which what are known as 'secondary victims' can recover damages for psychiatric injury. The difference between 'primary' and 'secondary' victims was addressed in the Hillsborough Stadium football ground disaster case of football ground disaster case of *Alcock v Chief Constable of the South Yorkshire Police* [1992] 1 AC 310. A 'primary victim' was defined as someone 'who is involved either mediately or immediately as a participant in an accident' and a secondary victim as someone who is 'no more than a passive and unwilling witness of an injury to another'.

The Control Mechanisms

The limits set as a matter of policy are known as 'control mechanisms' (Box 8.5). They exist to control the floodgates without which 'the number of secondary victims who would be able to bring successful nervous shock claims would be virtually limitless' (*Shorter v Surrey and Sussex Healthcare NHS Trust* [2015] EWHC 614). But the reasoning in some of the decisions is odd, resulting in 'a patchwork quilt of distinctions which are hard to justify' (*White*).

The term 'nervous shock' is somewhat unfortunate, as the courts recognise: 'The term "nervous shock" can be misleading. It does not mean that the "shock" is the psychiatric injury caused to the claimant; what it means is that the claimant is claiming damages for the psychiatric injury caused by the shocking event' (*Shorter*).

So, the issue is not just diagnosis as such, but also as to aetiology and causation. The essential causal elements are the suddenness of the experience, its horrifying nature and its direct perception through senses such as sight, hearing or touch, which is not dissimilar to the exceptionally threatening or catastrophic nature of the threshold criterion in PTSD, as the courts have recognised: 'To describe an event as shocking in common parlance is to use

Box 8.5 The Control Mechanisms

1. The claimant must have a close tie of love and affection with the person killed, injured or imperilled ('the dearness test')
2. The claimant's illness must have resulted from a sudden and unexpected shock to the claimant's nervous system ('the nervous shock test')
3. The claimant must have been either personally present at the scene of the incident or witnessed the aftermath shortly afterwards ('the nearness test')
4. The claimant must have directly perceived the incident rather than, for example, heard about it from a third person ('the perception test')
5. The injury suffered must have arisen from witnessing the death of, extreme danger to, or injury and discomfort suffered by, the primary victim ('the causation test')
6. There must have been a close temporal connection between the incident and the claimant's perception of it ('the temporal test')
7. The claimant must have suffered frank psychiatric illness or injury ('the diagnostic test')

Rix and Cory-Wright 2018

an epithet so devalued that it can embrace a very wide range of circumstances. But the sense in which it is used in the diagnostic criteria for PTSD must carry more than that colloquial meaning' (HHJ Simon Hawkesworth QC in *Ward v Leeds Teaching Hospitals NHS Trust* [2004] EWHC 2106).

Suddenness

The suddenness criterion is not satisfied where the person has some warning and gradually cumulative events will not satisfy. In *Sion v Hampstead Health Authority* [1994] 5 WLUK 348, the claimant failed to recover damages when his son died fourteen days after a road traffic accident. He stayed at his son's bedside, watched his deterioration, and saw him fall into a coma and die. He witnessed a process that continued for some time. When death occurred, it was not surprising, but expected. Likewise, in another unsuccessful case, where a 14-year-old boy died following an accident, his parents experienced 'a dawning consciousness that they were going to lose him' (*Taylorson v Shieldness Produce Ltd* [1994] 2 WLUK 173). In *Alcock*, it was held that nervous shock was yet to include psychiatric illness caused by the accumulation over a period of time of more gradual assaults on the nervous system.

Lewis (2006), however, has observed that in *Sion* there did appear to have been some discrete, 'shocking' events, including a sudden deterioration, sudden respiratory difficulties, cardiac arrest and transfer to the intensive care unit. So, the judgment in *Sion* is to be contrasted with that in *Tredget v Bexley Health Authority* [1994] 5 Med LR 178, where the judge held that the two-day period beginning with the traumatic birth of a fatally injured baby and culminating in its death was a single, frightening and harrowing event. Likewise, in *North Glamorgan NHS Trust v Walters* [2002] EWCA Civ 1792, it was held that 'there was an inexorable progression . . . a seamless tale with an obvious beginning and an equally obvious end . . . played out over a period of 36 hours . . . one drawn-out experience'.

Horrifying

The horrifying criterion is not satisfied where the distressing experience does not agitate the mind violently. In *Ward*, the claimant's descriptions of what she witnessed did not strike the judge as shocking at the time, although, undoubtedly, they were distressing. The experience had to be wholly exceptional: 'An event outside the range of human experience does not encompass the death of a loved one in hospital unless accompanied by circumstances which were wholly exceptional in some way so as to shock or horrify.'

Thus, in *Liverpool Women's Hospital NHS Foundation Trust v Ronayne* [2015] EWCA Civ 588, the court found that 'the appearance of Mrs Ronayne on this occasion must have been both alarming and distressing to the Claimant, but it was not in context exceptional and it was not I think horrifying in the sense in which that word has been used in the authorities'. Furthermore, what is 'horrifying' has to be judged by objective standards and by reference to persons of ordinary susceptibility (*Owers v Medway NHS Foundation Trust* [2015] EWHC 2363 (QB)). What Mr Ronayne saw was not horrifying by objective standards.

Perception

Hearing about the event in a telephone call will not satisfy the direct perception criterion (*Brock v Northampton General Hospital Trust* [2014] EWHC 4244). The shock must come through sight or hearing of the event or of its immediate aftermath.

Sudden and Shocking

The frank psychiatric injury and nervous shock elements go together to form the requirement, (1) that the event should be not just sufficiently sudden and shocking, but that it should also in fact cause the psychiatric injury and (2) that it should do so because of its sudden and shocking nature.

Foreseeability

A further control mechanism is reasonable foreseeability. In *Page v Smith* [1996] AC 155 (albeit a case of psychiatric injury suffered by a *primary* victim – that is, as a result of perceived danger to himself), reasonable foreseeability was specifically defined as a control mechanism. Thus, for there to be a breach of duty, the circumstances must be such that a person of what the law terms 'normal fortitude' or 'ordinary phlegm' might suffer psychiatric injury by shock. So, it must have been reasonably foreseeable that a person of normal fortitude would be affected by what occurred. However, someone who is not of normal fortitude or ordinary phlegm may recover damages (whether as a primary or as a secondary victim) because 'once it is established that a person of normal phlegm would suffer psychiatric injury, then the fact that the victim has suffered unusually badly because of previous vulnerability means that the normal "eggshell skull" or "thick skull" rule of remoteness of damage applies, so that the susceptible plaintiff may recover for the full extent of the illness' (Marshall *et al.* 2012).

Normal Fortitude

Thus, the person of normal fortitude test is used to establish the threshold in terms of *breach*. If the threshold is reached, a person who is not of normal fortitude may have a claim albeit that but for their vulnerability they might not have suffered psychiatric injury. If they have suffered more injury as a result of their vulnerability, their damages are not limited to those which a person of normal fortitude would have been awarded.

Causation

Causation is often problematic. It is easy for defendants to argue, and difficult for claimants to disprove, that the psychiatric harm has been caused by the death of the loved one and

Box 8.6 Guidance for Expert Psychiatric Witnesses in Secondary Victim Cases

- Explore the claimant's reaction to past traumatic experiences.
- Explore the claimant's relationship with the primary victim, paying particular attention to close ties of love and affection.
- Create a timeline and explore experiences, thoughts and feelings step by step, noting any changes in the claimant's mental state as they describe these.
- Look for evidence that the perception has been conditioned or informed by information received in advance and by way of preparation.
- Identify as far as possible the cause of any shock – the triggering event (taking into account the content of nightmares and intrusive phenomena, such as flashbacks).
- Consider whether the triggering event is sufficiently sudden and shocking – an objective test – would it be expected to cause psychiatric injury to a person of 'customary phlegm' and 'normal fortitude'?
- Is there evidence of susceptibility to psychiatric harm?
- Is there a frank psychiatric disorder? If so, what is the diagnosis?
- Ask whether the psychiatric illness can be ascribed to (1) a particular sudden, unexpected and shocking event and (2) the sudden, unexpected and shocking nature of that event.
- Consider and, if necessary, take into account, the possibility that it was some other response, such as extreme grief, that caused the illness.
- Be able to 'subtract' what would have occurred if there had been no sudden, horrifying event.

would have occurred in any event, whether or not they had witnessed the tragedy or its immediate aftermath. Causal analysis depends in part on knowing the normal reactions, for example, of parents to a stillbirth, an early neonatal death, the sudden accidental death of a 2-year-old child or the death of an 18-year-old child. It depends in part on understanding the unique history of the claimant so as to explain, if it be possible, why they have reacted the way in which they have.

Assessment

Box 8.6 sets out the guidance for the assessment of secondary victim cases.

History

The claimant's previous psychiatric history and personality has to be explored. A secondary victim has to show that he was not unusually susceptible to psychiatric harm of the kind in question (*Bourhill v Young* [1943] AC 92) unless the trigger event would have caused psychiatric harm in a person of normal fortitude.

Some of the most important facts in the case will usually be the claimant's experiences following the tortious event. So, when the claimant is sufficiently settled, carefully obtain a chronological account of what they experienced, paying attention to what they actually perceived by sight, sound or through other senses at the time rather than what they later learned (the event or its components), the suddenness or otherwise of the perception, through what senses (sight, hearing, touch, etc.) the event or component was perceived and whether directly or indirectly, and what effect the perception had on them at the time. The thoughts and feelings, physical (such as autonomic manifestations of anxiety) as well as emotional, may assist as to the extent to which the mind was violently agitated, affronted or insulted. Where events are played out over a period of time, establish how the claimant was affected at each point in time. This may form part of a forensic analysis of the different accounts that the claimant gives of their experiences. Take into account the claimant's reaction, or otherwise, to previous shocking experiences and if the case goes to trial the claimant's mental state when giving evidence in court as to their experiences.

Diagnosis

Diagnosis needs very careful attention: 'Close attention to diagnostic criteria is in my view likely ... to be of assistance in resolving what are often complex questions of causation' (*Ronayne*). A clear distinction should be made between positive psychiatric illness and states of anxiety, depression, stress, grief, etc. that do not amount to a psychiatric disorder.

Causal Analysis

By reference, if possible, to psychopathology such as the content of nightmares, flashbacks or other intrusive phenomena, it will be necessary to give an opinion as to whether, on a balance of probabilities, it was the sudden, unexpected and shocking nature of that event, or one or more of its components, that caused the identified psychiatric injury. In the alternative, the opinion may be that it was some other response such as extreme grief that caused the psychiatric injury. These are not mutually exclusive scenarios. A claimant may suffer PTSD as a consequence of the nervous shock and a complicated grief reaction which would have occurred even if they had not been exposed to the shocking event or events. The causal analysis may be further complicated by the need to take into account pre-existing vulnerability, adverse events and circumstances coincidental with, or subsequent to, and independent of, the index event and non-tortious aspects of the index event, such as, for example in an obstetric case, the 'ordinary' stress and anxiety associated with childbirth.

Such a complex aetiology can be a particular challenge because, in theory at least, the court needs to know whether the psychiatric injury was caused simply by the shocking nature of the events, or by other factors, or by some combination. Each case currently has to be resolved on its own facts and merits. One possible answer would be for the law to adopt and apply here the concept of 'material contribution'. So, the claimant would recover if they can show that the sudden shock of the objectively shocking event made a material contribution to their psychiatric condition, even where it is impossible to disentangle the strands of the complex aetiology concerned.

In answering questions as to causation, it should then be possible to identify one or more sufficiently shocking or horrifying events. If part or all of the psychiatric injury would have occurred even in the absence of the shocking event or events, this needs to be made clear. However, it may be sufficient for the claimant to show no more than that the event or events made a material contribution to the psychiatric illness.

Mere Mental or Emotional Distress

There are a number of circumstances in which compensation may be awarded for what has been termed 'mere mental or emotional distress' (Handford 2006). The torts of trespass to the person – battery and false imprisonment – can attract compensation for the mental distress occasioned. Examples are: anger and indignation at unnecessary dental treatment (*Appleton v Garrett* [1995] 7 WLUK 344); the reaction to being forcibly ejected from *Harrods* (*Corr v Harrods Ltd* [1999] EWCA 2381 Civ); manhandling and assault by police officers followed by wrongful detention in a police cell for four hours (*Thompson v Commissioner of Police for the Metropolis* [1998] QB 498); and a ship's steward wrongly accused of indecently assaulting a child and locked up until the *Queen Elizabeth* docked in New York (*Hook v Cunard SS Co. Ltd* [1953] 1 WLR 682). The hurt feelings of tenants wrongly evicted by their landlords can attract damages (*Drane v Evangelou* [1978] 1 WLR 455). In *Khodaparast v Shad* [2000] 1 WLR 618, damages were awarded to a woman whose former lover caused her distress by using photographs of her in advertisements in pornographic magazines. In *Batty v Metropolitan Realisations Ltd* [1978] QB 554, damages were awarded for injury to a householder's peace of mind caused by the imminent collapse of the house.

Damages can also be awarded for mental distress resulting from a breach of contract. In *Jarvis v Swans Tours Ltd* [1973] QB 233, a solicitor was compensated for the injured feelings brought about by a disappointing holiday. A case in which a photographer failed to turn up to take photographs of the pursuer's wedding led to a successful award for mental distress (*Diensen v Samsom*, 1971 SLT 49). Damages have even been awarded for the distress caused by selling someone a faulty car (*Bernstein v Pamson Motors (Golders Green Ltd)* [1987] 2 ALL ER 220). They may also be awarded for a breach of constitutional rights (*Sullivan v Boylan (No. 1)* [2012] IEHC 389; *Sullivan v Boylan (No. 2)* [2013] IEHC 104).

The PHA provides for an award for any anxiety caused by what is now the tort of harassment.

It is arguable that when it comes to ordinary feelings, hurt or upset or 'mere mental or emotional distress', the courts should not turn to experts in psychiatry. Arguably, these are matters within the experience of judges (and juries). If an expert is needed, it should be a psychologist who is an expert on normal human behaviour. However, expert psychiatric evidence may be necessary if only to make the distinction between mere mental or emotional distress and actual psychiatric illness.

Exaggeration and Malingering

In England and Wales, under the Criminal Justice and Courts Act 2015, s 57, and *in Ireland*, under the Civil Liability and Courts Act 2004, s 26, a claimant will not recover any damages if they are found to have been dishonest in relation to their claim. However, some lawyers have been known to advise their clients about the symptoms of PTSD. It is therefore necessary to give some careful consideration to exaggeration and malingering.

The credibility of the claimant is a matter for the court. Furthermore, 'malingering' is not a diagnosis or mental disorder and it has no legal definition. In *Turner v Jordan* [2010] EWHC 1508 (QB), the judge said of one expert that it was 'to her credit, as it seems to me, [that she] does not agree that malingering is a psychological condition' and he observed: 'All the DSM-IV-TR definition of malingering appears to do is expand the dictionary definition and to classify what is in fact dishonest behaviour as a psychological condition.' Psychiatrists have no special skills enabling them to tell whether someone is genuine. So, avoid describing the claimant as appearing genuine or commenting that she did not seem to be exaggerating. To state that the claimant has endorsed symptoms and psychological problems in a manner which is highly consistent with individuals honestly reporting their difficulties may be no more than testimony to their skills in deception. Sooner or later, you will be provided with conclusive evidence that what appeared to be a genuine case is nothing but the sort. How often is it the case that incontrovertible covert surveillance evidence of malingering is disclosed in cases described as 'genuine' by medical experts!

The psychiatrist's role is to assist the court in deciding whether a disorder is manufactured, exaggerated or otherwise misrepresented. This is more difficult than for other experts, as most psychiatric disorders encountered in personal injury litigation depend for their diagnosis entirely or mainly on reported symptoms rather than objective signs. Psychiatrists, however, do have expert knowledge and experience of the natural history of psychiatric disorders, in particular the evolution, onset and course of symptoms, typical and atypical presentations, patterns of symptomatology and co-morbidity, the relationship between symptoms and signs and their usual impact on personal, social and occupational functioning.

Dr Ian Bronks has regard to: (1) whether the symptoms of which complaint is made are inherently improbable; (2) discrepancies between the statements made by the claimant and the facts or probable facts as revealed by other evidence; (3) discrepancies between statements made by the claimant at different times about their condition; (4) their demeanour on interview – this last area probably being the least important.

Similar points are made by Rogers (2008): (1) a tendency to endorse more blatant than subtle symptoms; (2) a tendency to endorse an unlikely number of symptoms with extreme and unbearable severity; (3) difficulty distinguishing symptoms that are infrequent in psychiatric populations from those that are more common and often endorsing many rare symptoms; (4) unawareness of the incongruities between their actual presentation and reported impairment, which is similar to the point in DSM5 about a '[m]arked discrepancy between a person's claimed stress or disability and the objective findings and observations'; (5) an eagerness to discuss, or an elaboration of, symptoms or an obvious response set; (6) difficulty remembering symptoms previously endorsed and their severity so repeating a set of clinical enquiries, even in the course of a single consultation, measures the stability of the response set.

Other suggested indicators are lack of cooperation with assessment, particularly a significant difference between how the claimant cooperates with his own and the defendant's experts, and failure to accept treatment or comply with treatment recommended or prescribed. However, the vast majority of those who exaggerate or misrepresent their psychiatric condition are just as pleasant and cooperative with assessment and treatment as others. Furthermore, allowance has to be made for the attitude of an expert which can persuade a claimant to be awkward and also for the effects of brain damage.

Reliance on the claimant's demeanour can be problematic in other respects. Some experts rely on: hostility from the claimant; refusal to answer simple questions; responses in history-taking that are defensive or unelaborated; frequent 'don't know' answers; disparaging remarks; and refusal to attempt certain tests. However, there is no evidence to justify reliance on these and such behaviour may be a consequence of the adversarial litigation process.

Evidence from other experts may assist, in particular psychologists. Psychological testing may include symptom validity tests, tests with internal symptom validity indicators, and tests of effort and malingering, but performance can be influenced by memory impairment, dementia, education, IQ and age. Psychological expertise is necessary to interpret such test results. Leave to the psychologists the tests which only they are qualified to administer, score, interpret and defend in cross-examination. But you can refer to the opinions of other experts as being consistent, if they are, with your opinion on fabrication or exaggeration. Hints as to fabrication may be found in unexpected places. In an industrial accident case, the claimant's credibility was called into question when filed in his medical records, without comment by his general practitioners, was a report on his 'kidney stone': 'Appearance: rock-hard brown pebble fragment. Composition: Non-biological in origin; probably early Jurassic'!

Conclude any opinion as to fabrication or exaggeration by pointing to the subjectivity and fallibility of such an opinion and acknowledge that this will be an ultimate issue for the parties or the court and your role is no more than to assist. Aim 'to assist the court with a dispassionate, logical, sequential account of those factors that support, and those that go against, a true diagnosis, and their relative strengths; actively identifying confounders and areas of conflict, ambiguity, and uncertainty; and accepting the limitations of one's knowledge and expertise' (Rix and Tracy 2017).

Beware that some lawyers are deeply uneasy about experts giving evidence as to malingering. This is especially in circumstances where the claimant does not know that this is what is being examined by specialised testing, where the accredited tester is under an obligation to those by whom he is licensed to administer the tests not to reveal the test details, thus preventing their necessary scrutiny by the parties, other experts and the court, and where tests cannot be challenged as to validity, sensitivity, specificity or confounding variables.

What you cannot do is to ignore the issue or side-step it by stating boldly that it is a matter for the court. Ultimately, all facts, inferences and opinions are a matter for the court. However, some of these require expert assistance.

Further Reading

Buchan, A. (gen. ed) (2019) *Lewis and Buchan: Clinical Negligence. A Practical Guide*, 8th edn (Bloomsbury Professional).

Handford, P. (2006) *Mullany and Handford's Tort Liability for Psychiatric Damage*, 2nd edn (Lawbook Co).

Marshall, D., Kennedy, J. and Azib, R. (2012) *Litigating Psychiatric Injury Claims* (Bloomsbury Professional).

Powers, M. and Barton, A. (2015) *Clinical Negligence*, 5th edn (Bloomsbury Professional).

Reports for Family Proceedings Relating to Children

Keith Rix, Rajan Nathan and Karl Rowley QC

Family judges deal with increasingly difficult child cases and are much assisted in their decision-making process by professionals from other disciplines: medical, wider mental health and social work among others. The courts pay particular attention to the valuable contribution from paediatricians and child psychiatrists as well as others, but it is important to remember that the decision is that of the judge and not of the professional expert.

Butler Sloss LJ in *Re. B (A Minor) (Care: Expert Witnesses)* [1996] 1 FLR 667

Public Law Proceedings

In England and Wales, public law proceedings, sometimes also known as care proceedings, usually involve an application by a local authority to take a child or children temporarily or permanently into its care. To do so, threshold conditions have to be met. Pursuant to the Children Act 1989, s 31(2), the court has to be satisfied that the child was suffering, or was likely to suffer, 'significant harm' which was attributable to the parent(s). If so satisfied, it has to be better for the child to make an order, than to make no order, and it has to be in the child's best interests.

Re L (A Child) (Care: Threshold Criteria) [2007] 1 FLR 2050 (Fam Div) illustrates how the threshold criteria were applied in a case involving intellectually disabled parents (Box 9.1). In such cases, the critical issue is 'significant harm'. In *Buckinghamshire CC v CB* (Family Court, unreported, 23 July 2015), it was held that continual care by the intellectually disabled mother would be harmful to, and the level of support required by the mother to care for, her child, who had a global developmental delay, would have been so extreme as to be detrimental to his welfare.

Commenting on *Re L (A Child) (Care: Threshold Criteria)*, Dimopoulos (2009) has expressed concern 'that the judicial reasoning focused selectively on specific facts of the case in relation to the harm the children were suffering, rather than addressing the parents' disability' and has submitted that 'the element of disability requires a different approach from the court'. Such an approach, he submits, is suggested by the case of *Kutzner v Germany (46544/99)* [2003] 1 FCR 249 (ECHR). Therefore, the first step should be to provide intensive and individually tailored support to intellectually disabled parents and if this fails the second step is for social care to take a more active role in the children's upbringing and care in order to avoid compulsory intervention. Only where harm to their welfare is so great that it disturbs the balance between the competing interests of the parents exercising their parental care, free of interferences, and harm to the children's welfare should judicial intervention occur with the possibility of removal from parental care.

Box 9.1 Application of the 'Threshold Criteria' to Parenting by Intellectually Disabled Parents

The intellectually disabled parents received support from social services for a number of years. The family came to their attention when the elder child was sexually assaulted by an offender whom the father had invited to stay at the family home. Subsequently, there were allegations of domestic violence inflicted on the mother by the father and an allegation that the father had been beating the children with a belt. So the children were removed from the family home under an emergency protection order. There was also evidence of worrying instances of lack of boundaries between parents and children; bad language and bad behaviour of the children seemed to go unchecked by the father; and the children were encouraged to kick their mother. In quashing the order, the court concluded that, although there was evidence that the children had suffered harm, and were likely to suffer harm in the future, the threshold criterion of 'significant harm' had not been satisfied. The court found that: 'Significant harm is fact specific and must retain the breadth of meaning that human fallibility may require of it . . . However, it is clear that it must be something unusual; at least something more than the commonplace human failure or inadequacy.' It therefore followed that society must be willing to tolerate very diverse standards of parenting, including the eccentric, the barely adequate and the inconsistent. It was also observed that it is not the provenance of the state to spare children all the consequences of defective parenting.

Re L (A Child) (Care: Threshold Criteria) [2007] 1 FLR 2050 (Fam Div)

Such an approach would uphold the right to respect for the family life of intellectually disabled parents. Likewise, Booth *et al.* (2004) have concluded that:

> The application of the threshold criteria and the provision of supports to parents are intimately connected, vitally so in the case of parents with learning difficulties whose problems in parenting can be traced back to their disability . . . adequate supports protect against parenting breakdown . . . the additional difficulties parents with learning difficulties encounter in providing good-enough care . . . can be offset by compensatory services. Against this background, the failure to deliver support sets the family up to fail the threshold criteria.

There is the further complication that the standard for proving 'likely significant harm' is a lesser standard than the 'balance of probabilities' standard that is necessary for proving actual significant harm. However, the mere satisfaction of the threshold criteria will not necessitate or warrant separation of child and parents; it is a gateway into the exercise of judicial discretion. Sir James Munby P, in *Re D (A Child (No. 3)* [2016] Fam Law 272, endorsed some key points of principle established in *Re G and A (Care Order: Freeing Order: Parents with a Learning Disability)* [2006] NI Fam 8 for dealing with cases involving parents with learning disability. Of crucial importance is 'parenting with support'. Sir James Munby P stated that this concept imposes a broad obligation on the local authority to provide such support as will enable the child to remain with their parents. The test is then whether the parents, if provided with all the necessary support and services, would be able to provide the child with adequate care and parenting in a setting which promotes the child's welfare and does not cause harm.

In Ireland, these are simply called childcare or secure care proceedings. They are initiated by the Child and Family Agency (CFA). The threshold question is whether: (1)

the child has been, or is being, assaulted, ill-treated, neglected or sexually abused; or (2) the child's health development or welfare has been or is being avoidably impaired or neglected; or (c) the child's health, development or welfare is likely to be avoidably impaired or neglected and the child requires care or protection which (s)he is unlikely to receive unless a care order is made (CCA 1991, s 18). A supervision order may be considered appropriate (CCA 1991, s 19).

An application may also be made by the CFA for a 'special care order' for the detention of a child over the age of 11 years (1) where there is reasonable cause to believe that the behaviour of the child poses a real and substantial risk of harm to life, health, safety, development or welfare, (2) having regard to that behaviour and risk of harm, there is reasonable cause to believe that ordinary care provision and treatment and mental health services by reference to the MHA 2001 will not adequately address the behaviour and risk of harm and care requirements, and (3) there is reasonable cause to believe that the child requires special care to address the behaviour and risk and care needs which it cannot provide without an order of the High Court (CCA 1991, s 23F). A family welfare conference assists in deciding if a child is in need of special care and protection which they are unlikely to receive otherwise.

In all proceedings *in Ireland*, the court, having regard to the rights and duties of parents, is required to regard the child's welfare as the first and paramount consideration and insofar as is practicable, give due consideration, having regard to their age and understanding, to the wishes of the child (CCA 1991, s 24). The proceedings are heard *in camera*.

There is also a wardship jurisdiction *in Ireland* in respect of minors (Courts (Supplemental Provisions) Act 1961, s 9), which is often exercised in respect of children with significant mental health difficulties (e.g. anorexia nervosa).

Private Law Proceedings

In England and Wales, usually there is no local, or other public, authority involvement. The orders made are now called 'child arrangement orders' rather than residence and contact orders. In such cases, the Children and Family Court Advisory and Support Service (CAFCASS) may be invited to investigate and provide evidence for the court.

The inherent jurisdiction of the Family Division of the High Court is a power to override the parents so as to safeguard children who are incapable of caring for themselves. Most often, this occurs when the parents and child are in disagreement as to whether the child should have some particular treatment.

As some of these proceedings take place in public, in response to a preliminary enquiry about being instructed, the expert should make any representations they wish as to being named or otherwise identified in any public judgment given by the court.

In Ireland, the language of 'custody and access' is still used. Where, in any proceedings before any court, the guardianship, custody or upbringing of, or access to, a child is in question, the best interests of the child are the paramount consideration (Guardianship of Infants Act 1964, s 3). Section 31 of the same Act sets out the factors to be taken into consideration, which include the physical, psychological and emotional needs of the child; their social, intellectual and educational upbringing and needs; any special characteristics; any harm which the child has suffered or is at risk of suffering; and the protection of the child's safety and psychological well-being.

Issues in Family Proceedings

There may be an issue as to whether an adult party, or intended party, to the proceedings lacks capacity, within the meaning of the MCA, to conduct the proceedings. An adult who lacks capacity is a 'protected party' and must have a representative, such as a 'litigation friend', 'next friend' or guardian. There may be a related issue as to whether a protected party who is competent to give evidence should give evidence having regard to their 'best interests' and having regard to the implementation of any 'special measures' to assist them.

Similarly, in the case of a child, who is nearing their 18th birthday and who is a party to the proceedings, but not subject to them, there may be an issue as to their capacity to conduct the proceedings.

The court may require an assessment of a child or children in terms of health, development and functioning (Box 9.2). Where there are problems or difficulties, the court needs to know their aetiology and their prognosis, the latter having regard to whether or not their problems or difficulties are addressed. The short-term and long-term needs of the child or children have to be considered with regard to the nature of care-giving, education and treatment.

Parents (or primary caregivers) may need to be assessed (Box 9.3). Such assessment is likely to include exploration of the presence of psychiatric disorder and its potential impact on relevant issues such as the adult's (1) interactions with the child or children, (2) ability to safely meet the needs of the child or children, (3) capacity to accept agreed concerns about

Box 9.2 Questions in Letters of Instruction to Child Mental Health Professional or Paediatrician in Children Act 1989 Proceedings

A. The Child[ren]

1. Please describe the child[ren]'s current health, development and functioning (according to your area of expertise), and identify the nature of any significant changes which have occurred
   - Behavioural
   - Emotional
   - Attachment organisation
   - Social/peer/sibling relationships
   - Cognitive/educational
   - Physical
     - Growth, eating, sleep
     - Non-organic physical problems (including wetting and soiling)
     - Injuries
     - Paediatric conditions
2. Please comment on the likely explanation for/aetiology of the child[ren]'s problems/difficulties/injuries
   - History/experiences (including intrauterine influences, and abuse and neglect)
   - Genetic/innate/developmental difficulties
   - Paediatric/psychiatric disorders
3. Please provide a prognosis and risk if difficulties not addressed above.

4. Please describe the child(ren)'s needs in the light of the above

   - Nature of care-giving
   - Education
   - Treatment

   in the short and long term (subject, where appropriate, to further assessment later).

B. The parents/primary care-givers

5. Please describe the factors and mechanisms which would explain the parents' (or primary care-givers') harmful or neglectful interactions with the child(ren) (if relevant).
6. What interventions have been tried and what has been the result?
7. Please assess the ability of the parents or primary care-givers to fulfil the child(ren)'s identified needs now.
8. What other assessments of the parents or primary care-givers are indicated?

   - Adult mental health assessment
   - Forensic risk assessment
   - Physical assessment
   - Cognitive assessment

9. What, if anything, is needed to assist the parents or primary care-givers now, within the child(ren)'s time scales and what is the prognosis for change?

   - Parenting work
   - Support
   - Treatment/therapy

C. Alternatives

10. Please consider the alternative possibilities for the fulfilment of the child(ren)'s needs.

   - What sort of placement
   - Contact arrangements

   Please consider the advantages, disadvantages and implications of each for the child(ren).

Annex to FPR Practice Direction 25C, *Children Proceedings – The Use of Single Joint Experts and the Process Leading to an Expert Being Instructed or Expert Evidence Being Put Before the Court*

interactions with, or parenting of, the child or children, (4) capacity to work constructively with social care professionals and (5) risk to others, including the child or children. Where a psychiatric disorder is identified, the expert is often instructed to comment on appropriate evidence-based interventions, the means of accessing these interventions, the likelihood that treatment would result in positive change and the anticipated timescale within which sustained improvement would occur. The expert may also be instructed to consider whether other assessments (e.g. forensic assessment, cognitive assessment) or non-clinical interventions (e.g. parenting intervention, support) are indicated.

Box 9.3 Questions in Letters of Instruction to Adult Psychiatrists and Applied Psychologists in Children Act 1989 Proceedings

1. Does the parent/adult have – whether in his/her history or presentation – a mental illness/disorder (including substance abuse) or other psychological/emotional difficulty and, if so, what is the diagnosis?
2. How do any/all of the above (and their current treatment if applicable) affect his/her functioning, including interpersonal relationships?
3. If the answer to Q1 is yes, are there any features of either the mental illness or psychological/emotional difficulty or personality disorder which could be associated with risk to others, based on the available evidence base (whether published studies or evidence from clinical experience)?
4. What are the experiences/antecedents/aetiology which would explain his/her difficulties, if any (taking into account any available evidence base or other clinical experience)?
5. What treatment is indicated, what is its nature and the likely duration?
6. What is his/her capacity to engage in/partake of the treatment/therapy?
7. Are you able to indicate the prognosis for, time scales for achieving, and likely durability of, change?
8. What other factors might indicate positive change?

(It is assumed that this opinion will be based on collateral information as well as interviewing the adult.)

Annex to FPR Practice Direction 25C, *Children Proceedings – The Use of Single Joint Experts and the Process Leading to an Expert Being Instructed or Expert Evidence Being Put Before the Court*

When addressing capacity to engage in or partake of therapy, bear in mind that parents 'are more likely to be motivated to change if they receive early support services as part of the assessment process' (Horwath and Morrison 2001) and ensure that the process of reporting goes hand in hand with interventions. When addressing treatment, response to treatment and timescales, bear in mind that therapeutic optimism, if not justified, can lead to a child or children staying longer with a mentally ill, personality-disordered or substance misusing parent and suffering more harm before the court decides that their interests are best met by removing them from the care of the parent. Such therapeutic optimism has probably resulted in the caution urged upon the courts 'in receiving supportive testimony from adult psychiatrists called on behalf of patients, who may be unused to the child-focused, as opposed to patient-focused, approach of the court' (Hershman *et al.* 1991).

In family cases, experts should expect to receive, in their letter of instruction, a synoptic view of the proceedings, the background to them and a set of specific questions that are within the ambit of their expertise, do not contain unnecessary or irrelevant detail, are kept to a manageable number and are clear, focused and direct. The letter should identify any other expert instructed and other relevant people, such as a treating clinician. You have a right to talk to these people provided that you keep an accurate record and indicate in your report that such discussion has taken place. The documentation that accompanies the letter should be indexed and paginated. With very few exceptions, unless the court gives permission, the documents cannot be disclosed to third parties. This does not preclude the expert from using them in discussions with other experts or professionals in the case. Nor does it preclude the expert from making them available to an expert who is peer-reviewing their report or evidence.

Documents Seen

In England and Wales, you are required by FPR 25B PD 9.1(b) to list all of the documents you have seen.

The 'court bundle' of documents in care proceedings is often extensive. Whilst there may be significant overlap between different documents, study the full bundle as information therein supplements the data arising from the clinical assessment. A comprehensive description of the history leading to the initiation of the proceedings and subsequent progress is usually offered by the social worker's initial statement, which is presented in the standardised Social Work Evidence Template and contains a chronological account of noteworthy events and concerns. The 'Threshold Statement' summarises the evidence on which the local authority will rely to satisfy the threshold criteria (Children Act 1989, s 31(2)). Documents that specifically relate to the respondents include medical records, statements, police disclosures (including the official list of offences, the Police National Computer record), parenting assessment reports, and drug and alcohol test results. With regard to documents that only become available after your report is submitted, you may be instructed to confirm whether sight of this new information causes you to alter the opinions expressed in an earlier report. This can be addressed in the form of an addendum report.

Credibility

A parent with a history of substance misuse may deny having used drugs for some time. There may be witness evidence, for example, to the effect that they have been seen using drugs. They may deny this. The court will decide whether the parent has continued to use drugs, but it needs alternative opinions to match its alternative findings. Do not say which set of facts you prefer unless you are relying on psychiatric expertise. It is not enough to say that you believe the parent in preference to the witnesses. The credibility of parties and witnesses is for the judge. If, on psychiatric grounds, you have a view as to the parent's credibility you can say so, but be thorough and balanced in your reasoning and, even if you think that your argument is compelling, you should be prepared for challenge by the parent's advocate. Beware that the Court of Appeal has ruled that psychometric testing has no place where the credibility of an adult witness is an issue (*Re S (Care: Parenting Skills: Personality Tests)*; *Re L (Children)*).

Outcome

Within ten days of the final hearing, the solicitor instructing the expert should inform the expert of the outcome of the case and the use made of the expert's opinion. Furthermore, within ten days of receiving the court's written reasons for its decision, the instructing solicitor or lead solicitor should send the expert a copy. Experts, however experienced, ought to find much to learn and much that shapes practice if these two directions are strictly followed. As Lord Justice Wall (2007) says: 'if your work is conscientiously undertaken, your report and oral evidence honest, fair and well-reasoned, and provided that you have worked within the area of your expertise, you have nothing to fear, and much to gain from participating in family proceedings as an expert witness'.

Further Reading

Wall, N. (2007) *A Handbook for Expert Witnesses in Children Act Cases*, 2nd edn (Jordan).

Chapter 10

Reports in Cases Involving Capacity Issues

Keith Rix

Autonomy entails the freedom and the capacity to make a choice.
Baroness Hale in *R v C* [2009] UKHL 42

Since 2000, several jurisdictions have codified a considerable amount of case law relating to capacity, but interpretation of the statutory law is informed by the earlier case law and with which you should be familiar. In short, 'it is a general rule of English law, whatever the context that the test for capacity is the ability to understand the nature and quality of the transaction' (*Sheffield City Council v E* [2004] EWHC 2808 (Fam)). Common law, as to such matters as testamentary and capacity to marry, has not been affected. In *James v James* [2018] EWHC 43 (Ch), it was held that the test for judging capacity retrospectively in relation to a will already made did not fall within the scope of the MCA.

Capacity is issue-specific and time-specific. It 'depends on time and context . . . inevitably a decision as to capacity in one context does not bind a court which has to consider the same issue in a different context' (*Masterman-Lister v Brutton & Co.* [2002] EWCA Civ 1889) and 'the Court must focus on the matters which arise for decision now, and on the Claimant's capacity to deal with them now' (*Saulle v Nouvet* [2007] EWHC 2902 (QB)). A person may lack the capacity to make a gift at one time and have the capacity to do so at a later date. A person may have the capacity to marry at 11.30 a.m. (*In the Estate of Park deceased, Park v Park* [1954] P 89), but not have the capacity to make a will early in the afternoon of the same day (*Re Park, Culross v Park*, Times, 2 December 1950). The test is not monolithic, but tailored to the task in hand (*Perrins v Holland* [2009] EWHC 1945 (Ch)). It is also tailored to the gravity of the decision: a person need only have such capacity as is 'commensurate with the gravity of the decision' (*Re T (Adult: Refusal of Medical Treatment)* [1993] Fam 95).

The Statute Law

Legislation began with the Adults with Incapacity (Scotland) Act 2000 (AI(S)A), followed by the MCA and then, more recently, the Capacity and Self-Determination (Jersey) Law 2016 (CSD(J)L) and, yet to be commenced, Northern Ireland's MCA(NI) and Ireland's ADM(C)A. The MCA, the MCA(NI), the CSD(J)L and the ADM(C)A have much in common, but there are subtle differences. Readers preparing reports to which such legislation applies should consult the online version of the appropriate act. There is a common principle that someone is not to be treated as unable to make a decision unless all practicable steps have been made to help and support them to do so without success, such as ensuring that they receive appropriate explanation and ensuring that this happens at a time or times, or in an environment, likely to help. Another common principle is that a person is not to be treated as unable to make a decision merely because they make an unwise decision.

The MCA, the CSD(J)L and the MCA(NI) define lack of capacity in terms of impairment or disturbance in the functioning of the mind or brain, but the AI(S)A and the ADM(C)A do not. The MCA, the CSD(J)L, the MCA(NI) and the ADM(C)A have a four-part 'test', so a person lacks capacity to make a decision for himself if he is unable:

- to understand the information relevant to the decision;
- to retain that information;
- to use or weigh that information as part of the process of making the decision; or
- to communicate their decision (whether by talking, using sign language or any other means).

Information relevant to a decision may include information about the reasonably foreseeable consequences of deciding one way or another or failing to make the decision.

In Scotland, under the AI(S)A, 'incapable' means incapable of: (1) acting; (2) making decisions; (3) communicating decisions; (4) understanding decisions; or (5) retaining the memory of decisions.

In Ireland, in the meantime, there is a wardship jurisdiction regulated, subject only to the Constitution, by the Lunacy Regulation (Ireland) Act 1871. The test, in relation to adults, is simple: is the person an idiot, a lunatic or of unsound mind and incapable of managing his person or property? *FD v Registrar of Wards of Court* [2004] IEHC 126 established that the term 'person of unsound mind', in the context of the case, 'means no more than that the person is incapable of managing his affairs', albeit a statutory tautology.

In most jurisdictions, the standard of proof is the balance of probabilities and although the ADMCA is silent on this, in *Fitzpatrick v FK* [2009] 2 IR 7, the court stated:

> In assessing capacity . . . the assessment must have regard to the gravity of the decision, in terms of the consequences which are likely to ensue from the acceptance or rejection of the proffered treatment. In the private law context this means that, in applying the civil law standard of proof, the weight to be attached to the evidence should have regard to the gravity of the decision, whether that is characterised as the necessity for 'clear and convincing proof' or an enjoinder that the court 'should not draw its conclusions lightly'.

Irresponsibility and Vulnerability

Issues that have probably troubled experts the most are 'irresponsibility', in the sense of making rash or irresponsible decisions, and 'vulnerability' in the sense of risk of exploitation. This is because, in *Masterman-Lister*, the trial judge rejected the submission that a finding of incapacity was required 'if the effect of the injury to his brain renders [the plaintiff] vulnerable to exploitation or at the risk of the making of rash or irresponsible decisions' and in the Court of Appeal Chadwick LJ confirmed this: 'It is not the task of the courts to prevent those who have the mental capacity to make rational decisions from making decisions which others may regard as rash and irresponsible.' In *Lindsay v Wood* [2006] EWHC 2895 (QB), the court acknowledged that '[m]any people of full capacity make rash decisions, or cannot be trusted to use their money sensibly' and concluded that 'these qualities or deficiencies do not necessarily lead to a finding of incapacity'. It was acknowledged that medical practitioners understood Chadwick LJ to mean that vulnerability to exploitation is irrelevant to questions of capacity and must be ignored when deciding on the issue of capacity. However, the court did not regard this as correct:

> When considering the question of capacity, psychiatrists and psychologists will normally wish to take into account all aspects of the personality and behaviour of the person in question, including vulnerability to exploitation. However, vulnerability to exploitation does not of itself lead to the conclusion that there is lack of capacity ... The issue is ... whether the person has the mental capacity to make a rational decision.

Furthermore, other cases confirm the relevance of vulnerability and irrationality. In *Mitchell v Alasia* [2005] EWHC 11 (QB), reliance was placed on qualities such as impulsiveness and volatility when deciding whether the claimant was, by reason of mental disorder, incapable of managing and administering his property and affairs. Irresponsibility and vulnerability are relevant, but not determinative. In *MB (An Adult: Medical Treatment)* [1997] 2 WLUK 313, the court held that '[a]lthough it might be thought that irrationality sits uneasily with competence to decide, panic, indecisiveness and irrationality in themselves do not as such amount to incompetence, but they may be symptoms or evidence of incompetence'. The test is about comprehension and decision-making and not about wisdom, but where someone repeatedly makes unwise decisions that put them at significant risk of harm or exploitation or makes a particularly unwise decision that is obviously irrational or out of character, this may be evidence of lack of capacity.

Capacity Issues

It is impossible to list and consider here all the decisions about which a capacity issue might arise. This chapter includes only some of them. Over the years, I have learned a lot from instructing solicitors and counsel about what is required for different decisions. The chapter reflects this.

Appointment of an Appointee to Act in respect of Department for Work and Pensions Proceedings

Whether someone requires an appointee in DWP proceedings calls for consideration of their ability to:

- understand the basis of probable entitlement to benefits;
- understand and complete the claim form;
- respond to correspondence relating to social security benefits;
- collect or receive benefits;
- know what the money is for;
- choose whether to use it for its intended purpose.

Making a Will

Testamentary Capacity

The leading case on testamentary capacity is *Banks v Goodfellow* (1869–70) LR 5 QB 549. John Banks lived with his teenage niece, Margaret Goodfellow. He had paranoid schizophrenia; he believed that a grocer, long since dead, was pursuing and persecuting him and that he was being chased by evil spirits. He left his entire estate of fifteen properties to his niece. On his death, his testamentary capacity was challenged. The court recognised that where a testator is deluded 'a will should be regarded with great distrust, and every presumption should in the first instance be made against it', a presumption which 'becomes additionally strong when the will is . . . one in which the natural affection and the claims of near relationship have been disregarded'. However, it was held that, as there was no connection between his delusions and the disposition of his property, he was not incapable of validly disposing of his property by will:

> It is essential . . . that a testator shall understand the nature of the act and its effects; shall understand the extent of the property of which he is disposing; shall be able to comprehend and appreciate the claims to which he ought to give effect; and, with a view to the latter object, that no disorder of mind shall poison his affections, pervert his sense of right, or prevent the exercise of his natural faculties – that no insane delusion shall influence his will in disposing of his property and bring about a disposal of it which, if the mind had been sound, would not have been made.

By contrast, in *Smee v Smee* [1879] LR 5 PD 84, where the testator wrongly believed that he was the son of George IV, who had built Brighton Pavilion, and therefore left a reversionary interest in his estate to fund a free library for the people of Brighton, it was held that his delusion had drastically affected his testamentary wishes and his will was pronounced invalid.

The threshold for testamentary capacity has been and remains low (*James*). In *Sharp v Adam* [2006] EWCA Civ 449, the court quoted with approval *Den v Vancleve* (1819) 2 Southard, and upon which *Banks* had relied: 'By the terms "a sound and disposing memory" it has not been understood that a testator must possess these qualities of mind in highest degree.' In *Banks*, the court recognised that 'want of intelligence occasioned by defective organisation, or by a supervening physical infirmity or the decay of advancing age' resulting in 'the mental power [being] reduced below the ordinary standard' might not be sufficient to prevent the understanding and appreciation of 'the testamentary act in all its different bearings'. Furthermore, '[t]he simpler the estate and the fewer the claimants, the less difficult it is to dispose of, and accordingly the less acute the faculties required to do so successfully' (*James*).

Assessment should address the ability of the testator to understand the nature of a will – that is, that they will die, that the will will come into operation on their death, but not before, and that they can change or revoke it at any time subject to having the capacity to do so. They must understand the effects of making a will and making choices with regard to: who the executors should be and, perhaps also, why they should be appointed; who gets what; whether a beneficiary's gift is outright or conditional, such as the right to occupy a property only during their lifetime; that if they spend their money or dispose of their properties, the beneficiaries might lose out; a beneficiary might die before them; and whether they have already made a will, in which case they need to understand how the new one differs from the old one.

The testator must comprehend broadly the extent of their property (that is, what the will will 'bite' on) and so must the expert. Actual knowledge of a value is unnecessary (*Blackman v Man* [2007] EWCA 3162 (Ch)); the value of property can change – rapidly in unstable economic times and in the lifetime of the testator. It is not 'a requirement that a person actually understand the extent of his property, only that he have the capacity to do so' (*Simon v Byford* [2014] EWCA Civ 280).

There may be property that is jointly owned and will pass to the joint owner irrespective of anything that is said in the will. There may be benefits payable, such as pension rights, that the will cannot determine. There may be debts and the testator should understand how these are to be paid.

In order to understand the claims to which the testator ought to give effect, you need to know who the testator's family members are, along with others who might have a claim on the estate. 'A testator with a complex estate and many potential beneficiaries may need a greater degree of cognitive ability than one with a simple estate and few claimants' (*Parker v Felgate and Tilly* (1883) 8 PD 171). The testator should be able to take into account the extent to which possible beneficiaries may already have received adequate provision, be better off financially than others, have been more attentive and caring or may be in greater need of assistance according to their particular circumstances. You need to be informed about such matters by the instructing solicitors.

Sometimes, incapacity supervenes after a will has been made and before it is executed. Then, three questions have to be answered (*Parker*):

1. When the will was executed, did she remember and understand the instructions she had given to her solicitor?
2. If it had been thought advisable to stimulate her, could she have understood each clause of the will when it was explained to her?
3. Was she capable of understanding, and did she understand, that she was executing a will for which she had previously given instructions to her solicitor?

As these questions have to be answered in order and a positive response to any of them indicates that the will is valid, the bottom line is that the testator should understand that she is executing a will for which she had previously given her solicitors instructions. This is important where there has clearly been a deterioration in the testator's condition between giving their instructions and signing the will. *Perrins v Holland* has established that no more is required than that the testator believes that it gives effect to their instructions and that they continue to represent their wishes.

Bear in mind that a testator can still act in an unorthodox way: 'But the law does not say that a man is incapacitated from making a will if he proposes to make a disposition of his property moved by capricious, frivolous or even bad motives' (*Boughton v Knight* [1873] LR 3 PD 64). The testator does not have to behave 'in such a manner as to deserve approbation from the prudent, the wise or the good' (*Bird v Luckie* (1850) 8 Hare 301).

In Ireland, however, where a spouse or civil partner has statutory rights to a share of the estate, there is a limit to the extent to which an otherwise 'perverse' will can be made. Where a court considers that the testator failed in his moral duty to make proper provision for a child in accordance with his means, whether by his will or otherwise, it may order that such provision be made out of the estate. The court considers the application from the point of view of a prudent and just parent, taking into account, *inter alia*, the position of each of the children of the testator and any other circumstances in arriving at a decision that will be as fair as possible to the child in question and to the other children (Succession Act 1965, s 117).

In *Kostic v Chaplin* [2007] EWHC 2909 (Ch), Zoran Kostic's father left most of his £8.2 million estate to the Conservative Party. Zoran Kostic's challenge to the two wills made by his father was on the basis that he suffered from an undiagnosed and untreated mental illness which had resulted in a delusional belief that there was a worldwide conspiracy of dark forces and he was included in the conspiracy. In pronouncing against the wills, the court held that, as a result of his mental illness, Kostic was unable to appreciate his son's claims on the estate. In *Ritchie v National Osteoporosis Society* [2009] EWHC 709, the testator left nothing to her children on the basis of their maltreatment of her. The court found that these allegations were untrue and as the medical evidence suggested that she may have omitted her children from her will on account of 'paranoid delusions', her will was declared invalid. In *Walters v Smee* [2008] EWHC 2029 (Ch), the court found that the dispositions of the testatrix in her 2004 will, made a month before she died, were motivated largely, if not wholly, by 'misapprehensions' that were the result of her dementia and its effect on her cognitive faculties.

Undue Influence

Related to testamentary capacity is 'undue influence'. *Wingrove v Wingrove* (1885) 11 PD 81 established that in law 'under influence' could be summed up in one word – 'coercion' and: 'The coercion may ... be of different kinds ... (a) person in the last days of life may have become so weak and feeble, that a very little pressure will be sufficient to bring about the desired result.' It is for the court, not the expert, to decide if undue influence was brought, but expertise may be needed to identify the nature and cause of a state rendering the testator vulnerable or susceptible to coercion and as to the likelihood of the undue influence alleged being sufficient coercion in the circumstances revealed in the lay witness evidence. In *Gill v Woodall* [2009] EWHC 3778 (Ch), where the issue was the undue influence of the deceased's husband, the court had regard to the fact that the testator was a shy and timid person who suffered from agoraphobia and was very, and unusually, dependent on her husband and concerned not to lose his support. The diagnosis of agoraphobia, of which there was no evidence in medical records, was based on the evidence of the lay witnesses. It is dementia which is more often identified as increasing vulnerability to the influence of others.

Burden of Proof

Although there is a rebuttable presumption in favour of the testamentary capacity of a testator whose will is duly executed, where a claimant raises a real doubt as to testamentary capacity, the burden of proof shifts to the propounder of the will to prove, on a balance of probabilities, that the testator did in fact have testamentary capacity (*Key (Deceased)* [2010] EWHC 408 (Ch)), but with a degree of flexibility appropriate to the seriousness of the case (*Borman v Lel* [2001] 6 WLUK 189). So, the psychiatrist instructed by those acting for the party challenging the will needs to analyse the evidence to see if it casts real doubt on the testator's testamentary capacity; the psychiatrist instructed by those acting for the party propounding the will needs to carry out the analysis to see if, on a balance of probability, the testator possessed testamentary capacity.

Investigation of the Case

You should be provided with the disputed will and any relevant earlier wills. If it has not been provided, you should ask if there is a *Larke v Nugus* letter and its response. This is a letter to the solicitors responsible for drafting the will and sent in response to enquiries about the circumstances surrounding its drafting and execution pursuant to the principles set out in the case of *Larke v Nugus* (1979) 123 SJ 327. It may reveal whether a testamentary capacity assessment was undertaken and, if so, by whom; if there were concerns on the part of the will drafter, how they dealt with them; and whether 'the golden rule' was followed, that is, did a medical professional act as a witness to the testator's signature. The information provided should extend to the preparation of the will and the circumstances in which it was executed. It may be accompanied by copies of the will drafter's notes, including a copy of any telephone notes or attendance notes made by the will writer. These should reveal the instructions that were given, the advice that was provided and how the final will came to be as drafted. You will also need a family *dramatis personae* so that you can understand the potential claims on the testator's estate.

The starting point in a retrospective assessment of capacity is a chronology. It may include entries in medical or care home records that refer to the mental state of the testator, medication prescribed, side effects, illnesses that cause pain, distress or agitation that may affect cognitive functioning, results of cognitive tests, observations of family and friends and references to other decisions that have been made. Evidence as to mental state before and after the drafting and execution of the will can be used to form an opinion as to the mental state at the time it was drafted and/or executed. In *Bishop v Bishop* [2009] 4 WLUK 329, the issue was whether the testator lacked testamentary capacity as a result of alcoholic dementia when he executed his will on 3 November 1995. On 9 and 22 November 2005, the testator was assessed by a consultant physician who assessed his cognition on a 10-point scale, finding that it increased from 2–3 out of 10 to 8–9 out of 10. The court found that these results and the physician's evidence were '"fatal" to the dementia view' as 'it would not have been possible for [the testator] to obtain the test score of 9/10 on 22nd November 2005 if he had dementia'.

Revoking a Will

Re Sabatini (1970) 114 SJ 35 established that capacity to revoke a will requires:

- understanding the nature of the act of revoking a will;
- understanding the effect of revoking a will (including perhaps a greater understanding of the operation of the intestacy rules than is necessary for the purpose of making a will);
- understanding the extent of their property; and
- comprehending and appreciating the claims to which they ought to give effect.

Capacity to Make a Lasting Power of Attorney

In England and Wales, under the MCA, s 9(1), a lasting power of attorney (LPA) allows the donor to confer on the donee/s authority to make decisions about all or any of the following: the donor's personal welfare or specified matters concerning their personal welfare and the donor's property and affairs or specified matters concerning their property and affairs, including the authority to make such decisions in circumstances where the donor lacks capacity.

For this particular decision, the person has to be able to answer the following questions:

- What is a lasting power of attorney?
- Why do they want to make a lasting power of attorney?
- Who are they appointing as attorney(s)?
- Why have they chosen that/those person(s) as attorney(s)?
- What are the nature and scope of the powers being given to the attorney (the attorney will be able to assume complete authority over the donor's property and finances and will be able to do anything with them that the donor could have done)?

The donor will also need to appreciate that their attorney's authority to make decisions will apply as soon as the LPA is registered, unless they specify that it should only apply when they lack capacity to make a relevant decision, and will continue should they lose mental capacity, but they can revoke the LPA at any time if they have the capacity to do so. This contrasts with a power of attorney as to welfare, rather than property, where the attorney can only make decisions on welfare if the donor lacks capacity. Also, the donor will need to understand the reasonably foreseeable consequences of making or not making the LPA or of making one on different terms or appointing different attorneys.

In Ireland, the ADM(C)A, Pt 7 will introduce a new enduring power of attorney scheme which, unlike the old regime, may also extend to healthcare decisions other than relating to refusal of life-sustaining treatment. This will require a report from a doctor and another healthcare professional that the donor had the capacity to understand the implications of creating, varying or revoking the power at the relevant time (ADM(C)A, ss 60 and 73). Currently, only a single medical opinion is required that the donor had the mental capacity, with the assistance of such explanations as may have been given, to understand the effect of creating the power (Powers of Attorney Act, 1996, s 5).

Capacity to Make a Personal Injury Trust

Personal injury trusts are important in the settlement and resolution of personal injury claims. They ensure that the funds or property are used for the claimant's benefit. They are important where the claimant has no experience of handling a large sum of money. They can protect the claimant from exploitative relatives. They relieve the claimant of the responsibility of financial administration. They allow the claimant to retain, or if eligible for them in the future, to qualify for, means-tested benefits. The income earned from capital held on trust is tax-free.

To create a personal injury trust, the person needs to be able to answer the following questions:

- What is a personal injury trust?
- Why do they want to create a personal injury trust?
- Who are they appointing as trustee(s)?
- Why have they chosen that/those person(s) to act as trustee(s)?

Capacity to Marry and to Assume Marital Cohabitation

The issue of capacity to marry is particularly likely to call for evidence from experts in intellectual disability. *Sheffield City Council* is the leading case. Munby J held that: (1) the question is about the capacity to marry and not, specifically, the capacity to marry a particular person; (2) it is not necessary to show that the person has capacity to take care of their own person and property; (3) whether it is wise to marry or wise to marry a particular person is not relevant; (4) the issue is not whether it is in the best interests of the person to marry or to marry a particular person; (5) the test remains that in *Park v Park* [1954] P 89, that the person is mentally capable of appreciating the responsibilities that normally attach to marriage; (6) it is not enough to understand that they are taking part in a marriage ceremony as there must also be an understanding of the duties and responsibilities that normally attach to marriage.

Setting out a modern view of marriage, including the duties and responsibilities that ordinarily attach to marriage, Munby J. referred to how, '[i]nsofar as the concept of consortium – the sharing of a common home and a common domestic life, and the right to enjoy each other's society, comfort and assistance – still has any useful role to play, the rights of husband and wife must surely now be regarded as exactly reciprocal'. He summarised the duties and responsibilities:

> Marriage, whether civil or religious, is a contract, formally entered into. It confers on the parties the status of husband and wife, the essence of the contract being an agreement between a man and a woman to live together, and to love one another as husband and wife, to the exclusion of all others. It creates a relationship of mutual and reciprocal obligations, typically involving the sharing of a common home and a common domestic life and the right to enjoy each other's society, comfort and assistance.

He also identified the potential danger of setting 'the test to marry too high, lest it operate as an unfair, unnecessary and indeed discriminatory bar against the mentally disabled'.

Consent to marriage includes the capacity to consent to sexual intercourse, which is regarded as an ordinary consequence of the celebration of marriage (*Westminster City Council v C* [2008] EWCA Civ 198) (see below, 'Capacity to Engage in Sexual Activity') and without which there is no capacity to marry (*Local Authority v H* [2012] EWHC 49 (COP)).

Notwithstanding a person's capacity to give valid consent to marry, it is a ground for annulment of a marriage, under the Matrimonial Causes Act 1973, ss 11–13, that, as a result of mental disorder (as defined in the MHA 1983), the party was 'unfitted' to marriage, which means being unable to carry out the duties and obligations of marriage. It is not enough that it is difficult to live with the spouse (*Bennett v Bennett* [1969] 1 WLR 430).

In *PC v City of York Council* [2013] EWCA Civ 478, the issue was whether a woman with significant learning difficulties, and an IQ of 66 to 69, had the capacity to decide to take up married life, upon his release from prison, with the husband she had married during his prison sentence for sexual offences. The Court of Appeal decided that she was capable of making that decision and distinguished it from her inability to understand the potential risk that her husband presented and her inability to weigh up all of the information relating thereto. It was acknowledged that her decision might be regarded by professionals as extremely unwise, but it reiterated that 'people are free to make unwise decisions, provided that they have the capacity to decide'.

In Ireland, nullity of marriage and of civil partnerships may arise where there is unfitness for marriage (or civil partnership) as a consequence of mental disorder. It is dealt with disjunctively from consent.

Capacity to Separate, Divorce or Dissolve a Civil Partnership

There have been no reported court decisions in the UK concerning the capacity to separate, divorce or dissolve a civil partnership. The courts are likely, however, to have regard to the Canadian case of *Calvert (Litigation Guardian) v Calvert* (1997) 32 OR (3d) 281:

> Separation is the simplest act requiring the lowest level of understanding. A person has to know with whom he or she does or does not want to live. Divorce, while still simple, requires a bit more understanding. It requires the desire to remain separate and to be no longer married to one's spouse. It is the undoing of the contract of marriage . . . If marriage is simple, divorce must be equally simple . . . the mental capacity required for divorce is the same as required for entering into a marriage . . . While Mrs Calvert may have lacked the ability to instruct counsel, that did not mean she could not make the basic personal decision to separate and divorce.

Capacity to Decide Whether to Use Contraception

In *Re A (Capacity: Refusal of Contraception)* [2010] EWHC 1549 (Fam), the court had to decide whether a woman with an IQ of 53 had the capacity to make decisions regarding contraception. The court held that the test for capacity should be so applied as to ascertain her ability to understand and weigh up the immediate or proximate medical issues surrounding contraception, including:

- The reason for contraception and what it does (which includes the likelihood of pregnancy if it is not in use during sexual intercourse);
- The types available and how each is used;
- The advantages and disadvantages of each type;
- The possible side-effects of each and how they can be dealt with;
- How easily each type can be changed; and
- The generally accepted effectiveness of each.

It was not necessary to ascertain her understanding of what bringing up a child would be like in practice, how she would be likely to get on, or whether any child would be likely to be removed from her care. The judge was also against a broad reading of 'reasonably foreseeable consequences' as required by the MCA, s 3(4) so as to require her to understand the social consequences, such as the parenting of a child, as it would 'set the bar too high and would risk a move away from personal autonomy in the direction of social engineering'.

In *NHS Trust v DE* [2013] EWHC 2562 (Fam), a man with an IQ of 40 was found to lack capacity to consent to a vasectomy and it was ruled to be in his best interests. However, the psychiatrist was of the opinion that he lacked capacity to consent to sexual relations. Nevertheless, after intensive work by a clinical psychologist and community learning disability nurse, he achieved that capacity.

Capacity to Engage in Sexual Activity

In England and Wales, Southwark LBC v KA [2016] EWCOP 20 has confirmed that the information it is necessary to understand to consent to sexual activity is rudimentary: (1) the mechanics of the act; (2) that it can lead to pregnancy; and (3) that there are health risks involved. The second is not applicable to someone who is homosexual (*Local Authority v TZ* [2013] EWHC 2322 (COP)). An understanding of the emotional consequences of having sexual relations has also to be considered (*Local Authority v TZ*). The capacity to decide more complex questions about long-term relationships is not a requirement (*Local Authority X v MM* [2007] EWHC 2003 (Fam)). Knowledge and understanding does not need to be complete or sophisticated; rudimentary knowledge may be sufficient (*X City Council v MB* [2006] EWHC 168 (Fam)). The person has to understand that they have a choice and can refuse and there has to be an understanding of the need to use contraception to avoid pregnancy and sexually transmitted disease (*Local Authority v H*). Although sexual intercourse will usually be a private activity with one other person, appropriate advice, support and assistance from others on these various matters can 'enable' capacity.

Do not apply too high a threshold. 'Most people faced with the decision whether or not to have sex do not embark on a process of weighing up complex, abstract or hypothetical information' (*Local Authority v TZ*). Further, morality is to be ignored (*Local Authority v H*).

The SOA may also have to be considered. Section 74 states that 'a person consents if he agrees by choice, and has the freedom and capacity to make that choice'. Section 30 applies to people who are 'unable to refuse because of or for a reason related to a mental disorder' (as defined in the MHA 1983, s 1). It may be either the inability to choose (s 30(1)(a)) or the inability to communicate the choice made (s 30(2)(b)). In such cases, it is necessary to consider whether the person would have capacity to consent if only minor threats or inducements were made by a person seeking sexual intercourse. In other words, what level of threat or inducement would be so overbearing as to invalidate 'consent'? It may also be necessary to assist as to whether the accused knew, or could reasonably be expected to know, that the complainant has a mental disorder and that because of it, or for a reason related to it, he is likely to be unable to refuse (s 30(1)(d)).

In Ireland, likewise, a person lacks the capacity to consent to a sexual act if they are 'by reason of a mental or intellectual disability or a mental illness, incapable of (a) understanding the nature, or the reasonably foreseeable consequences, of that act, (b) evaluating relevant information for the purposes of deciding whether or not to engage in that act, or (c) communicating his or her consent to that act by speech, sign language or otherwise' (Criminal Law (Sexual Offences) Act 2017, s 21). The ingredients of the offence are also slightly different: the defendant must know, or be reckless as to whether, the other is such a person and there is a rebuttable presumption, in this regard (s 21(3)).

R v C was the case of a man who was found guilty of, but successfully appealed against, his conviction for sexual touching (oral intercourse) under the SOA 2003, s 30. The complainant had a history of schizoaffective disorder, an emotionally unstable personality disorder, an IQ of less than 75 and a history of harmful alcohol use. The Crown successfully appealed to the House of Lords, where Baroness Hale held that (1) a lack of capacity to choose can be person- or situation-specific and (2) an irrational fear that prevents the exercise of choice can be equated with a lack of capacity to choose. She also explained that the words 'for any other reason' in s 30 'are clearly capable of encompassing a wide range of circumstances in which a person's mental disorder may rob them of the ability to make an autonomous choice, even though they have sufficient understanding of the information relevant to making it'. She held that it was not the case that to fall within s 30(2)(b) a complainant must be physically unable to communicate by reason of his mental disorder. She held that Parliament clearly had in mind an inability to communicate that was the result of, or associated with, a disorder of the mind.

Capacity to Decide the Matter of Contact

MM (see above, 'Capacity to Engage in Sexual Activity'), who had schizophrenia, an IQ of 56, a moderate learning disability and poor cognitive functioning, was held to have capacity to decide about having sexual relations, but not to have capacity to decide about contact with her partner KM. It was held that contact is 'a potentially complex concept involving a range of considerations arising in the context of a potentially wide variety of situations, for example, from having a cup of tea with someone to going away with them for a long holiday'.

Capacity to Consent to Medical Treatment

In England and Wales, the court decided that 'in serious or complex cases involving difficult issues about the future health and well-being, or even the life of the patient', the issue of capacity should be examined by an independent psychiatrist, ideally one approved under the MHA, s 12(2) (*St George's NHS Trust v S* [1999] Fam 26).

The test remains fundamentally that proposed by Professor Nigel Eastman, adopted by the court in *Re C (Adult: Refusal of Treatment)* [1994] 1 WLR 290, and now embodied in the MCA: (1) comprehending and retaining treatment information; (2) believing it; and (3) weighing it in the balance to arrive at a choice. It is only necessary to retain the information temporarily. Treatment information refers to the nature, purpose and effects of the treatment, the last including 'the benefits and risks of deciding to have or not to have one or other of the various kinds of [treatment], or of not making a decision at all' (*Heart of England NHS Foundation Trust v JB* [2014] EWHC 342 (COP)). However, following *Montgomery v Lanarkshire Health Board* [2015] UKSC 11, it is now necessary to recognise that patients' information needs vary; the doctor has to judge the significance that 'a reasonable person in the patient's position would be likely to attach . . . to the risk' or that the doctor is, or should be reasonably, aware that 'the particular patient would be likely to attach' to it. Although more recent formulations of the test do not refer to 'belief', this is 'subsumed in understanding and the ability to use and weigh information' (*Local Authority X v MM*).

The required capacity has to be 'commensurate with the gravity of the decision' (*Re T (Adult: Refusal of Medical Treatment)*); '[t]he graver the consequences of the decision, the commensurately greater the level of competence is required to take the decision' (*X City Council v MB*). Consistent with this, the threshold capacity required to consent to treatment is lower than the threshold capacity to refuse treatment.

The MCA and the ADM(C)A preserve the patient's right to take unwise decisions. However, in *Mental Health Trust v DD* [2014] EWCOP 11, a case concerning a pregnant woman with a complex obstetric history, learning difficulties and an autism spectrum disorder, the judge found that although her 'decision-making is undoubtedly "*unwise*"', it was not 'just "*unwise*"; it lacks the essential ingredient of discrimination which only comes when the relevant information is evaluated and weighed . . . in relation to each of the matters under consideration her impairment of mind (essentially attributable to her autistic spectrum disorder, overlaid with learning disability) prevents her from weighing the information relevant to each decision' (emphases in the original). In *Kings College NHS Foundation Trust v C* [2015] EWCOP 80, C's decision to refuse dialysis was one which could be characterised as unwise, unreasonable, illogical or even immoral, but the court found that she was 'entitled to make her own decision . . . based on the things that are important to her, in keeping with her own personality and system of values and without conforming to society's expectations of what constitutes the "normal" decision in this situation [if such a thing exists]'.

Refusal of treatment for anorexia nervosa commonly arises. In *Local Authority v E* [2012] EWHC 1639 (COP), the court found that there was strong evidence that E's fear of weight gain made her incapable of weighing the advantages and disadvantages of eating in any meaningful way. The compulsion to prevent the calories entering her system had become the card that trumps all others. The need not to gain weight overpowered all other thoughts. However, in *NHS Trust v L* [2012] EWHC 2741 (COP), it was decided that L had the capacity to decide whether to take antibiotics for her pneumonia, which would in all likelihood kill her, as the antibiotics were not calorific. Likewise, in *NHS Trust v X* [2014] EWCOP 35, X, who lacked capacity in relation to the treatment of her anorexia, because she believed that she was larger than she was and was therefore unlikely to understand how ill she was, was regarded as having the capacity to make decisions about her drinking, which was relevant to her alcoholism and end-stage liver cirrhosis, including weighing such information as the calorific content of alcohol.

In the case of children, *Gillick v West Norfolk and Wisbech AHA* [1986] AC 112 established that a person under 16 years of age may achieve a state of maturity, intelligence and understanding sufficient to take a decision as to medical treatment without the need for parental consent. However, in *Re S (A Minor: Consent to Medical Treatment)* [1994] 2 FLR 1065, where a 15-year-old girl no longer wanted to undergo monthly blood transfusions for thalassaemia, it did not seem to the judge that her capacity was commensurate with the gravity of the decision and although she seemed to understand that she would die, she did not sufficiently understand the manner of her death, the pain and the distress. Similarly, in *Re E (A Minor) (Wardship: Medical Treatment)* [1993] 1 FLR 386, where E, also 15 years old, suffered from leukaemia and wished to refuse a blood transfusion because he was a Jehovah's Witness, the court overrode his, and his parents', decision because he did not have:

> . . . any sufficient understanding of the pain he has yet to suffer, or the fear that he will be undergoing, of the distress not only occasioned by that fear but also – and importantly – the distress he will inevitably suffer as he, a loving son, helplessly watches his parents' and his family's distress . . . as to the manner of his death and to the extent of his and his family's suffering I find he has not the ability to turn his mind to it nor the will to do so.

The level of competence expected of children who refuse treatment is very high.

In *Re JA (A Minor) (Medical Treatment: Child Diagnosed with HIV)* [2014] EWHC 1135 (Fam), a 14-year-old boy who was regarded as Gillick-competent for some decisions was found to be not Gillick-competent to decide whether to take antiretroviral treatment as he did not accept his diagnosis, lacked the understanding of the consequences of not having the treatment and therefore the understanding needed to weigh up the pros and the cons. But even in the case of a Gillick-competent child, although their refusal is a very important factor in the doctor's decision whether or not to treat, this does not prevent the necessary consent being obtained from another competent source (*Re R (A Minor) (Wardship: Consent to Treatment)* [1992] Fam 11 (CA)).

In Ireland, there is no authority by reference to which it could safely be stated that *Gillick* is part of Irish law. However, art 42A of the Constitution – the Children's Rights Amendment – provides for securing, as far as practicable, that in all proceedings, brought by the state, as guardian of the common good, for the purpose of preventing the safety and welfare of any child from being prejudicially affected, in respect of any child who is capable of forming their own views, due weight is to be given to the child's views having regard to their age and maturity.

Capacity to Consent to Termination of Pregnancy

Where capacity to consent to termination of pregnancy has been addressed by the Court of Protection in the light of the MCA, the court has criticised psychiatrists and hospitals for setting the bar too high. In *NHS Trust v P* [2013] EWHC 50 (COP), the court commented that 'the intention of the Act is not to dress an incapacitous person in cotton wool but to allow them . . . to make the same mistakes that all other human beings are at liberty to make'. In *Re SB (A Patient) (Capacity to Consent to Termination)* [2014] EWHC 1417 (COP), the court observed that 'autonomy includes the autonomy to make a decision which may be unwise'.

Capacity to Litigate

In England and Wales, under CPR 21.9, a person who by reason of mental disorder within the meaning of the MHA is incapable of managing and administering their affairs must have a 'litigation friend' to conduct proceedings on their behalf.

The most important relevant judgments are those in the case of *Masterman-Lister*, where the judge at first instance relied considerably on *White v Fell* (unreported, 12 November 1987) (Rix 1999). This concerned a woman who was seriously injured in a road traffic accident at the age of 18 years and sought to bring her action against the defendant more than three years later when it was statute-barred. There was no dispute that she had suffered significant brain damage, had suffered a fall in intellectual level from 'normal' to 'borderline subnormal' and was substantially less capable of managing her own affairs and property than she would otherwise have been. However, the judge decided that she had capacity to litigate, taking into consideration how she had divorced her husband, lived alone in sheltered accommodation, provided for her dog, arranged to visit a friend by taxi, could find her way about town, managed her benefits and took her oral contraceptive regularly. He found that, first, she had 'insight and understanding of the fact that she has a problem in respect of which she needs advice', second, as her involvement in divorce proceedings indicated, having identified the problem, she could seek an appropriate advisor and instruct him with sufficient clarity to enable him to understand and advise appropriately, and, third, she had sufficient mental capacity to understand and to make decisions based upon, or otherwise she was able to give effect to, such advice as she might receive.

In *Masterman-Lister*, the judge at first instance approved the approach in *White* and he was upheld on appeal. The Court of Appeal confirmed that in addition to the actual medical evidence, 'that element has to be considered in conjunction with any other evidence that there may be about the manner in which the subject of the enquiry actually has conducted his everyday life and affairs' and with 'capacity at other times and in other contexts'. The Court of Appeal approved the test, now on a statutory basis in the MCA, as being that the person should 'be able to absorb and retain information [including advice] relevant to the matters in question sufficiently to enable him or her to make decisions based on such information'.

It was also held that the focus should be on the capacity or ability of the individual and not the actual outcome. Outcomes are, however, relevant as they 'can often cast a flood of light on capacity' (Kennedy LJ in *Masterman-Lister*), but they are not determinative. This 'functional' test is to be contrasted with an 'outcomes' test or one based on 'diagnosis'. It does not follow that because someone has a condition, such as dementia or schizophrenia, they lack the capacity to make some particular decision.

In personal injury litigation, the following are matters that are relevant to the claimant's capacity to litigate (and where appropriate qualified by 'with the assistance of such proper explanation from legal advisers and experts' and/or 'if necessary with suitable help from someone who knows him well'):

- knowing that potentially he has a case, not necessarily a cast-iron case, and being able to understand the issues in the case;
- knowing about the chances of not succeeding and about the risk of an adverse order as to costs;
- knowing who the case is against;

- understanding evidence as to the nature and severity of the injuries for which compensation is sought;
- appreciating the need for legal advice;
- the ability to seek, understand and act on legal advice to investigate and bring the claim;
- understanding how the proceedings are to be funded;
- the ability to give proper instructions to solicitors;
- the ability to make decisions in the course of the proceedings:
    - o to authorise proceedings to be issued;
    - o to approve the particulars of claim;
    - o to approve the disclosure of witness statements and expert evidence;
    - o to approve an offer to settle;
    - o to accept a suitable offer to settle made by the defendants;
    - o to compromise the claim, whether on a percentage basis or in monetary terms, taking into account what is being given up and what would happen in the event of a refusal to accept the offer of compromise;
    - o to proceed to trial;
    - o to withdraw the claim if there is evidence that the defendants acted lawfully;
- the risks involved in rejecting an offer that the claimant is reasonably advised to accept, that is:
    - o withdrawal of Legal Aid Authority or insurance funding for the claim;
    - o being awarded by the court less than the offer that was rejected;
    - o being ordered to pay the other side's costs from the date the offer was rejected;
- the advantages and disadvantages of a lump sum payment versus a periodical payment.

This is not an exhaustive list. Sometimes, instructing solicitors point out the particular decisions for which the claimant will need to have capacity. This list relates to a personal injury action. There are other proceedings where people bring or defend a case. Instructing solicitors should provide sufficient information as to the nature and extent of those proceedings for the psychiatrist to assess the person's capacity to bring or defend the case. *Lindsay* is worth reading as an example of how the court approaches capacity to litigate.

Sometimes, the expert is instructed after the claimant has already commenced proceedings, in which case it is advisable to find out what instructions they have already given.

The claimant in *Dunhill v Burgin* [2014] UKSC 18 settled her road traffic accident personal injury claim for £12,500 on the basis of a gross undervaluation of her claim and ignorant then of the fact that subsequently it was valued at over £2 million. The court found that it did not matter that she understood matters well enough to make the decision to compromise her claim for the total sum of £12,500 with costs upon the advice of her then legal advisors; what mattered was that she did not have the capacity to conduct the larger and much more complicated claim which should have been brought. As '[t]he proceedings ... may take many twists and turns [and] may develop and change as the evidence is gathered and the arguments refined', be prepared to revisit an opinion as to litigation capacity in a case where, as it progresses, the size of the claim or the complexity of the litigation changes.

Since 2005, in compensating for injury and related financial losses, there have been provisions for 'periodical payments' as well as 'lump sum' payments. Choosing between them involves a mixture of practical, financial and legal considerations.

The first advantage of periodical payments is that, as they are guaranteed for life, they more accurately meet the claimant's needs by providing for them until they die, regardless of what the estimate was of their life expectancy, whereas a lump sum is based on an estimate of life expectancy which, if it is a significant underestimate, leaves the claimant with insufficient funds for their needs and possibly just when those funds are needed most. The second advantage is that the responsibility for ensuring investment sufficient to make the periodical payments is transferred from the claimant, or his trustees, to the insurer, who will be better placed to protect the funds against inflation. Lump sums that are invested may perform poorly or fail to keep up with inflation. The third advantage of a periodical payment is that it is free of tax. The disadvantage of the periodical payment is that, in order to achieve the annual income, the claimant has to give up a substantial part of his lump sum so that, in effect, the defendant can buy an insurance policy to cover the claimant. Also, the tax and benefit advantages may be changed by future legislation; there are no beneficiaries following the claimant's death; the funds cannot be used as security for a loan; and they are inflexible.

The advantages of the lump sum are that it is final, simple and offers flexibility to the claimant who can decide how to prioritise his various needs and wants (*Tameside and Glossop Acute Services NHS Trust v Thompstone* [2008] EWCA Civ 5). The claimant, or his trustees, has/have the power to make plans for the whole of the award at the outset. There is also the advantage, for the family-minded claimant, that if they die much sooner than expected, their family can benefit from the residue of the compensation. Significant problems with the lump sum are that the amount of income generated will depend on the element of risk the claimant is prepared to take. Also, although the lump sum itself is not taxed, income and capital gains from the investments are taxable, which may become a more important consideration if tax rates rise.

What is best for the claimant will depend on a number of factors. If the experts disagree about life expectancy, periodical payments may be particularly appropriate. Whether it is a short- or long-life expectancy can make a difference. If it is long, there is more time for investment of a lump sum to achieve a better than average result; if it is short, it may not be possible to do well by investing a lump sum (Braithwaite and Waldron 2010). If there is a significant deduction for contributory negligence on the part of the claimant, a lump sum may be more appropriate (Braithwaite and Waldron 2010). A similar consideration applies if the claim is compromised at less than 100 per cent liability because the claimant's legal advisors feel that there is a risk that if the case goes to trial the claimant might lose entirely.

A settlement meeting can last for several hours. There will usually be several heads of damage, with pros and cons for each, and one figure based on the claim, a second based on the counter schedule (the defendant's proposed settlement for the head of damage) and the third, counsel's compromise. Each one has to be explained in simple enough terms for the claimant to understand. Life expectancy may be disputed. At the end of the meeting, in order to decide whether to accept or reject the offer, the claimant has to remember all of the issues, blend them together, take account of the risks on each, understand what is meant by an offer to settle and make a judgement.

In Ireland, RSC Ord. 15, r 17 provides that a 'person of unsound mind' may sue as plaintiff by his committee or next friend, and may defend by his committee or guardian appointed for that purpose. This is not linked with 'mental disorder' within the meaning of the MHA 2001. The consent of the wardship court is required in the case of a ward of court. The question of periodic payments only arises in Ireland in the case of catastrophic injury claims. As to tax on lump-sum awards, in the case of a person who is permanently and totally incapacitated from maintaining himself, where the income from the award is the sole or main income of the individual, it is exempt.

Capacity to Manage and Administer Property and Affairs

Capacity to manage and administer property and affairs particularly arises in personal injury cases where the claimant receives, or stands to receive, a significant amount of compensation and about which they may need investment advice. Experts are often instructed to deal with litigation capacity at the same time, but in *Masterman-Lister* it was held that someone can lack the capacity to litigate but possess the capacity to manage and administer their compensation and vice versa.

In the context of a personal injury claim, capacity in relation to financial affairs and property is the central issue. In most cases, the difficulty is that the amount of compensation awarded will be an amount that most people have never handled and never will handle. Although the assumption is that the person will have appropriate financial, legal and other advice, it is reasonable to explore the following areas:

- the purpose of compensation;
- the distinction between general damages and damages for care, loss of earnings, etc.;
- an understanding of the nature and purpose of investments;
- the ability to seek, understand and act on appropriate advice, which means having regard to the likelihood they would recognise their need for advice and the likelihood that, having so recognised it, they would do something about it;
- their understanding of their financial needs and responsibilities, including family and social responsibilities;
- the degree of support the person receives or could expect to receive from others.

The claimant must understand that compensation is intended to last for life.

It is necessary to explore how the claimant currently manages their property and affairs, so as to try to understand how they would do so in the future. This means being informed as to their current financial circumstances, such as the value of their home, their financial needs and responsibilities. Box 10.1 sets out examples of various activities and situations about which it is useful to make enquiry and Box 10.2 suggests an approach to exploring a claimant's current financial affairs.

Affairs extend beyond financial affairs. In a case where twenty-four-hour care will be needed for the rest of the person's life, issues may include, for example, job descriptions, the hiring and firing of staff, employer's liability insurance, rotas and contracts with agencies.

Capacity to Bring and Conduct Proceedings before the First-tier Tribunal in Its Mental Health Jurisdiction

In England and Wales, for a patient to bring proceedings before the First-tier Tribunal in its mental health jurisdiction, the test is: 'The patient must understand that they are being detained against their wishes and that the First-tier Tribunal is a body that will be able to decide whether they should be released' (*VS v St Andrew's Healthcare* [2018] UKUT 250

Box 10.1 Examples of Transactions or Situations to Be Considered under Capacity to Manage Property and Affairs

- open and close a bank account, including understanding what a bank account is and what the implications are of having a bank account;
- pay any bills for which responsible, including making payment by standing order or direct debit;
- work out a monthly budget to pay bills;
- remember to pay the car insurance, get a new MOT certificate and obtain a new tax disc;
- choose a holiday, book it, pay the deposit, organise insurance and, if necessary, save to pay the balance of the price of the holiday and spending money;
- deal with correspondence from the Inland Revenue, Benefits Agency, insurance companies, bank and utility services;
- appreciate the need to obtain household and buildings insurance and be able to submit a claim if anything went wrong with the property;
- know what to do with a letter offering the opportunity to take out credit or investments;
- be able to seek and accept advice in relation to tax, investments, savings and running a house on their own and all that that entails.

Box 10.2 Exploring a Claimant's Current Financial Affairs

- What is the claimant's weekly/fortnightly/monthly income?
- From what sources does the income come?
- How does the claimant access his money?
- Is the claimant able to go to a cashpoint to access his money and understand that this gets deducted from his account?
- Is the claimant able to write cheques and understand that this sum gets deducted from his account?
- On what does the claimant spend his money?
- Does the claimant save money?
- Can the claimant work out from a bank statement how much money he has left at the end of the month?
- Does the claimant understand that he should not spend more than his income?

(AAC)). This is less demanding than the capacity to conduct such proceedings as set out in *YA v Central and North West London NHS Mental Health Trust* [2015] UKUT 37 (AAC). To conduct proceedings, the detained patient has to be able sufficiently to understand, retain, use and weigh the following factors:

i) the detention, and so the reasons for it, can be challenged in proceedings before the tribunal who, on that challenge, will consider whether the detention is justified by the provisions of the MHA 1983,
ii) in doing that, the tribunal will investigate and invite and consider questions and argument on the issues, the medical and other evidence and the legal issues,
iii) the tribunal can discharge the section and so bring the detention to an end,

iv) representation would be free,
v) discussion can take place with the patient and the representative before, and so without the pressure of, a hearing,
vi) having regard to that discussion a representative would be able to question witnesses and argue the case on the facts and the law, and thereby assist in ensuring that the tribunal took all relevant factual and legal issues into account,
vii) he or she may not be able to do this so well because of their personal involvement and the nature and complication of some of the issues (e.g. when they are finely balanced or depend on the likelihood of the patient's compliance with assessment or treatment or relate to what is the least restrictive available way of best achieving the proposed assessment or treatment),
viii) having regard to the issues of fact and law his or her ability to conduct the proceedings without help, and so
ix) the impact of these factors on the choice to be made.

Capacity to Bring Proceedings in the Court of Protection

The capacity to bring proceedings in the Court of Protection 'simply requires P to understand that the court has the power to decide that he/she should not be subject to his/her current care arrangements. It is a lower threshold than the capacity to conduct proceedings' (*Re D (Incapacitated Person) (Representatives and Advocates: Duties and Powers) v Herefordshire Council* [2016] EWCOP 49).

Capacity to Make a Gift

The leading case on the capacity to gift is *Re Beaney (Deceased)* [1978] 1 WLR 770. The testatrix signed a deed of gift transferring her house to her older daughter a few days after being admitted to hospital with advanced dementia. It was held that:

> In the case of a contract, a deed made for consideration or a gift inter vivos, whether by deed or otherwise, the degree required varies with the circumstances of the transaction. Thus, at one extreme, if the subject matter and value of the gift are trivial in relation to the donor's other assets a low degree of understanding will suffice. But, at the other extreme, if its effect is to dispose of the donor's only asset of value and thus, for practical purposes, to pre-empt the devolution of his estate under his will or on his intestacy, then the degree of understanding is as high as that required for a will, and the donor must understand the claims of all potential donees and the extent of the property to be disposed of.

Thus, the assessment of capacity should include (The British Medical Association (BMA) and Law Society 2015):

- Understanding what a gift is: not a loan or something that the donor can ask to be returned
- Whether they expect to receive anything in return
- When the gift is to take effect
- Who the recipient is
- Whether the donor has already made substantial gifts to the recipient or others
- Whether it is a one-off gift or part of a larger series of transactions
- The underlying purpose of the transaction

Capacity to Engage in Social Media

Re A (Capacity: Social Media and Internet Use: Best Interests) [2019] EWCOP 2 is the case of a young man with an intellectual disability who used social media to share images and videos of his genitals with unknown men and searched compulsively for pornography – some of which was illegal. In determining capacity to consent to social media use, the court found that the relevant information to be understood was:

i) Information and images (including videos) which you share on the internet or through social media could be shared more widely, including with people you don't know, without you knowing or being able to stop it;
ii) It is possible to limit the sharing of personal information or images (and videos) by using 'privacy and location settings' on some internet and social media sites …
iii) If you place material or images (including videos) on social media sites which are rude or offensive, or share those images, other people might be upset or offended …
iv) Some people you meet or communicate with ('talk to') online, who you don't otherwise know, may not be who they say they are ('they may disguise, or lie about, themselves'); someone who calls themselves a 'friend' on social media may not be friendly;
v) Some people you meet or communicate with ('talk to') on the internet or through social media, who you don't otherwise know, may pose a risk to you; they may lie to you, or exploit or take advantage of you sexually, financially, emotionally and/or physically; they may want to cause you harm;
vi) If you look at or share extremely rude or offensive images, messages or videos online you may get into trouble with the police, because you may have committed a crime.

The Assessment

The overriding principle is that the person should be assessed when at their highest level of functioning (Ashton *et al.* 2006, p. 84). The assessing psychiatrist has a responsibility to maximise or enhance the person's mental capacity (Braithwaite and Waldron 2010). Consider assessing the person in their own environment, because taking all practicable steps to enable the person to make a decision (MCA, s 1(3), ADM(C)A, s 8(3)) includes making sure that the person is in an environment in which they are comfortable. Braithwaite and Waldron (2010) suggest that it should 'probably not [be] in circumstances which might create nervousness or tension (such as hospital, surgery or office)'. 'Practicable' means the exercise of common sense, otherwise known as the combination of sound judgment with compromise (*Dedman v British Building and Engineering Appliances Ltd* [1974] 1 WLR 171). Just as it was recognised in *Re T (Adult: Refusal of Medical Treatment)* that, when making a decision about treatment, someone who is 'very tired, in pain and depressed will be much less able to resist having his will overborne, than one who is rested, free from pain and cheerful', so far as is practicable, the subject should be assessed when they are rested, when analgesia is at its optimal level and their mental state is as settled as possible. Also, presentation of information in a user-friendly manner can make all the difference as to whether a person has capacity. Other considerations are the time of day, the assistance of a speech therapist or interpreter and any cultural, ethnic or religious factors that may influence the person's functioning.

Always take into consideration the actual assistance available, or likely to be available. It can make a critical difference between the person having and not having capacity. Thus, it may be appropriate for part of the assessment to take place with the assistance of someone such as a family member. But some people function better when seen without family present. Ask the subject which they would prefer. But be alive to the case where assistance is actually influence, or even undue influence, as 'where the influence is that of a parent or other close dominating relative, and where the arguments and persuasions are based upon personal affection . . . the influence may . . . be subtle, insidious, pervasive and powerful' (*Re SA (Vulnerable Adult with Capacity: Marriage)* [2005] EWHC 2942).

No capacity assessment should begin without knowing precisely the decision which the person is to make and the relevant information. Although it is not necessary for the person to understand all the peripheral information, a view will need to be taken as to the salient information which needs to be understood. This should be clear either from the information provided by the instructing solicitors or by reference to the literature and case law or a combination of these. An assessment of capacity must include questions that reveal how the person responds to being asked to consider the decisions specific to the issue in question, such as those that arise in a settlement meeting. When the claimant says that he will do whatever his solicitor advises, this must lead to an exploration of how, and with what information, they will evaluate and weigh in the balance what their solicitor advises.

It will usually be necessary to have some knowledge of the subject's background history and premorbid personality. In deciding whether current thinking and behaviour reflects an abnormal mental state, information about their previous patterns of behaviour, values and goals from those with professional or personal knowledge of the person and their circumstances may assist. In a head injury case, it may be 'intrinsically difficult to separate conduct and patterns of behaviour that might bear upon the relevant assessment, that were wholly or mainly attributable to psychological explanation rather than wholly or mainly attributable to the organic brain injury' because '[i]n simple terms many young men, who suffer no brain injury at all, are indolent, unmotivated and prone to make financial, and other, decisions that are unwise or even calamitous' (*Loughlin*).

All relevant medical records should be available. If the issue is the testamentary capacity of someone who was in hospital at the relevant time, it will be necessary to see the nursing and any other records for the day, or even the part of the day, when the instructions were given or the will executed.

Usually, assessment is best approached as if the person lacked capacity and conducting the examination so as to enable them to prove, if they can, that they have capacity (Rix 2006). This means starting with as limited an introduction as possible and then asking them why they have attended. It may be obvious, and confirmed by asking about 'your case', 'solicitors' and 'court', that the person has no idea that they have a case. Care has to be taken in the way questions are put and capabilities tested. You do not ask, 'How would you compromise your claim?' Ask a simple question like the 'car boot sale' question: 'You want £40 for your clock and you are offered only £20. What could you do to make sure you sell it?' If the person has been accompanied, or if someone else is present, find out what, if anything, they were told about the purpose of the consultation and when they were told. This assists in understanding ability to understand and retain relevant information. It will almost always be necessary to include in the mental state examination at least a rudimentary cognitive assessment and in many cases some tests of cognitive functioning.

As capacity is time-specific, the person's mental state at the consultation is important. However, it is important to analyse carefully the documentary evidence as this will indicate how the person functions on a day-to-day basis. For example, daily in-patient rehabilitation and nursing or care home records can provide a wealth of information relevant to capacity to manage property and affairs. Likewise, reliable evidence from family and friends can provide good examples of capacity or the lack of it.

Particularly in cases involving brain injury or intellectual disability, there is likely to be a neuropsychological assessment. But allow for the fact that 'neuropsychological testing makes it almost inevitable that an external structure will be provided for the undertaking of tasks, including those tasks considered to fall under the rubric of executive functioning' and without which structure there may be 'substantial impairments in [the subject's] ability to structure and organise activities by and for himself' (*Loughlin*). Similarly, in *Lindsay*, the judge identified a 'discrepancy between the general picture given by Mrs Lindsay and that given by the medical evidence [which was] largely explained by the difference between "real life", as it is described, and the artificial conditions of a medical assessment'.

Where the assessment is retrospective and entirely based on papers, set out as your chronology the evidence from medical and other records, correspondence, witness statements, etc. in strict chronological order in a table so that the day, hour or even minute when the decision is taken can be seen in context. Distinguish non-contemporaneous information, such as that from witness statements, with *italic* type. Be prepared for the rival members of the family giving conflicting accounts of the mental abilities of the person whose capacity is in question. If the case goes to trial, the judge will decide on the factual evidence and unless one side's version is so obviously at odds with the contemporaneous documentary evidence, it may be necessary to give alternative opinions depending on which account is accepted.

Further Reading

Ashton, G., Letts, P., Oates, L. and Terrell, M. (2006) *Mental Capacity: The New Law* (Jordans)

British Medical Association and the Law Society (2015) *Assessment of Mental Capacity: A Practical Guide for Doctors and Lawyers*, 4th edn (Law Society).

Clancy v Clancy [2003] EWHC 1885 (Ch).

Jackson, E. (2019) *Medical Law: Text, Cases and Materials*, 5th edn (Oxford University Press).

Jones, R. and Piffaretti, E. (2018) *Mental Capacity Act Manual*, 8th edn (Sweet & Maxwell).

Chapter

11 Reports for the First-tier Tribunal (Health, Education and Social Care Chamber) Mental Health

Chris Jones and Srikanth Nimmagadda

There is . . . no canon of construction which presumes that Parliament intended that people should, against their will, be subjected to treatment which others, however professionally competent, perceive, however sincerely and however correctly, to be in their best interests.
McCullough J in *R v Hallstrom (ex p W) (No. 2)* [1986] 2 All ER 306

Psychiatrists testifying as expert witnesses before mental health tribunals (MHTs) and review boards face specific challenges which would be unusual in other judicial settings. These relate both to the inquisitorial nature of the tribunal and its inherent expertise. Consider carefully your role if your evidence is to be both effective and appropriate.

In England and Wales, independent psychiatric testimony is now largely confined to cases of long-term detention under the MHA 1983, s 3, s 37 or, most commonly, ss 37/41. It is also almost exclusively commissioned on behalf of the patient, but very similar considerations apply where the detaining authority or Secretary of State commissions it.

In Ireland, the Mental Health Commission automatically commissions an independent report for the purpose of the tribunal hearing in every case. But patients detained pursuant to the MHA 2001 can also commission an independent report and are most likely to do so in the context of a proposal for transfer to the CMH or for psychosurgery, but most patients do not, in the context of ordinary tribunal reviews, have the financial means or the cognitive wherewithal to do so. Likewise, patients detained pursuant to the Criminal Law (Insanity) Acts 2006 and 2010 whose cases fall to be considered by the Mental Health (Criminal Law) Review Board can commission their own independent report.

The Inquisitorial Tribunal

Tribunals are unusual in explicitly adopting an inquisitorial rather than an adversarial stance. The rules of evidence on matters such as hearsay are more relaxed, but the basic rules for an expert witness still apply.

As an inquisitorial forum, there is wide discretion over the evidence admitted. MHTs may refuse the parties permission to call certain witnesses whose evidence the tribunal is not persuaded would be relevant. While this is less likely now that there is an explicit duty of fairness to the parties, the party calling an expert, and the expert themselves, may well be expected to demonstrate why expert evidence is required.

Similarly, the tribunal will take the lead in questioning witnesses and in determining the relevant areas of evidence. While patients' representatives are entitled to ask further questions, this is often limited in scope. While representatives are usually given leeway in exploring further issues, the tribunal can be expected to identify the issues which it considers relevant for the admission of expert evidence, and pursuing lines of evidence which the tribunal has not itself raised, even if admitted, may have limited impact.

Finally, note that although the parties will present their views of the case, unlike an adversarial forum, the tribunal can take evidence and raise issues that the parties do not (see below).

The Tribunal Rules and Procedures

In England and Wales, familiarise yourself with the Tribunals Procedure (First-tier Tribunal) (Health, Education and Social Care Chamber) Rules 2008 (TP(FTT)(HESCC) 2), which govern both the procedure and the content. The following are important:

- the overriding objective of any tribunal is to deal with the case before it 'fairly and justly';
- procedural decisions of the tribunal must always seek to give effect to these objectives;
- parties may be permitted or required to provide expert evidence and the tribunal may direct that a single expert is jointly appointed (TP(FTT)(HESCC) 15); and
- the tribunal has wide discretion to admit or exclude evidence, and to limit the issues, nature of evidence and number of witnesses (TP(FTT)(HESCC) 15).

In Ireland, there are written procedures for the Criminal Law (Mental Health) Review Board, promulgated by the Board (Criminal Law (Insanity) Act 2006, s 11 and First Schedule, para. 13), but these largely reflect the statutory provisions. There are no written rules for MHTs: a tribunal determines its own procedures, subject only to the MHA 2001.

The Statutory Criteria

Tribunals often hear wide-ranging evidence about a patient's psychiatric condition, life history, circumstances and future plans, and not uncommonly are invited to make comments and recommendations based on this. But remember that ultimately a tribunal is bound to reach its decision in line with statutory criteria. Other considerations may influence a tribunal's views, but the decision itself must be expressed in response to specific tests, and all evidence should ultimately aim at establishing the appropriate answer to these specific questions (adapted from the MHA 1983, s 72, applicable to s 3 and, with minor (but important) alterations, to other sections and other jurisdictions):

- Does the patient suffer from a mental disorder?
- Is that mental disorder of a nature or degree that makes it appropriate for the patient to be detained in hospital for treatment?
- Is that treatment necessary for the health of the patient or the safety of the patient or the protection of other persons?
- Is appropriate treatment available?

In Ireland, for patients detained pursuant to the MHA 2001, specific questions are:

- Is transfer of a detained patient to the CMH in the best interest of the health of the patient concerned?
- Is psychosurgery in the best interest of the health of the patient concerned?

In Ireland, for patients detained pursuant to the Criminal Law (Insanity) Acts 2006 and 2010, specific questions are:

- Unfitness to plead: Does the patient, although still unfit to be tried, still require in-patient care or treatment in the designated centre?
- Not guilty by reason of insanity: Does the patient still require in-patient care or treatment in the designated centre?
- Variation of Conditions of Discharge: Is it appropriate to vary or remove one or more of the conditions of the conditional discharge order?
- Unconditional Discharge: Is it proper to make an order for an unconditional discharge?
- Breach of Condition of Discharge: All of the foregoing fall for consideration.

Reports and the Practice Direction

Psychiatrists *in England and Wales* will be familiar with the *Practice Direction: First-tier Tribunal Health Education and Social Care Chamber: Statements and Reports in Mental Health Cases*, which specifies the information that must be included in reports submitted by responsible clinicians (and also by the detaining authority, nursing staff and those providing social circumstances reports). This has been developed in response to perceived failings of reports to cover relevant topics, but inevitably reports can become dense with irrelevant information.

Expert witnesses have wider discretion to tailor reports individually. You would not be likely to be criticised for following the Practice Direction format, but we suggest that a report limited to directly relevant issues may be more effective.

The points detailed in the Practice Direction will only be relevant to a tribunal's decision if they speak to the statutory criteria in a particular case. We therefore suggest that your report would usefully be structured along the lines of the statutory criteria outlined above, clearly delineating sections of the report dealing with the diagnosis (or not) of mental disorder, the appropriateness of detention, the risks of non-treatment, and the appropriateness and availability of treatment.

We also suggest that your report does not need to repeat issues that are common ground. Focus on the contested areas, but be prepared to address any points raised by the tribunal. A tribunal has the power to require the production of evidence not originally presented by the parties, and to adjourn if necessary for this purpose (*R (X) v MHRT* [2003] EWHC 1272 (Admin)). This could potentially include directing expert opinion on a specific issue (TP(FTT)(HESCC) 5 and 16).

The Tribunal's Inherent Expertise

Like some other tribunals, MHTs are constituted deliberately to possess inherent expertise in their subject matter. Panels include a medical member, almost invariably a current or retired consultant psychiatrist, further selected for their knowledge and experience and trained specifically in psychiatric and legal issues relevant to the tribunal. Second, the specialist lay members are appointed from a range of professional backgrounds, again based on considerable knowledge and experience of mental health, such as mental health nursing or psychiatric social work. Finally, legal members of the tribunal, while not having clinical experience, are often appointed with years of experience of practising mental health law – often in front of tribunals – and even those appointed from other jurisdictions have specialist training and considerable experience of mental health issues. The inherent expertise 'is an important contribution to the equality of arms, thereby reducing the need ... for the patient to have their own expert evidence' (*MD v Nottinghamshire Health Care NHS Trust* [2010] UKUT 59 (AAC)).

In consequence, while evidence from the responsible clinician and from experts will carry significant weight, '[i]t is open to a Tribunal, provided that they act rationally, to disagree with the view of *any* psychiatrist whose evidence is put before them' (*R v London South & Southwest Region Mental Health Review Tribunal, ex p Moyle* [2000] Lloyd's Rep Med 143) (emphasis added). The duty to consider cases fairly and rationally requires reasons to be explicit: 'while the Tribunal was under no obligation to accept the conclusions of the experts, it was under an obligation to explain clearly why it rejected their opinion' (*DL v South London & Maudsley NHS Trust* [2010] UKUT 455 (ACC)). Likewise, *in Ireland*, the duty to give reasons is required by the MHA 2001.

While significant, the inherent expertise should not be overestimated. Tribunals hear cases from a wide range of clinical settings, reviewing patients with many different disorders and in widely differing circumstances. However, panel members' expertise is specific to their own practice, and while many concepts will generalise across different cases, medical members are not selected as clinical experts in particular areas of psychiatry. The tribunal has established specific Child and Adolescent Mental Health Services panels, comprising members considered to have particular knowledge of child and adolescent psychiatry, but even within this subgroup, experience of the specific patient's individual presentation may be limited.

Further to the tribunal's own expertise, evidence will usually be presented by the patient's responsible clinician or less commonly another senior member of the medical staff. As well as being experienced clinicians in their own right, responsible clinicians will generally have the advantage of knowledge of the patient over a considerable length of time, compared to the expert's brief involvement. Evidence is also likely to be heard from several other members of the clinical team, all of whom have the advantage of extended acquaintance with the patient.

The Role of Expert Evidence

Tribunals and boards appreciate a well-written independent psychiatric report because it brings a new perspective and because the author has more time available than a busy clinician. Independent experts should make sure that they cover in their report the patient's strengths and any other positive factors of which the tribunal should be aware.

Given the considerable experience and detailed clinical knowledge already available within the tribunal and from existing witnesses, we suggest that the expert has broadly two legitimate functions: to provide highly specialist knowledge or to provide alternative interpretations.

Although psychiatry is a broad field, services are often stratified by age group or level of security as much as or more than by clinical presentation. So, where a patient is being managed by a psychiatrist with limited clinical experience of their condition, an expert may possess knowledge that will genuinely increase the level of clinical understanding available to the tribunal.

Also, psychiatry is a field in which opinions can vary widely, and in which objective clinical facts are subject to interpretation and dispute. The responsible clinician will present a particular view of the patient's condition and needs which, given the setting, inevitably focuses on continuing detention. Clinical teams rarely lack for dissenting views, but the evidence presented by members of the team at a tribunal will typically support or even repeat the responsible clinician's views. A patient challenging detention lacks the professional's clinical credibility and may be dismissed as lacking understanding or insight.

Perhaps the most valuable role for expert evidence, therefore, is to provide professional respectability to an alternative perspective on the patient's situation.

This does not mean taking the patient's view uncritically. Whereas a legal representative's duty is ultimately to present the client's case, experts must remain true to their own professional integrity and give an honest opinion, even if unwelcome to the party instructing them. But that honest opinion can serve to introduce options which a tribunal might not consider solely based on a patient's own wishes.

Confidentiality

The tribunal rules give discretion to the tribunal not to allow disclosure of information if this would be likely to cause serious harm (TP(FTT)(HESCC) 14(2)). The question has arisen whether the patient or his or her legal representative can prevent the disclosure of any unfavourable report that they have commissioned for an MHT. The seminal case highlighting these issues is *W v Egdell* [1990] 1 All ER 835.

W was a detained patient in a special hospital with a restriction order authorised by the MHA 1959, ss 60/65 (equivalent to the MHA 1983, ss 37/41) having been convicted of the manslaughter of five people. Dr Egdell was commissioned by W's solicitors to prepare an independent psychiatric report for an MHT. His report suggested that the patient was more dangerous than the responsible medical officer or hospital managers thought and he stressed a number of factors relevant to W's treatment and dangerousness that had not previously been identified by his clinical team. W did not want the report to be disclosed to the MHT and withdrew his application. However, Dr Egdell disclosed the report to the Secretary of State and the hospital authorities and was sued for breach of confidence.

The Court of Appeal held that the value of the information with regard to public safety was so great that it outweighed the usual duty of confidentiality. It was held that the expert was entitled to disclose the report if, in their professional opinion, this was necessary in the public interest to protect against possible harm to others.

Presenting Expert Evidence

So, these are some practical suggestions for psychiatrists preparing and presenting expert evidence to MHTs:

- Be respectful and mindful of the expertise inherent in all the members of the tribunal, not just the medical member.
- Acknowledge the unique position of the responsible clinician in relation to longitudinal knowledge of the patient, ongoing responsibility for care and treatment, and also their difficulties presenting evidence unwelcome to the patient while maintaining a therapeutic relationship.
- Explicitly justify the relevance of expert evidence and what you aim to add to the tribunal's deliberations.
- Structure written and oral evidence to address the statutory criteria.
- Avoid lengthy repetition of background information which the practice direction requires other reports to cover.

Reports in Immigration and Asylum Cases

Cornelius Katona, Andrew Leak and David Rhys Jones

The consideration given to a report depends on the quality of the report and the standing and qualifications of the doctor.

Ouseley J in *HE v Secretary of State for the Home Department* [2004] UKIAT 321

The majority of requests for reports in immigration and asylum cases arise in the asylum context. However, issues of mental health will frequently come up in human rights applications and may give rise to similar requests. Here, we provide an outline of the asylum legal process, identifying the relevance of expert psychiatric evidence within that process and the duties of the psychiatric expert, and providing guidance on the conduct of such assessments and the preparation of reports.

The Asylum and Appeal Process and the Potential Functions of Expert Psychiatric Reports within that Process

A refugee is a person who meets the definition in the UN 1951 *Convention Relating to the Status of Refugees* ('the Convention'), art 1A. An asylum seeker is a person who has left their country of origin and formally applied for recognition as a refugee.

An asylum seeker is required to demonstrate a well-founded fear of persecution due to their race, religion, nationality, political opinion or membership of a particular social group, and inability or unwillingness to seek protection from the authorities in their own country. The perspective is forward-looking as what determines whether asylum should be granted is risk on return, not demonstration of past persecution, although, in the absence of evidence of a significant or major change of circumstances, it can substantially support the well-foundedness of the present fear and be considered probative of future risk. This is an important consideration when considering the use of medical evidence in support of asylum applications. Furthermore, as the UN 1999 *Manual on Effective Investigation and Documentation of Torture and Other Cruel, Inhuman or Degrading Treatment or Punishment* ('the Istanbul Protocol'), para. 261 makes clear:

> Psychological evaluations provide useful evidence for medico-legal examinations, political asylum applications, establishing conditions under which false confessions may have been obtained, understanding regional practices of torture, identifying the therapeutic needs of victims and as testimony in human rights investigations. The overall goal of a psychological evaluation is to assess the degree of consistency between an individual's account of torture and the psychological findings observed during the course of the evaluation. To this end, the evaluation should provide a detailed description of the individual's history, a mental status examination, an assessment of social functioning and the formulation of clinical

> impressions . . . A psychiatric diagnosis should be made, if appropriate. Because psychological symptoms are so prevalent among survivors of torture, it is highly advisable for any evaluation of torture to include a psychological assessment.

Decisions on asylum applications made in the UK rest with United Kingdom Visas & Immigration (UKVI). The asylum seeker will have at least two interviews with officials from UKVI. The first is the 'screening interview', in which the UKVI official takes the personal details of the applicant and an account of their journey to the UK. The second 'substantive interview' is the opportunity for the applicant to describe their past experiences and their fear for the future if returned to their country of origin.

UKVI officials then consider the account of persecution and further supporting evidence, including medicolegal reports, in order to decide whether the applicant has met the criteria for a grant of asylum under the Convention. To be recognised as a refugee under the Convention, a person must demonstrate, *inter alia*, that their fear is well-founded and related to a Convention-specified reason, that they are unable to seek protection from their own state and that, if the persecutor is a non-state actor, it would be unreasonable for them to seek protection in another part of their country of origin.

One consequence of the asylum seeker's fear may be a risk of suicide and this may be created by a genuine fear even if lacking objective foundation (*Y (Sri Lanka) v Secretary of State for the Home Department* [2009] EWCA Civ 362). However, the test is not just of a significantly increased suicide risk, but of a real risk; merely more than 'not fanciful' is not enough (*J v Secretary of State for the Home Department* [2005] EWCA Civ 629).

A particular issue may be vulnerability to harm in immigration detention as the Immigration Act 2016, s 59 has created a statutory duty for the Secretary of State to take this into account. The Home Office (2018) has issued *Guidance on adults at risk in immigration detention*. Paragraph 11 lists conditions or experiences which may indicate such vulnerability, including 'a mental health condition or impairment (this may include more serious learning difficulties, psychiatric illness or clinical depression, depending on the nature and seriousness of the condition)' and PTSD. The corollary is that only in very exceptional circumstances will someone be considered suitable for detention if suffering from a serious medical condition which cannot be satisfactorily managed within detention. However, it is not sufficient to diagnose a mental disorder within the meaning of the MHA 1983. Whether the person is 'suffering' means having regard to the effects of the condition on the individual and the effect of detention on them. Consideration of 'satisfactory management' means having regard to such matters as the medication they are taking, their demonstrable needs and whether they can be met in detention, the facilities available at the centre where they are, or are to be, detained and the expected period of detention (*R (Das) v Secretary of State for the Home Department* [2014] EWCA Civ 45). In *OM (Nigeria) v Secretary of State for the Home Department* [2011] EWCA Civ 909, regarding OM, who suffered from a recurrent depressive disorder and emotionally unstable personality disorder and had attempted suicide, the court accepted the balance of expert opinion that she could be managed appropriately in detention. If for some reason the standard of care in detention was not equal to the standard of care which would be available to the detainee if released, this could call into question how satisfactorily their condition could be managed in detention.

What Constitutes Relevant Evidence?

The UNHCR *Handbook and Guidelines on Procedures and Criteria for Determining Refugee Status under the 1951 Convention and the 1967 Protocol Relating to the Status of Refugees*

(December 2011) ('the Handbook') explains that persecution has no 'universally accepted definition' (Handbook, para. 51), but that:

> The subjective character of fear of persecution requires an evaluation of the opinions and feelings of the person concerned. It is also in the light of such opinions and feelings that any actual or anticipated measures against him must necessarily be viewed. Due to variations in the psychological make-up of individuals and in the circumstances of each case, interpretations of what amounts to persecution are bound to vary. (Handbook, para. 52)

An assertion of persecution therefore needs to be understood in the overall context of the evidence given, which may include medical evidence.

The standard of proof in asylum matters is very low (a 'reasonable degree of likelihood'), but the burden of proof in asylum matters is upon the asylum seeker. The Handbook (para. 37) explains that:

> No documentary proof as such is required in order for the authorities to recognise a refugee claim, however, information on practices in the country of origin may support a particular case. It is important to recognise that in relation to gender-related claims, the usual types of evidence used in other refugee claims may not be as readily available. Statistical data or reports on the incidence of sexual violence may not be available, due to under-reporting of cases, or lack of prosecution. Alternative forms of information might assist, such as the testimonies of other women similarly situated in written reports or oral testimony, of non-governmental or international organisations or other independent research.

Thus, while objective evidence is a requirement, information on the political and human rights situation in the asylum seeker's country of origin is usually presented in the form of generic country reports. On occasions, a specific report will be produced to substantiate particular aspects of the asylum seeker's allegations by a person recognised as a country expert.

Paragraph 208 of the Handbook explains that:

> The examiner should, in such cases, whenever possible, obtain expert medical advice. The medical report should provide information on the nature and degree of mental illness and should assess the applicant's ability to fulfil the requirements normally expected of an applicant in presenting his case (see paragraph 205(a) above). The conclusions of the medical report will determine the examiner's further approach.

However, in the UK, medical reports are never commissioned by UKVI in relation to first instance decision-making, and are therefore generally prepared on the instructions of, and provided through, the asylum seeker's legal representative. Medical reports, invariably described as medicolegal reports, may also be commissioned to consider the asylum seeker's mental and physical health in order to determine the degree of consistency between the presented mental and physical trauma and their attributed cause. Other evidence will often include legal jurisprudence from the UK and around the world.

The UKVI official will then assess all this evidence to make a decision. As set out in the Handbook at para. 195: 'The relevant facts of the individual case will have to be furnished in the first place by the applicant himself. It will then be up to the person charged with determining his status (the examiner) to assess the validity of any evidence and the credibility of the applicant's statements.'

Credibility is frequently a critical feature. For example, if an asylum seeker states that they were a citizen of, and were a political activist in, Cameroon, but were then unable to provide information about the geography, economy or politics of Cameroon, it is unlikely that it would be accepted that they were from Cameroon or that they were politically active. However, if the same person instead claims to be in need of protection because they are homosexual, then having established that they are from Cameroon, the emphasis will be on their subjective experiences in Cameroon alongside country information as to how Cameroon treats homosexuals. Evidence always needs to be carefully curated so as to best assist the UKVI in reaching the correct decision. The Handbook explains (para. 52) that: 'Due to variations in the psychological make-up of individuals and in the circumstances of each case, interpretations of what amounts to persecution are bound to vary.'

Asylum Decisions

Positive decisions will be made where UKVI finds the asylum seeker to be credible and to have a well-founded fear of persecution. A person recognised as a refugee will be granted five years' leave to remain in the UK. That decision is reviewed upon application and the refugee may be granted indefinite leave to remain following the completion of their initial five years.

Negative decisions normally arise where no Convention reason or well-founded fear is established or where the asylum seeker is found to be not credible. In most circumstances, following a negative decision, a right of appeal is available which can be exercised from within the UK. Some decisions carry no right of appeal from within the UK, but in certain circumstances this may be challenged by judicial review.

Appeals against Negative Decisions

Appeals can be heard within the Immigration and Asylum Chambers of the First-tier Tribunal and the Upper Tribunal. An immigration judge hears the appeal within the First-tier Tribunal. Their decisions may be appealed to the Upper Tribunal, but only on an error of law. There are limited rights of appeal to the higher courts.

Where an Application Is Refused and No Further Applications or Appeals Are Pending

Asylum seekers who have received a negative decision and have no further appeal rights are expected to make arrangements to leave the UK. Persons considered not to be taking steps to remove themselves from the UK may face further difficulties in the community, such as having to meet the cost of any healthcare they are receiving, being denied welfare support and subsistence, and/or access to private accommodation.

The Duties of the Expert in the Immigration and Asylum Context

The duties of an expert in the tribunal are set out in Practice Direction 10 of the Immigration and Asylum Chambers of the First-tier Tribunal and the Upper Tribunal. Box 12.1 sets out those duties as summarised in *MOJ and Others (Return to Mogadishu) Somalia CG* [2014] UKUT 442 (IAC).

Box 12.1 The Duties of an Expert

(i) to provide information and express opinions independently, uninfluenced by the litigation;
(ii) to consider all material facts, including those which might detract from the expert witness' opinion;
(iii) to be objective and unbiased;
(iv) to avoid trespass into the prohibited territory of advocacy;
(v) to be fully informed;
(vi) to act within the confines of the witness's area of expertise; and
(vii) to modify, or abandon one's view, where appropriate.

As summarised by the Upper Tribunal in *MOJ and Others (Return to Mogadishu) Somalia CG* [2014] UKUT 442 (IAC)

A medical expert producing a medicolegal report for the tribunal will also be expected to be familiar with the Istanbul Protocol, specifically para. 162: 'A medical evaluation for legal purposes should be conducted with objectivity and impartiality. The evaluation should be based on the physician's clinical expertise and professional experience. The ethical obligation of beneficence demands uncompromising accuracy and impartiality in order to establish and maintain professional credibility.'

Questions that a Psychiatric Expert Might Be Instructed to Answer

Questions often included in the 'instructions' that solicitors issue to psychiatric experts include the following:

- Does the individual have any mental health condition such as PTSD?
- If so, please specify and state how severe it is.
- If so, describe the particular symptoms and offer opinion on the possible cause(s).
- Does the individual suffer from depression? If so, how severe?
- Does the individual suffer any anxiety symptoms?
- Might there be a learning disability?
- Are there any other mental health problems, for example, bipolar disorder/personality disorder/head injuries/dementia, etc.?
- Explain how you have reached your diagnosis and what diagnostic system you used. Were any validated scales used? If so, explain them.
- If there is no diagnosis, what is the level of suffering of traumatic events and discuss at length the person's vulnerability?
- Is the overall presentation clinically plausible and in keeping with the account of trauma given? In this context, it is important to remember that it is not for the psychiatric expert to give an opinion as to the *credibility* of the account – that is a matter for the decision-maker (UKVI or court).
- What mental health consequences (if any) have there been as a result of past or current immigration detention?

Experts may also be routinely requested to assess the following:

- Whether the individual's mental health problems affect their ability to give evidence in an interview setting (stressful and private) and/or a court situation (stressful and public).
- What effect will continual recounting of traumatic experiences in a non-therapeutic setting have on them?
- Is their memory impaired in any way?
- Are they likely to avoid discussing traumatic experiences?
- Is the individual likely to underplay their symptoms and, if so, how have you structured your assessment accordingly to take this into account?
- How is the individual currently coping with the process of claiming asylum and having to deal with UKVI officials, lawyers and courts? Is the individual able to trust the necessary people involved in their asylum claims or is an inability to trust causing problems?
- The impact upon the individual's mental health of removal and/or return to their country of origin.

Where there is an issue of the satisfactory management of the detainee in detention, establish exactly what treatment the detainee is receiving, what treatment is available and how that compares with what would be available to the detainee if released.

Where instructions expect you to provide opinions outside your field of expertise, discuss this in advance. Do not feel obliged to reach conclusions beyond your field of expertise – for example, about the causes of alleged psychological sequelae, or about the standard of healthcare in a particular country of origin of which you have no direct experience. Such matters should be left to an expert in the appropriate field.

There is no requirement to set out instructions in reports before the immigration courts, but many experts find this useful. Where an instruction poses a question which is not straightforward, setting out the question often provides context for the answer.

Conducting a Psychiatric Interview in order to Prepare an Expert Report

The Istanbul Protocol, para. 136 recommends that a detailed history should be taken and that 'the examiner should enquire into the person's daily life, relations with friends and family, work or school, occupation, interests, future plans and use of alcohol and drugs. Information should also be elicited regarding the person's [post-trauma] psychosocial history.' A history of the traumatic events should then be sought. In taking a history, the Istanbul Protocol, para. 142 points out that:

> Torture survivors may have difficulty recounting the specific details of the torture for several important reasons, including:
>
> (a) Factors during torture itself, such as blindfolding, drugging, lapses of consciousness, etc.;
> (b) Fear of placing themselves or others at risk;
> (c) A lack of trust in the examining clinician or interpreter;
> (d) The psychological impact of torture and trauma, such as high emotional arousal and impaired memory, secondary to trauma-related mental illnesses, such as depression and post-traumatic stress disorder (PTSD);

(e) Neuropsychiatric memory impairment from beatings to the head, suffocation, near drowning or starvation;
(f) Protective coping mechanisms, such as denial and avoidance;
(g) Culturally prescribed sanctions that allow traumatic experiences to be revealed only in highly confidential settings.

Paragraph 143 of the Istanbul Protocol continues:

> Inconsistencies in a person's story may arise from any or all of these factors. If possible, the investigator should ask for further clarification. When this is not possible, the investigator should look for other evidence that supports or refutes the story. A network of consistent supporting details can corroborate and clarify the person's story. Although the individual may not be able to provide the details desired by the investigator, such as dates, times, frequencies and exact identities of perpetrators, a broad outline of the traumatic events and torture will emerge and stand up over time.

In *R (PA (Iran)) v Upper Tribunal (Immigration and Asylum Chamber)* [2018] EWCA Civ 2495, the court found that psychiatric evidence provided 'an explanation for the infelicities and inconsistencies in the Appellant's account'.

As above, although determining credibility, and indeed the objective basis upon which any fears of persecution are themselves determined, fall outside the remit of the expert psychiatric witness, clinical plausibility based on the above issues remains an important factor. Paragraphs 105(f), 287(vi) and 290 of the Istanbul Protocol all ask the report writer to consider whether a false allegation of torture has been made. It is important to distinguish clinical plausibility from credibility. Findings of fact and credibility are for the decision-maker – not the medical expert.

Take a detailed account of the symptoms of which the individual complains, how long they have lasted, any past mental health problems, any past or current medical problems, the individual's current psychosocial circumstances, any past or present use of prescribed drugs and/or substance abuse, and any history of criminal behaviour or convictions. Corroborative evidence from general practitioner medical records, reports by other HCPs and, on occasion, from witnesses such as friends, a partner or a parent should be considered. For example, avoidant behaviour, dissociation or poor sleep patterns may be witnessed by others. General practitioner records are particularly useful and should be summarised, but bear in mind that many asylum seekers, despite their health needs, are unable to access healthcare in the UK.

An important aspect of the report-writing process is preparation. You need to have a clear understanding of the issues in advance of the assessment. This involves a holistic approach to discussions with those instructing you to produce the report, carefully reading the specific instructions and background papers, including the UKVI interviews, and preparing a list of the issues, including any instances where the individual may have given inconsistent statements.

Be mindful that the Istanbul Protocol, para. 164 makes clear that:

> Trust is an essential component of eliciting an accurate account of abuse. Earning the trust of someone who has experienced torture or other forms of abuse requires active listening, meticulous communication, courtesy and genuine empathy and honesty. Physicians must have the capacity to create a climate of trust in which disclosure of crucial, though perhaps very painful or shameful, facts can occur. It is important to be aware that those facts are

sometimes intimate secrets that the person may reveal at that moment for the first time. In addition to providing a comfortable setting, adequate time for the interviews, refreshments and access to toilet facilities, the clinician should explain what the patient can expect in the evaluation. The clinician should be mindful of the tone, phrasing and sequencing of questions (sensitive questions should be asked only after some degree of rapport has been developed) and should acknowledge the patient's ability to take a break if needed or to choose not to respond to any question.

On mental state examination, you will be documenting and attending closely to the subject's facial expression, speech tone, non-verbal gestures, general behaviour and cognitive function, as well as to the content of what you are being told. Any inconsistencies contribute to the conclusions drawn.

Differential Diagnoses

It is important to demonstrate that other possible causes for a mental health condition have been considered. For this reason, a detailed history of pre- and post-trauma mental health should always be taken. Corroborative evidence of the trauma history will usually not be available, so you should ask yourself to what extent the subject's presentation is consistent with such a history.

Consideration should also be given to the possibility that any pre-existing trauma (prior to the history of persecution) was exacerbated by later traumatic events and whether those prior events are likely to account, in whole or in part, for the presented symptomatology and diagnosis. The difficulty, from a clinical perspective, of apportioning the symptomatology between the prior event(s) and the event(s) which is/are pertinent to the asylum claim should be rehearsed and a recognition of the difficulty in distinguishing causation discussed.

Further Reading

Hameed, Y. and Katona, C. (2019) 'Migrants, refugees and asylum seekers' in R. Butler and C. Katona (eds), *Seminars in Old Age Psychiatry*, 2nd edn (Cambridge University Press).

Waterman, L. Z., Katona, C. and Katona, C. (2019) 'Assessing asylum seekers, refugees and undocumented migrants', *BJPsych Bulletin*, DOI: https://doi.org/10.1192/bjb.2019.67.

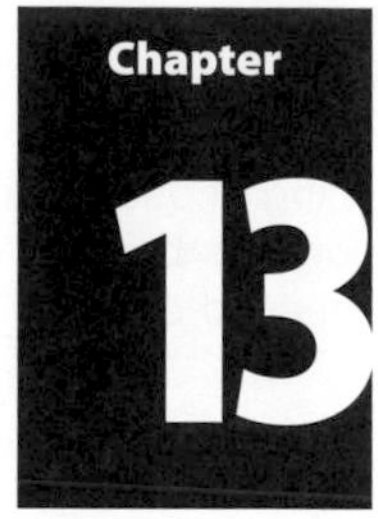

Reports in Employment, Disability Discrimination and Pension Cases

James Briscoe, Gareth Vincenti and Keith Rix

However elastic the notion of execution of duty might be, it cannot be stretched wide enough to encompass stress related illness through exposure to discipline procedures.
Simon Brown LJ in *R (Stunt) v Mallett* [2001] EWCA Civ 265

Here, along with consideration of expert psychiatric evidence in cases of disputes between employers and employees and in pension cases, we deal with its relevance to disability discrimination in the context of employment, but expert psychiatric evidence may also be sought where the issue is disability discrimination in other contexts.

General Considerations

Find out for whom the report is intended, particularly if it is a non-clinician, as this will influence how informed consent is obtained and the report's structure and content.

What Is Required in Preparation?

This can vary considerably. An OHP may refer an employee and provide no more documentation than a brief letter, in which case the report should make clear the opinion's limitations. A solicitor in employment tribunal proceedings will provide a range of records and other relevant evidence.

The Instruction

An OHP will almost always require an opinion as to an employee's ability to render efficient service consequent upon any mental disorder. Likely questions are set out in Box 13.1.

Consent and Confidentiality

Health professionals as a general rule should not disclose confidential information to a third party without the patient's informed consent. The common law also imposes a duty of confidentiality, as does the Human Rights Act 1998. There are exceptions, including where there is a statutory duty, where there is a court or tribunal order and where public interest overrides the duty of confidence (e.g. *W v Egdell* [1990] 1 All ER 835 – see Chapter 11, 'Confidentiality').

Consent must be informed (see Chapter 5, 'Introducing Yourself, Explaining and Obtaining Consent'). If the employee lacks capacity to give consent, a discussion should take place with the instructing party. It may be that a report should still be provided in the best interests of the employee, subject to the provisions of the MCA or equivalent legislation, or, if there is prospect for improvement, delayed until such improvement manifests and consent can be given.

Box 13.1 Typical Instruction from Occupational Health Physician

1. What is the current diagnosis under the ICD/DSM?
2. What is the prognosis for the condition(s) identified above?
3. Has treatment for the above condition(s) to date been optimal? What could be done to improve the condition(s)?
4. Are there any maintaining factors, particularly work-related, which are preventing recovery? What can be done to remove them?
5. How long will it take to bring about a substantial improvement in the condition(s) if further changes to the treatment plan are suggested?
6. What additional obstacles to recovery remain and what can be done to remove them (including likely timescales for possible return to work)?
7. Is a return to work likely and, if so, when and in what capacity? What adjustments are likely to be required in the short, medium and longer term?

The GDPR need cause no difficulty. The Faculty of Occupational Medicine's *Ethics Guidance for Occupational Health Practice* (FOM 2018) advises that GDPR provides a number of different justifications for processing personal data; consent is only one. It is perfectly feasible to register under an alternative justification, such as a legitimate interest or public health. The fact that consent is not given as a lawful basis for processing personal data does not mean that you do not need to obtain the data subject's consent because the common law and the ethics of the health professions are still in force and require consent other than exceptionally.

There is debate about whether the doctor in the UK should show the report to the subject before sending it to the commissioner, so it is wise to explain your approach to consent when first accepting instructions, so as to avoid later disappointment. *In Ireland*, there is no provision for advance disclosure.

Where the Report Is Required for Litigation

Where you are an expert witness with a primary duty to the court or tribunal and the person has agreed through their solicitor for the report to be made, it is unnecessary to show it to them before sending it to the instructing solicitor. In *Kapadia v Lambeth LBC* [2000] 6 WLUK 180, Kapadia claimed that the Council, his employer, had discriminated against him because of a disability. The employer was not convinced of his disability and asked for an examination by a consultant OHP, to which Kapadia consented. The Court of Appeal held in passing that the physician, as an expert witness, was not required to disclose the report to Kapadia or his solicitor for their approval before sending it to the employer's solicitor and giving evidence in the tribunal, as he had consented to examination on behalf of the employers.

Where an OHP is instructed as an expert not previously involved to report to the employer for the purpose of actual or contemplated litigation, the OHP needs the employee's consent to interview them, and/or review their records and report to their employer's solicitors. Such consent, which includes consent for the report's disclosure to the employers, does not impose a duty to show it to them before sending it to the employer's solicitors. If the employee later demands this, as in *Kapadia*, the employer's solicitors should raise the issue with the tribunal judge, who has power to order the employee to agree to disclosure and to strike out the claim if he or she refuses.

Where the Report Is Requested for Employment or Insurance Purposes

Where a report is requested for employment or insurance purposes, the Access to Medical Reports Act 1988 provides that written consent must be obtained from the patient, who must be allowed to ask for access to it before it is sent to the employer or insurance company and at that stage to withdraw consent. This only applies to a request for a report from a doctor who is, or has been, responsible for the patient's clinical care; it does not apply to a report from a doctor not responsible for clinical care, such as an expert witness or an OHP.

Where the OHP Is Reporting, or an Independent Expert Is Advising the OHP, after a Management Referral in the UK

In 2009 (GMC 2009), and repeated in 2017 (GMC 2017a; GMC 2017b), the GMC advised that occupational physicians, before reporting to management, should offer patients a written copy of their report and allow a reasonable time for them to consider it before submitting it to management unless:

- they have already indicated that they do not wish to see it;
- disclosure would be likely to cause serious harm to the patient or anyone else; or
- disclosure would be likely to reveal information about another person who does not consent.

This is also included in the FOM's guidance. However, Tamin (2010) has argued that offering sight of the report to the subject *before* the commissioner, thereby providing the opportunity to suppress it, is morally wrong. Nevertheless, there is a counter-argument that this ignores the fiduciary obligation to put the patient's interest first. However, 'the GMC appears to be the only professional body in the world that has introduced a new guidance that enables patients to gain privileged access to their occupational health reports in advance of the commissioning parties' and its stance 'also stands in stark and striking contrast to that in many other jurisdictions' (Wong and Choong 2013).

Where the OHP is reporting after a management referral in the UK, or an independent expert is advising the OHP, the GMC and FOM guidance should be applied. A patient who refuses to sanction the report's release can be advised that an employer is entitled to proceed without the benefit of medical advice in the best interests of the business (*O'Donoghue v Elmbridge Housing Trust* [2004] EWCA Civ 939) and that although legally obliged to make reasonable efforts to obtain medical advice where there seems good cause to do so, that duty ends if the employee prevents this.

As to the extent to which the subject may wish to amend or comment upon the report, correction of factual errors is clearly appropriate, but long, detailed commentary on the facts or opinions may entail significant redrafting. This may be disproportionate or irrelevant. Where there is a risk of consent being withdrawn if the expert refuses amendment, a compromise, if the subject consents, is to send the report with the commentary appended.

Recent ethical guidance from the FOM (2018) advises that where an employee has asked to see the report before agreeing its release, a standard opt-out approach permits release after two to three days if nothing is heard. However, in the more contentious case, the prudent clinician will obtain additional written or email consent to its release after amendment. However, no consent is needed to tell an employer that the subject has withdrawn consent, or indeed failed to attend the appointment. However, some occupational health providers have contracts to provide a medical report within a tight timetable that does not sit comfortably within the legal requirements of consent. Resist bending the rules on consent to accommodate these pressures and inappropriate expectations.

Where the Report Is Required in Relation to a Pension Scheme

Difficulty arises where reports are requested by an OHP on behalf of a pension scheme, or its trustees for advice on suitability for ill-health retirement, the award of an enhanced pension, or on whether retired police officers are eligible for an injury on duty award. Such reports are not part of litigation, employment tribunal or other legal proceedings, but equally are not advising their employer on the management of an employee's state of health.

Where expert medical evidence is required in relation to an ill-health retirement pension, especially when the procedure is laid down in statutory regulations, the opinion of Kloss (2015) is that this is a special case: arguably the medical expert may be in a position analogous to that of an expert witness. As Wong and Choong (2013) have observed: 'The right [to veto release] would . . . introduce bias. A patient who has been assessed not to meet the medical criteria for an early pension release due to ill-health . . . could choose to veto its release . . . and seek a more favourable opinion from another doctor.' An employee applying for a pension ought not be able to withdraw consent to the report's submission because they disagree with it. In any event, many schemes provide that assessment and review of entitlement is subject to submission of reports; the default position usually being the refusal or cesser of entitlement in the event of non-compliance.

But the expert in such cases is in a difficult position. The position of the GMC is unclear and experience shows that often commissioners lack sufficient knowledge of these matters. Most experts will not want to be the test case where a complaint is made to the GMC that consent has been breached by reporting to pension trustees without allowing them to withdraw their consent for the report's release. You have three options: (1) find out from the commissioner if the report is to be furnished without prior review and/or approval, (a) if it is, and the subject refuses, there is no consent to prepare the report, (b) if the commissioner is agnostic on the point or is satisfied that a report be furnished subject to prior review and/or approval, there can be no complaint if it is not then furnished; (2) offer the subject a written copy of their report and allow a reasonable time for them to consider it, but make it clear to the commissioner that you will be doing so; (3) do not take on such cases.

The consequences of (1) refusal of consent *simpliciter*, (2) refusal of consent to furnishing the report without prior review and/or approval, if the commissioner insists otherwise and (3) refusal of consent to furnishing the report, following prior review and/or approval, are quintessentially matters for the commissioner and the relevant scheme. If the subject refuses to consent to an unsupportive report being sent to the pension trustees, the answer is for the trustees to refuse the pension or the application for the award.

Where the Report Is Commissioned by Another Medical Practitioner Exercising Quasi-Judicial Functions

When an expert psychiatrist is instructed by a 'selected medical practitioner' (SMP) (or the 'duly qualified medical practitioner') under police pensions regulations to provide a report in relation to permanent disablement and injury on duty, fair procedures will require that it be disclosed to the subject of the report, in any event. However, the expert should still adopt the approach set out above in relation to pension scheme reports. Specific guidance for SMPs regarding report provision does not apply to experts providing reports to assist SMPs.

The Assessment

You may have to decide to assess the subject alone or accompanied, particularly if brought by a union representative. Although it is generally considered good practice to allow someone of the subject's choice in certain circumstances (see Chapter 5, 'Should Anyone Else Be Present?'), have regard to the effect that this may have on the consultation because:

- A psychiatric assessment explores an individual's personal history, revealing sensitive information which may be unknown to others. In the presence of another, the subject may be reticent to provide relevant information. Alternatively, information revealed at interview may cause embarrassment subsequently.
- A psychiatric assessment and exploration of mental state can be hampered by the presence of a third party.
- A third party can be distracting.

Formulating the Case

Most letters of instruction ask specific questions, each of which requires a response or an explanation for the omission. Where one exists, provide a diagnosis based upon either ICD or DSM (see Chapter 8, 'Diagnosis'). Make a clear distinction between distress and disorder. Employment cases commonly bring forward individuals with disparate emotional symptoms and associated illness behaviour and sickness absence who do not meet the diagnostic threshold for mental disorder.

Emotions such as anger, antipathy and embitterment towards an employer may be the consequence of perceived bullying or harassment or the result of a long unresolved period of sickness absence. Embitterment has been proposed as a condition in its own right (Linden 2003). It is linked to some perceived organisational injustice, and a breakdown in the abstract contract of trust between employer and employee. It carries a very poor prognosis as recovery, or the prospect thereof, requires a formal acknowledgement of wrongdoing by an employer who may see the facts quite differently.

In employment cases, there may be a hidden agenda. The employee will often furnish a detailed account of their perceived mistreatment or the context to their sickness absence, but there may be other facts which have not been disclosed. It is preferable to concentrate on the development of symptoms of psychological distress or mental disorder and their significance, rather than get drawn into any of the proposed causes. If there are relevant employment issues, include consideration of the role of management, alongside any specific treatment, in the report.

An understanding of the job role, informed by the job description, can inform your opinion as to what reasonable adjustments it may prove practical to suggest.

The report should summarise the treatment to date. Sometimes, a subject's account will include CBT, but in fact they have only had supportive counselling, or CBT delivered too infrequently to be effective. Be precise on these issues. They can also impact on ill-health retirement criteria and pension applications. Treatment recommendations should be based on mainstream guidance and the literature. An employee may decline treatment. Where this is understandable and due to lack of insight from mental illness, state this clearly, otherwise there can be adverse consequences. Employment law assumes that a sick employee will do all they can to recover; all claimants are expected to mitigate their losses.

When advising on prognosis, it is not just the recovery time from any current disorder, but the timescale for a return to work and then their likely future ability to render effective service. There are often powerful psychosocial/maintaining factors which can distort the normal prognosis for mental disorder and it is often useful to separate the two processes, emphasising that management intervention is needed for the latter for which clinical treatment can offer very little. Differentiate if possible between the prognosis of any diagnosed mental disorder and any maintaining factors which might affect that prognosis, such as alleged bullying at work.

It is particularly difficult to predict permanence when an employee is many years short of statutory retirement age. Most psychiatric disorders go into remission with adequate treatment, so a judgement must be made as to why someone with a potentially treatable disorder may be permanently unable to resume their employment. You will need to set out your reasoning in detail. Remember that the test is the balance of probabilities. There is no requirement for certainty, nor that the subject has exhausted every treatment possibility. You may also be asked to determine permanence in relation to the employee's current role or for any employment or until statutory retirement age.

Employment Tribunals and Disability Discrimination

Employment tribunals deal with disputes between employers and employees. The rules of procedure are broadly similar in Scotland, Wales and England. Joint experts are preferred.

Statutory Law

In England and Wales and Scotland, the Equality Act 2010 (Lockwood *et al.* 2012) brought all grounds of discrimination into one statute. Under the Equality Act 2010, s 6(1), 'a person has a disability if (a) P has a physical or mental impairment which has a substantial and long-term adverse effect on P's ability to carry out normal day-to-day activities'. As well as providing protection against discrimination in employment, the Act provides protection from discrimination in the provision of goods, services and facilities and in education.

In Northern Ireland, the Disability Discrimination Act 1995 (DDA) still applies, supplemented by the Disability Discrimination (Meaning of Disability) Regulations (Northern Ireland) 1996. It is therefore still necessary to show that the impairment has affected one or more of the following 'normal day-to-day activities': (a) mobility; (b) manual dexterity; (c) physical coordination; (d) continence; (e) ability to lift, carry or otherwise move everyday objects; (f) speech, hearing or eyesight; (g) memory or ability to concentrate, learn or understand; or (h) perceptions of the risk of physical danger.

In Ireland, the Disability Act 2005 defines disability as 'a substantial restriction in the capacity of the person to carry on a profession, business or occupation in the State or to participate in social or cultural life in the State by reason of an enduring physical, sensory, mental health or intellectual impairment'.

The Irish Equality Acts (the Employment Equality Acts 1998–2015 and the Equal Status Acts 2000–2015), which outlaw discrimination on grounds of disability, use a wider definition, and cover past as well as current disability: 'Disability' means (Employment Equality Act 1998, s 2):

(a) the total or partial absence of a person's bodily or mental functions, including the absence of a part of a person's body;
(b) . . .
(c) the malfunction, malformation or disfigurement of a part of a person's body;
(d) a condition or malfunction which results in a person learning differently from a person without the condition or malfunction; or
(e) a condition, disease or illness which affects a person's thought processes, perception of reality, emotions or judgement or which results in disturbed behaviour.

The prohibited grounds of discrimination are gender, civil status, family status, sexual orientation, religion, age, disability, race, membership of the traveller community, victim status and housing assistance.

In England and Wales and Scotland, psychiatric evidence may be sought where it is alleged that a person has been subject to discrimination based on a 'protected characteristic' under the Equality Act 2010, these being age, disability, gender reassignment, marriage and civil partnership, pregnancy and maternity, race, religion and belief, sex and sexual orientation. Where the issue of discrimination arises in the context of employment, a psychiatric report may be required for an employment tribunal, but other courts and tribunals also deal with discrimination, as, for example, when a person with a psychiatric disorder alleges discrimination in the provision of housing. The issue is usually disability and the expert evidence will go to that issue. Expert evidence may also be sought on the quantum of psychiatric damage once discrimination is established, as, for example, in the case of a Welshman of Somali extraction who developed clinical depression after being racially abused by his foreman when working on the construction of the Millennium Stadium in Cardiff (*Essa v Laing Ltd* [2004] EWCA Civ 2).

The focus in all cases should be on diagnosis, condition, causation, treatment and prognosis. Under the Equality Act 2010, the onus is on the claimant to prove impairment on the balance of probabilities.

In Ireland, expert psychiatric evidence will go to the issue of disability. Notwithstanding the statutory limits on compensation payable, it may also be useful on quantum. It is expressly provided that where facts are established by or on behalf of a complainant from which it may be presumed that there has been discrimination, it is for the respondent to prove the contrary. This is without prejudice to any enactment or rule in relation to the burden of proof in any proceedings which may be more favourable to a complainant.

Disability

Where the issue is 'disability', it is not the role of the expert to say whether the applicant is 'disabled'; this is for the tribunal (*Abadeh v British Telecommunications plc* [2000] 10 WLUK 529). However, you can and should comment on the likelihood that the employee has a disability by giving an opinion on the definition's component parts – for example, whether there is an impairment and how long it has lasted or is likely to last.

Impairment

The expert has to give an opinion on impairment. Physical symptoms, such as muscle weakness and wasting with no organic disease and resulting from psychological factors, have been sufficient to constitute physical impairment (*College of Ripon and York St John v Hobbs*

[2002] IRLR 185). Mental impairments can include personality disorders and some self-harming behaviour. They may be recurrent or fluctuating in nature. Conditions deemed not to be impairments include dependency on alcohol, nicotine or other non-prescribed substances, pyromania, kleptomania, a tendency to physical or sexual abuse of others, exhibitionism, voyeurism and hay fever. In *Edmund Nuttall Ltd v Butterfield* [2005] 7 WLUK 1007, although there was evidence that a businessman's indecent exposure offences, committed on a business trip, resulted from a depressive illness, it was held that his dismissal was solely on the basis of the offences for which he had no protection under the DDA 1995.

In Ireland, there is no requirement to prove 'impairment', merely that, insofar as psychiatric or cognate conditions are concerned, the condition *results in* a person learning differently or it *affects* a person's thought processes, perception of reality, emotions or judgement or results in disturbed behaviour. This guidance as it relates to impairment, and the guidance below as to 'substantial' impairment, proof of impairment, long-term adverse effects or normal day-to-day activities, is not immediately applicable in an Irish context in employment discrimination or equality matters. However, it is relevant insofar as the Disability Act 2005 and needs assessments are concerned, albeit the language is in terms of 'substantial restriction of capacity' by reason of an 'enduring . . . impairment'.

Substantial

'Substantial' means more than minor or trivial. Assessment involves considering the time taken to carry out an activity, the way in which it is carried out and the cumulative effects of activities which, on their own, would reveal no more than minor or trivial impairment. It is also necessary to consider the extent to which the person can reasonably modify their behaviour to reduce the effects; if they can, they no longer meet the criteria.

In deciding whether the impairment amounts to a substantial, long-term adverse effect on normal day-to-day activities, the effects of 'medical treatment' such as medication, psychological and other treatments, including counselling, have to be discounted. Disability will be decided on whether the claimant would be 'likely' to manifest a substantial long-term impact on normal day-to-day activities if they were not having the medication or treatment. Here, 'likely' does not mean 'more probable than not'; it is a deliberately lower threshold of just 'may well happen' (*SCA Packaging v Boyle* [2009] UKHL 37). This is called the 'deduced effect' because it is necessary to deduce that there would be a substantial adverse effect on normal day-to-day activities absent the medical treatment. Likewise, you have to disregard the successful coping strategies without which the claimant would have difficulty in carrying out normal day-to-day activities (*Vicary v British Telecommunications plc* [1999] 8 WLUK 231).

Whereas the onus is on the claimant to prove impairment on the balance of probabilities, the burden of proof lies with the employer to show that they met the requirements of the Equality Act 2010. Whether there is a substantial impairment is for the tribunal to decide. Therefore, you should set out the evidence that will assist the tribunal and then go no further than to say that you would expect that this is evidence of substantial impairment, but this is for the tribunal to decide.

Long-Term Adverse Effect

An effect is long-term if it has lasted, or is likely to last, at least twelve months, but including the cumulative effects of periods shorter than twelve months, or is likely to last for the rest of that person's life. If an adverse effect of an impairment ceases, it is treated as continuing if 'likely' to recur. Here, 'likely', taking account of *SCA Packaging*, means 'could well happen', which is a lower threshold than 'more probable than not'. The assessment is undertaken in a hypothetical untreated state (e.g. a bipolar patient without a mood stabiliser). Where the person has a recurrent condition which causes fluctuating impairments, they will be treated as long-term if the substantial adverse effect is likely to recur over a year or more. Medical evidence therefore has to address prognosis.

A retrospective opinion as to prognosis, specifically the likelihood of recurrence, must be based on the evidence available at the time of the alleged discriminatory act and not have regard to subsequent events because 'the statute requires a prophecy to be made' (*Richmond Adult Community College v McDougall* [2008] EWCA Civ 4). So ruled the court in a case where the psychiatrist had said at the time of her job application that a recurrence of the applicant's delusional and schizoaffective disorder was unlikely. An employment appeal tribunal, having regard to recurrences that occurred after her offer of employment was withdrawn, found in her favour, but the Court of Appeal overturned its judgment. Thus, the tribunal and the expert need to disregard the subsequent history.

Normal Day-to-Day Activities

Unlike its predecessor DDA, the Equality Act 2010 does not have a checklist of normal day-to-day activities. It provides for regulations and guidance to be published on this and on 'disability', the last being issued in 2011 and including an illustrative, non-exhaustive list of factors which it would be reasonable to regard as having a substantial adverse effect on normal day-to-day activities, such as persistent general low motivation or loss of interest in everyday activities, persistently wanting to avoid people or significant difficulty taking part in normal social interaction or forming social relationships and persistent distractibility or difficulty concentrating. Make sure that you are provided with any regulations or guidance and ask about any cases that assist.

Causation

In many employment tribunal cases, causation is complex. Tribunals will adjust compensation to reflect where an employer's contribution has been only partial, influenced by the expert's report. It will be for the tribunal to apply a proportionate percentage reduction. In *Thaine v London School of Economics* [2010] 7 WLUK 190, the employment appeal tribunal stated that:

> . . . the test for causation when more than one event causes the harm is to ask whether the conduct for which the [employer] is liable materially contributed to the harm . . . the extent of its liability is another matter entirely. It is liable only to the extent of that contribution. It may be difficult to quantify the extent of the contribution, but that is the task which the Tribunal is required to undertake.

This is reassuring for experts who struggle when asked for a fractional, or worse, percentage breakdown of causation. You can now with greater confidence qualify your opinion by referring to the difficulty of the exercise, go no further than comparing the likely impact of the different causes in general and leave the tribunal to undertake the quantification.

Causation is irrelevant to the issue of whether there is disability discrimination because there the issue is only whether the employee has a disability, not how it was caused, but it will arise if the claimant asks for compensation for psychiatric injury caused by discriminatory acts, as in *Essa v Laing* (above).

The Appropriate Time

You may be asked to consider whether, at the time of the alleged discriminatory act (and not the time when the impairment first became manifest, or the time of the medical consultation) – for example, a refusal to employ or a dismissal – the condition was more likely than not to last for at least twelve months.

Reasonable Adjustments

If it is alleged that the employer has failed to make reasonable adjustments, consider both (1) what effect, if any, would any specific adjustment have made and (2) what other adjustments, if any, would have materially mitigated the effect of what the tribunal may find was the disability. Examples are working part-time, working somewhere else in the company or business, having support, having more training, being better supervised and having scheduled meetings with supervisors or managers.

In Northern Ireland, there are different justification defences and different thresholds for making reasonable adjustments in the employment and non-employment fields (The Disability Discrimination (Providers of Services) (Adjustment of Premises) Regulations (Northern Ireland) 2003).

In Ireland, an employer is required to take 'appropriate measures, where needed, to enable a person with a disability to have access to, or participate or advance in, employment or undergo training, unless the measures would impose a disproportionate burden on the employer'. 'Appropriate measures' here means effective and practical measures, where needed in a particular case, to adapt the employer's place of business to the disability concerned, and includes the adaptation of premises and equipment, patterns of working time, distribution of tasks or the provision of training or integration resources, but does not include any treatment, facility or thing that the person might ordinarily or reasonably provide for themselves (Employment Equality Act 1998, s 16(3) and (4)).

In England and Wales, under the PHA, a course of conduct amounting to harassment is both a criminal offence and a civil wrong. Harassment related to a protected characteristic, like sex, race or disability, is also prohibited under the Equality Act 2010. Harassment at work so severe as to result in psychiatric damage can form a basis for a negligence action against the employer (*Green v DB Group Services (UK) Ltd* [2006] EWHC 1898 (QB)). Under both the PHA and the Equality Act 2010, compensation can be awarded for injury to feelings as well as actual psychiatric injury, but this is not possible under common law negligence. For a successful claim under the Equality Act 2010, as under the PHA, it is unnecessary to prove reasonable foreseeability (*Sheriff v Klyne Tugs (Lowestoft) Ltd* [1999] 6 WLUK 373), in contrast to the position at common law.

In Ireland, harassment is a criminal offence; in the employment context, harassment or sexual harassment constitutes discrimination and they are prohibited conduct for the purpose of the Equal Status Acts. Proof of psychiatric injury is not essential. A question of reasonable foreseeability may arise. Whereas a common law negligence action may be prosecuted in respect of harassment, usually associated with a claim for bullying, these are very difficult to maintain.

Pension Cases

The most comprehensive source of analysis of how an employee's mental health difficulties are evaluated in determining an ill-health retirement pension comes from the Police Pensions Regulations and judicial reviews arising from their application. This is a useful template upon which to base other ill-health retirement applications, as it addresses issues of infirmity, disablement and permanence. Each pension scheme is unique, but permanence is a common principle in determining whether an employee qualifies for ill-health retirement.

Police Pensions Regulations

Under the Police Pensions Regulations 1987 ('the 1987 Regulations'), an officer can retire on medical grounds if permanently disabled from undertaking the ordinary duties of a constable. Management and/or the officer can refer into the process. An independent SMP adjudicates.

Guidance as to the meaning of permanent disablement is provided by:

- the Police (Injury Benefit) Regulations 2006 ('the 2006 Regulations');
- court judgments;
- the Police Negotiating Board's *Joint Guidance – Improving the Management of Ill Health 2010* ('the PNB Guidance').

Disablement

The 1987 Regulations define 'disablement' at reg A12(2): 'disablement means inability, occasioned by infirmity of mind or body, to perform the ordinary duties of a . . . member of the force'.

The 1987 Regulations (as amended by the Police Pensions (Amendment) (No. 2) Regulations 2003) at reg A12(5) define 'infirmity' as a disease, injury or medical condition, physical or mental, which according to the PNB Guidance should if possible be described by reference to ICD or DSM.

The courts have ruled that in reg 12(2) of the 1987 Regulations, 'the police force' refers to the 'force for the area in which the officer was serving at the relevant time' (*R (Ashton) v Police Medical Appeal Board* [2008] EWHC 1833 (Admin)). The significance here is that in determining whether an officer is unable to perform the ordinary duties of a member of the force, the psychiatric condition causing the disablement may not apply to other police forces – for example, adjustment disorder due to bullying or PTSD resulting in avoidance of the location where the officer was traumatised. Thus, it could be argued that the officer is permanently disabled from returning to their current force, but not to an adjoining one.

'Ordinary duties' refers to the ordinary duties of the office of constable (*R v Sussex Police Authority, ex p Stewart* [2000] EWCA Civ 101). The court accepted that a constable cannot perform their ordinary duties unless they can run, walk reasonable distances, stand for reasonable periods and deploy reasonable physical force in exercising powers of arrest, restraint and retention in custody. In the context of duties, the PNB Guidance, para. 4.9 sets out in greater detail the view taken by the Court of Appeal in *Stewart*, listing the following as the ordinary duties of a constable:

- patrol/supervising public order;
- arrest and restraint;

- managing processes and resources and using information technology (IT);
- dealing with procedures, such as prosecution procedures, managing case papers and giving evidence in court;
- dealing with crime, such as scene-of-crime work, interviewing, searching and investigating offences;
- incident management, such as traffic and traffic accident management.

The PNB Guidance (para. 4.10) assists further, listing the key capabilities for each of the ordinary duties. Taking each of these duties in turn, inability, due to infirmity, as defined by the Regulations, in respect of *any* of the following key capabilities renders an officer disabled for the ordinary duties:

- the ability to run, walk reasonable distances and stand for reasonable periods;
- the ability to sit for reasonable periods, to write, read, use the telephone and to use (or learn to use) IT;
- the ability to exercise reasonable physical force in restraint and retention in custody;
- the ability to understand, retain and explain facts and procedures;
- the ability to evaluate information and to record details;
- the ability to make decisions and report situations to others.

An officer, who through infirmity (as defined) can perform the relevant activity to only a very limited degree or with great difficulty, is regarded as disabled.

Permanent

The Regulations do not define 'permanent', which is said to speak for itself. The PNB Guidance states that where an officer is in the early stages of a career, such a long-term view is difficult, and the test should be whether disablement is likely until at least the compulsory retirement age for his or her rank, that is 60 for ranks from constable up to and including chief inspector and 65 for superintendent and above. These judgements require careful analysis, and a sound knowledge of the prognosis of the disorder in question and the employment context in which it has arisen.

The 1987 and 2006 Regulations assume the administration of 'appropriate medical treatment'. This does not include medical treatment that it is reasonable in the opinion of the police authority for the officer to refuse. Conversely, to circumvent any unreasonable refusal of treatment, the Regulations also allow the proviso for assessing whether the disability is likely to be permanent.

Decisions require a judgement based on a balance of probability, and not certainty 'beyond reasonable doubt'. The issue relates to the time when the question arises for decision. There is no requirement to look at the case at an imaginary point in the future.

In Ireland, the Garda Síochána Pensions Orders 1925 to 1981, 'on a medical certificate', provide for retirement and a special (essentially a disability or ill-health) pension for life for a member of the force who is 'incapacitated for the performance of his duty by infirmity of mind or body' 'by an injury received in the execution of his duty without his own default'. This requires the evidence of some selected duly qualified medical practitioner or practitioners that the person is incapacitated, that the incapacity is likely to be permanent and that the infirmity was attributable to the injury. Medical evidence must determine whether the injury was accidental, as well as the degree of disablement (art 10(2)). Thereafter, medical evidence is generally required that the incapacity continues (art 10(3). If within five years of normal retirement age, or at any time before the pension is made permanent, there is medical evidence that the degree of disablement has substantially altered, the pension is reassessed according to the degree of disablement (art 10(6)). Where the medical evidence is that the infirmity was caused by the person's 'own default or his vicious habits', the pension or gratuity may be reduced by up to 50 per cent (art 11).

Also under the Garda Síochána (Compensation) Acts 1941 and 1945, an application can be made for compensation in respect of non-minor malicious personal injuries sustained in the course of the performance of a special risk duty.

The High Court, in fixing the amount of compensation, must take into consideration the detrimental effect which the injuries might reasonably be expected to have on the future earning power generally of the applicant and, in particular (if the injuries do not preclude the applicant from continuing to be a member of the Gárda Síochána), on his or her future career in that force, and have regard to the pain and suffering caused by the injuries and to any disease or tendency to disease caused by them.

In Ireland, similar provisions apply under the Army Pension Acts 1923 to 1980 and similar issues may arise under the Defence Forces Pensions Acts 1932 to 1975.

Although there are in Ireland (currently and historically) two police forces (An Garda Síoichána and the Police Service of Northern Ireland), for practical purposes, notwithstanding cooperation, they operate in different legal jurisdictions. Accordingly, the concerns that arose in *Ashton* do not apply in the context of the single force operating within the jurisdiction of the Irish courts. Although there is no guidance as to what 'performance of his duty' means, in the context of the Garda Pension regulations, it is, nevertheless, reasonable to adopt the criteria in *Stewart* and the PNB Guidance as a guideline, given that An Garda Síochána like the constabularies in England and Wales and Police Scotland are generally unarmed.

Two Illustrative Cases

R (Northumbria Police Authority) v Broome [2005] EWHC 2644 (Admin)

This judicial review of the decision of the SMP, that two police constables whom he had considered permanently disabled on grounds of their vulnerability to disorder, clarified further the definition of an 'infirmity'. The first was vulnerable to anxiety disorder/adjustment disorder, and to aggravation of mechanical spinal pain because of her enmity towards Northumbria Police. The second police constable's intractable antipathy towards her police role rendered her vulnerable to an anxiety/panic disorder with agoraphobia on return to a police role against her will.

It was held that a vulnerability to anxiety was neither a disease nor an injury nor a condition recognised by medicine and thus a claim to a disablement pension based on such a vulnerability failed:

> Vulnerability, enmity, and intractable antipathy do not appear in internationally authoritative guides available to doctors such as ICD-10 and DSM IV. A distinction must be made between a symptom and a condition. If a police officer is only 'vulnerable' there is in fact nothing wrong with him provided that the vulnerability has not in effect crossed the line into a condition. Regulation A12(5) of the Regulations defines infirmity, so far as the instant cases are concerned, as a medical condition. The word 'medical' is important because one must look to see if the 'condition' is a condition recognised in the medical world. For that purpose,

> there can be no better guide than by looking at internationally recognised, medical conditions. 'Vulnerability' is not within ICD-10 or DSM IV; indeed, so far as the evidence goes in the instant cases, it is not within any international, medical, authoritative guides. The same reasoning must apply to 'intractability' and 'enmity'.

Sharp v Chief Constable of West Yorkshire Police [2016] EWHC 469 (Admin)

This judicial review further addressed vulnerability. Mr Sharp suffered from recurrent depressive disorder, which at the relevant time was in remission. The psychiatric expert who provided a report to the PMAB described him as having a paranoid attitude which rendered him liable to develop psychiatric disorder under stress and without which his condition would have run a more benign course. It was, in the expert's view, inevitable that, if he returned to work, sooner or later he would again become unable to work or perform the ordinary duties of a constable due to a relapse of his recurrent depressive disorder.

The PMAB accepted that Mr Sharp suffered from a recurrent depressive disorder, which at the time of the hearing was in remission. The Board believed that the critical question was whether his paranoid attitude meant that he was permanently disabled and concluded that such an attitude did not equate to an infirmity, in line with the ruling in *Broome*. He was not permanently disabled within the meaning of the 1987 Regulations. On appeal, the court was:

> . . . satisfied that the PMAB ought to have held that Mr Sharp's recurrent depressive disorder was an infirmity . . . It was unnecessary and wrong to go on to consider whether his paranoid attitude was also an infirmity. It was a cause of the infirmity not the infirmity itself . . . I do not regard the question whether a paranoid attitude is an infirmity as relevant . . . The paranoid attitude was one of the causes of the severity of the recurrent depressive disorder . . . The question . . . was whether on the facts of this case Mr Sharp's recurrent depressive disorder was sufficiently serious to amount to a permanent disablement. That involves a consideration of the effect on Mr Sharp of previous incidents of recurrent depressive disorder, the likelihood of recurrence if Mr Sharp returns to work as a police officer, the likely effect on Mr Sharp of future incidents including the extent to which he is likely to recover from any further incidents.

This case illustrates the complexity of many pension applications, and the constantly changing environment facing experts in the field of employment, pension and disability cases.

Further Reading

Kloss, D. (2020) *Occupational Health Law*, 6th edn (Wiley Blackwell).

Chapter 14

Reports for Fitness to Practise, Conduct and Performance Proceedings

Gareth Vincenti

Trust in professionals is based on technical competence, gained through long, rigorous training, the mastery of specialised knowledge and skill, and the dedication to act responsibly in the patient's interests.

Quick 2006

Psychiatrists called upon to provide expert reports to regulatory bodies will in most cases be required to assist the regulator where there are concerns as to the practitioner's fitness to practise. Occasionally, where the issue is improper conduct or poor performance, a health examiner will be asked to assess whether poor health has contributed to the situation. In broad terms, the approach required mirrors that for psychiatric report-writing in general, but there are some important differences.

The timescale for the completion of these reports is often tight, but the amount of background reading is generally less than for a personal injury case, such as a road traffic accident or work injury. If a case proceeds to a formal tribunal hearing, there is a high likelihood of being called to give oral testimony. This can be challenging. MDOs have deep pockets which can fund the highest calibre QC. The stakes for the respondent practitioner are often high. Expect a robust challenge, not just of your report, but also your CV and experience in general, as happened in *Pool v General Medical Council* [2014] EWHC 3791 (Admin), where a paramedic challenged a psychiatrist's expertise in providing the Health Professions Council with an opinion on her fitness to practise. The maxim not to stray outside your area of expertise applies as much to fitness to practise proceedings as any other area of expert witness work.

Some regulators have a specific report framework which they require to be used, similar in principle to low-value whiplash claims. It is important to be aware of these and check first with instructing parties. Experts in fitness to practise cases rarely receive a full bundle of records. The increased emphasis on brevity can degrade an expert's ability fully to assist and has become a source of disquiet to some. Subjects under investigation cannot be relied upon to give an accurate history and without access to the medical records you are deprived of one of the sources of information that informs the assessment of the practitioner's clinical plausibility. Although you are less likely to have access to the medical records, you will often be expected to converse with treating clinicians by phone or via email. The GMC now requires that any notes from such conversations are appended to the report, so that the basis for any deductions can be scrutinised by the case examiners and possibly the tribunal too. The principle is one of increasing transparency and this requirement ought to be of general applicability.

The GMC now undertakes all testing, be that for blood samples, urine or saliva testing or hair testing, through a specialist commercial company which will arrange to visit the doctor under assessment. This ensures that there is no dispute over the chain of evidence. Other regulators will probably soon follow suit. It is a requirement usually to append the results of any tests to the report. The text of a report should discuss the results and any interpretation thereof. Where alcohol excess is an issue, be prepared to face questions, if subsequently called to give oral evidence, as to the lack of specificity of the standard clinical tools such as gamma-GT. Make sure you understand some of the theory behind hair sample analysis rather than learn this the hard way under cross-examination.

There are some other ways in which providing expert psychiatric opinion to regulators differs from other medicolegal practice. There can often be two psychiatrists commissioned by the regulator and there may be a third instructed by the practitioner's MDO. Joint statements are rare, but their use is slowly increasing. Concurrent evidence has yet to arrive. Direct collaboration between, say, two psychiatric experts instructed by the GMC is mostly forbidden; each examiner is meant to work independently. It is usually only at a tribunal that, in the case of a significant difference of opinion with a co-examiner, you are likely to be asked for specific comment on the other expert's findings. This can require you to think quickly on your feet.

The health regulatory bodies have in recent years become aware of, and concerned about, the stress imposed on health professionals by their investigation procedures. A landmark study in 2015 showed convincingly that being subject to a complaint had a measurable effect on the mental health of doctors in the UK (Bourne *et al.* 2015). The GMC itself commissioned a study examining the deaths of 114 doctors between 2005 and 2013 who had been under investigation at the time of death (Horsfall 2014) and found that twenty-eight had died through suicide. It concluded that a significant proportion of suicides were related to proceedings and might have been avoided. There has since been a welcome change of emphasis in the GMC's broad approach to investigating doctors, with an emphasis now on a more collaborative approach (Gerada 2019). The GMC has arranged for the provision of counselling through the BMA for all doctors referred to the regulator, whether or not BMA members. When writing reports for health regulatory bodies, psychiatric experts are now required to undertake a risk assessment looking at risk to self, risk to others, especially patients, and risk of relapse. Furthermore, *Hall v Egdell* (unreported, 2004) (see Chapter 6, 'Addressing Unidentified Issues') suggests that there is a duty to act if as an expert you see someone for a report and become aware that they have unmet treatment needs. With their agreement, a telephone discussion with the general practitioner will usually suffice, but safeguarding issues may require something more. The GMC has formalised these duties for its health examiners, who are now expected to take prompt and effective action if concerns about a doctor's safety are raised during an assessment interview. In addition, the GMC has introduced the concept of a 'vulnerable doctor'. Once identified as such, a communication plan is drawn up and published on GMC Connect (the GMC website and communication hub), which helps identify the doctor's preferred means of communication (e.g. through a partner or not at weekends) to keep stress to a minimum.

A crucial part of report writing for regulators involves providing advice as to fitness to continue professional practice. Again, the GMC has the most structured process and procedures, with other bodies following suit to some degree. It is vital to ensure that the criteria are fully understood before writing the report. The GMC requires the expert health examiner to advise one of three options for decision by the MPT:

- fit to practise generally;
- fit to practise with restrictions;
- not fit to practise.

Each case will turn on the facts and its risk assessment. The key areas for the latter are nature and degree of illness, insight, compliance, nature of work and support network. A doctor with a serious enduring mental illness, who lacks insight and refuses to engage in the health investigation process, and who lacks support and has limited access to help, is unlikely to be considered fit to practise. On the other hand, a doctor who has been under GMC supervision for several years and has cooperated fully, who has good support and a treating mental health team, and who has gained good insight, is likely to be permitted to resume unrestricted practice, in other words to practise generally with a revocation of any undertakings. No two cases are dealt with identically. Where a doctor is considered by the expert to require restrictions, these can be usefully combined with suggestions for support and treatment. The resulting framework is very often incorporated into the undertakings required of a doctor who agrees with the GMC or MPT to limit their practice. The GMC has a comprehensive bank of undertakings for experts to use in these situations. A doctor with a drug misuse disorder would be expected to submit to regular drug testing, to avoid self-medication with over-the-counter preparations, and not to prescribe or administer or have primary clinical responsibility for drugs listed in Schedules 1 to 4 of the Misuse of Drugs Regulations 2001. A doctor with an alcohol problem would be expected to abstain from alcohol, attend a support group as directed by their medical supervisor, and submit to regular tests of liver function and full blood count and hair testing.

In Ireland, where the Health Committee of the MC keeps sick doctors away from the disciplinary process, and a sick doctor will only get to a Fitness to Practise Inquiry if its processes have failed, a requirement for expert psychiatric evidence may arise at any or all stages of the processes of the Health Committee and the independent Practitioner Health Matters Programme, as it may in the context of allegations of professional misconduct or poor professional performance. There is no MPT in Ireland and fitness to practise enquiries are carried out by the Fitness to Practise Committee of the MC. The Committee merely decides the facts and whether they disclose professional misconduct or poor professional performance; although it may make a recommendation as to sanction, that is ultimately a matter for the Council and, in the case of the more serious penalties, affirmation by the High Court. Whereas in the UK the GMC has lowered the standard of proof in medical tribunals to a balance of probabilities, the standard of proof is still accepted as being that of beyond reasonable doubt. This is a crucial difference, albeit one that is difficult to reconcile.

Reports for Coroners Courts and Fatal Accident Inquiries

Laurence Mynors-Wallis and Keith Rix

It is the duty of the coroner as the public official responsible for the conduct of inquests ... to ensure that the relevant facts are fully, fairly and fearlessly investigated.

Lord Bingham MR in *R v HM Coroner for North Humberside and Scunthorpe, ex p Jamieson* [1995] QB 1

The role of the coroner has evolved since the office was formally established in 1194, from being a form of medieval tax gatherer to an independent judicial office holder charged with the investigation of sudden, violent or unnatural death. A coroner *in England and Wales* is appointed, but not employed, by the local authority and now has to have had a minimum of five years' legal experience. *In Ireland*, a barrister, solicitor or registered medical practitioner who has practised as such for not less than five years is eligible for appointment.

An inquest is the procedure used in all jurisdictions, *except Scotland*, to investigate certain forms of death. They may include sudden deaths for which the cause is unknown, violent or unnatural, suspicious deaths and deaths which have occurred in custody. The judicial officer who conducts what is essentially an inquisition is a coroner in *England, Wales, Northern Ireland* and *Ireland*, the Coroner of Inquests or Relief Coroner in the *Isle of Man* and the Deputy Viscount *in Jersey* (upon delegation by the Viscount who is responsible for inquests). In the other Channel Isles, inquests are conducted, following investigation by the law officers, HM Procureur or HM Comptroller, by a judge in the Magistrate's Court *in Guernsey* and by magistrates in the Court of *Alderney* and the Court of the Seneschal *in Sark*.

When to Hold an Inquest

In England and Wales, an inquest *must* be held if there is reason to suspect:

- the deceased has died a violent or unnatural death;
- the cause of death is unknown; or
- the deceased died whilst in custody or state detention.

An inquest may be held if the coroner believes that death may have been contributed to by neglect, failure of medical treatment, an otherwise natural death brought about by the deceased's employment or a death where consideration of ECHR, art 2 arises.

In Ireland, the coroner is under a duty to hold an inquest if of the opinion that the death may have occurred:

- in a violent or unnatural manner;
- suddenly and from unknown causes; or

- in a place or in circumstances which require that an inquest should be held by reference to any other enactment (this relates, essentially, to deaths in police, prison or military custody and industrial deaths).

An inquest may also be held where a medical certificate of the cause of death is not procurable and, following enquiry, it is not possible to ascertain the cause of death.

The Purpose of an Inquest

The purpose of an inquest is to answer four questions:

- who died – the identity of the deceased;
- where they died – the place of death;
- when they died – time of death; and
- how they died.

The answer to the first three is usually straightforward and does not require psychiatric expertise. 'How the deceased died', however, is a much more complex question and one in which psychiatrists are often involved as expert witnesses.

Inquest proceedings are inquisitorial. Their purpose is to assist the coroner in answering the above questions and to ascertain the truth about the death, not to apportion blame. The coroner leads questioning of witnesses.

How the deceased came by their death goes beyond the simple question of the medical cause. In *R v HM Coroner for East Sussex Western District, ex p Homberg* [1994] 1 WLUK 555, it was noted that although the word 'how' is to be widely interpreted, it means 'by what means', rather than in what broad circumstances. This ensures that the enquiry focuses on matters directly causative of death and is confined to these matters alone. This is also reflected in an Irish judgment:

> If a coroner's inquest were to extend its inquiries beyond the circumstances . . . in which the death occurred, it would become, in my view, an inquiry of a radically different nature and one which was not envisaged by the Oireachtas in enacting the 1962 Act [the Coroners Act 1962] . . . the formula 'how . . . the death occurred' in my opinion excludes matters not causally related to the process leading to death. (*Eastern Health Board v Farrell* [2001] 4 IR 627)

However, in *R v HM Coroner for Inner London West District, ex p Dallaglio* [1994] 4 All ER 139, it was noted that:

> . . . the Court . . . did not however rule that the investigation into the means by which the deceased came by his death should be limited to the last link in the chain of causation . . . It is for the coroner conducting an inquest to decide, on the facts of a given case at what point the chain of causation becomes too remote to form a proper part of his investigation.

Indeed, to limit it to the last link in the chain of causation would defeat the purpose of holding inquests at all.

Article 2, *Jamieson* and *Middleton* Inquests

There is a positive duty under ECHR, art 2 to protect life in certain circumstances, such as when the authorities knew, or ought to have known at the time, of the existence of a real and immediate risk to the life of an individual. This is known as the 'operational duty'. The test for real and immediate risk is a risk which is more than remote or fanciful and which is present and continuing. Where there are questions around this specific issue, it is likely that a coroner will hold an 'Article 2' or *Middleton* inquest, so named after *R (Middleton) v HM Coroner for Western Somerset* [2001] EWHC Admin 1043 to distinguish it from a *Jamieson* inquest named after *R v HM Coroner for North Humberside and Scunthorpe, ex p Jamieson* [1995] QB 1. In *Middleton*, the involvement of the state arose when the inquest jury communicated to the coroner that an agent of the state, in this case the Prison Service, had failed in its duty of care to the deceased. The deceased had hanged himself in prison, and whilst he had been identified as at risk, the proper safeguards were never put in place. In an Article 2 case, the process is 'a scheme in which limited issues are left to the jury, but a much wider power is given to the coroner, a professional adjudicator, to report on systemic failures' (*R (Lewis) v HM Coroner for the Mid and North Division of the County of Shropshire* [2009] EWHC 661 (Admin)).

Jamieson and *Middleton* inquests are, or were, distinguished in terms of their remit: a *Jamieson* inquest had a narrow remit of determining by what means the deceased died; and a *Middleton* inquest had a wider remit of determining by what means and in what circumstances the deceased died. However, the remit of a *Jamieson* inquest has expanded so much that the Court of Appeal has recognised that, in terms of inquisitorial scope, there is now practically little difference between them. That the scope of an inquest is as wide as the coroner deems necessary is illustrated by *R (Takoushis) v HM Coroner for Inner London North* [2005] EWCA Civ 1440. The deceased, who had a long history of schizophrenia, was an in-patient. He failed to return from ground leave and later the same day he was seen preparing to jump from a bridge into the River Thames. He was taken to a nearby hospital, where triage established that he was at high risk of self-harm and needed attention within ten minutes. He was not seen as intended and left the hospital to jump to his death in the River Thames. The Court of Appeal held that although his case did not engage EHCR, art 2, there had not been a proper investigation as to whether a systemic failure had allowed the circumstances of his death to occur. The coroner was found to have failed to 'investigate how the system was to work [after initial triage] and did not consider, for example, what was to be done and in particular what safeguards were in place if for some reason the patient could not be seen in the target time'. These are systemic issues which an expert psychiatrist should be prepared to address.

The Supreme Court, in *Rabone v Pennine Care NHS Foundation Trust* [2012] UKSC 2, decided that the operational duty under EHCR, art 2 applied not only to detained mental health patients, as established in *Savage v South Essex Partnership NHS Foundation Trust* [2008] UKHL 74, but also to non-detained mental health patients.

Since *Middleton*, there have been a small number of cases which illustrate other examples of state involvement. In *R (Hurst) v HM Coroner for Northern District of London* [2003] EWHC 1721 (Admin), the deceased was killed by a man known to be violent and potentially mentally ill and against whom he had given evidence in eviction proceedings. It was argued that the police and local authority could have foreseen the incident and that it was preventable, as both bodies were aware that Hurst was in danger from his eventual killer. In *Osman v UK (23452/94)* [1998] 10 WLUK 513, an individual was known to the police and education authorities to have been harassing and threatening students and their parents; he went on to kill one of the students' parents and a teacher.

Neglect

What used to be 'lack of care', now known as 'neglect', may be an issue (but not *in Ireland*, where it is not available as a verdict in the Coroners' Courts). It is open to the court to conclude that neglect has contributed to the death. The issue arose in *Jamieson*, a case in which a prisoner hanged himself. The family was concerned that his care in prison was poor and that adequate measures had not been taken by the prison authorities. They sought a verdict of 'lack of care' and when the case went to the Court of Appeal 'neglect' was thought to be a better term:

> Neglect . . . means a gross failure to provide adequate nourishment or liquid, or provide or procure basic medical attention or shelter or warmth for someone in a dependent position (because of youth, age, illness or incarceration) who cannot provide it for himself. Failure to provide medical attention for a dependent person whose physical condition is such as to show that he obviously needs it may amount to neglect. So it may be if it is the dependent person's mental condition which obviously calls for medical attention (as it would, for example, if a mental nurse observed that a patient had a propensity to swallow razor blades and failed to report this propensity to a doctor, in a case where the patient had no intention to cause himself injury but did thereafter swallow razor blades with fatal results). In both cases the crucial consideration will be what the dependent person's condition, whether physical or mental, appeared to be.

The key terms are 'gross' and 'basic'.

'Gross' has its everyday meaning: 'so bad as to be criminal' (*R v Adomako* [1995] 1 AC 171) or 'truly exceptionally bad' (*R v Misra* [2004] EWCA Crim 2375). The lack of care has to be total and complete. It is more than a simple error. The criterion is not met where care has been provided and what is alleged is no more than an incorrect judgement about the type of care or its manner of delivery. Neglect is not the same as negligence. Leaving a patient unattended on a trolley is neglect. Deciding incorrectly that a patient should have one particular approach to treatment as opposed to another may be negligent, but cannot be neglect, as care has been provided to the patient.

'Basic' has the effect of restricting the failure to provide attention, particularly medical attention, to a narrow range. So, complex decision-making cannot ever reasonably be considered to be a matter of 'basic' medical care and attention.

Thus, neglect has a much narrower meaning than negligence. As submitted by Dorries (2014):

> . . . neglect will often arise from a breakdown in communications rather than being the result of some deliberate act, and will sometimes flow from the combination of a series of small errors by different individuals . . . This verdict is now aimed at persons who ignore the plight of those in their care. An incorrect decision as to the proper course of action, even negligently made, will generally be insufficient.

Furthermore, it is non-transient; a single isolated mistake will not suffice.

It follows that for any failures you identify, you should determine whether these amount to a gross failure to provide or procure basic medical care, but adding if appropriate that ultimately this may be for the court to decide. For each, state whether the need for the care was known, or objectively should have been known, to those caring for the deceased and state whether the failure has directly caused the death. The test in a coronial case is whether there was anything done, or not done, which would have made a difference to the death, specifically anything which 'more than minimally, negligibly, or trivially contributed to the death' (*R v HM Coroner, ex p Douglas-Williams* [1999] 1 All ER 344).

For neglect or self-neglect to form any part of the court's conclusion, there will usually need to be established a clear and direct causal link between the conduct described and the cause of death.

Inquest Process

A coroner's inquest is a public hearing and the coroner must allow any 'interested person' the opportunity to question a witness, either in person or through a lawyer. This includes a spouse, civil partner, partner and various relatives. It means that an expert witness should be prepared to be directly questioned, for example, by family members. Families are not always legally represented, but one of the purposes of the inquest is 'to ensure so far as possible that the full facts are brought to light . . . and that those who have lost their relative may at least have the satisfaction of knowing that lessons learned from his death may save the lives of others' (*R (Amin) v Secretary of State for the Home Department* [2003] 1 UKHL 51).

The coroner may explore facts bearing on criminal and civil liability which may inevitably arise, but their determination must not be framed in such a way as to appear to determine any question of criminal liability by a named person or civil liability.

Any competent witness can be compelled to attend the coroner's court.

The Expert Report

A report for a coroner, because the body of the report may be read out at the inquest, should be easily understood by the family. Explain essential medical and technical terms, drugs, abbreviations and initials as they arise; a glossary will still assist. Aim for a sufficiently detailed, chronological account of the relevant history based on the totality of the information, with different sources distinguishable. Hearsay evidence is admissible, but it must be accurate, and its source identified. Do not omit information that could be upsetting for family members to hear. The coroner needs to be fully briefed.

Experts are warned about inquests that 'they should restrict themselves to questions of fact, diagnosis and opinion, refraining from argument or the expression of views which appear to usurp the function of the court' (*Re LM (A Child) (Reporting Restrictions: Coroner's Inquest)* (2007) EWHC 1902 (Fam)).

The coroner decides if it was suicide. So, avoid giving an opinion on a matter such as whether the patient enacted suicide. However, it may assist to draw attention to relevant information. Explain why, say what weight a psychiatrist would attach to it and explain how it would inform a clinical judgement as to suicidality. Acknowledge that this is only assistance and there is no intention to usurp the coroner's role.

The vast majority of inquests are heard by coroners sitting alone. When sitting with a jury, the number of jurors is seven to eleven. The jurors are allowed to ask questions of a witness.

Outcome

The CJA 2009 removed the word 'verdict' from use in the coroner's court and uses the following phrases:

- the determination – that is, the who, how, when and where questions;
- the findings – all the particulars required by the Births and Deaths Registration Act 1953;
- the conclusion – which either may be one of the traditional short forms of conclusion or a narrative conclusion.

In the short-form conclusions, one of the following may be adopted: accidental death, alcohol/drug related, industrial disease, lawful/unlawful killing, natural causes, open, road traffic collisions, stillbirth or suicide. A narrative conclusion enables the circumstances of the death to be described – for example: 'The deceased took his own life, in part because the risk of his doing so was not recognised and appropriate precautions were not put in place to prevent him doing so.'

The standard of proof for most conclusions is the balance of probabilities, now also including suicide following the judgment in *R (Maughan) v HM Senior Coroner for Oxfordshire* [2019] EWCA Civ 809. For unlawful killing, the standard is the criminal standard of 'beyond reasonable doubt' and this remains the standard of proof for suicide *in Ireland*.

The definition of suicide is: 'voluntarily doing an act for the purpose of destroying one's life while one is conscious of what one is doing. In order to arrive at a conclusion of suicide there must be evidence that the deceased intended the consequence of the act' (*R v HM Coroner for Cardiff, ex p Thomas* [1970] 1 WLR 1475).

The Fatal Accident Inquiry

The Fatal Accident Inquiry fulfils a similar function *in Scotland*. All sudden and unexpected deaths are investigated by the procurator fiscal. This is a common law power to which statutory authority is added by the Inquiries into Fatal Accidents and Sudden Deaths etc (Scotland) Act 2016. Following the consideration of the evidence of independent experts, if any, and as in a criminal investigation, the fiscal prepares a notice requesting the sheriff to order a hearing. In contrast to a coronial inquest, which is held in public, the fiscal's enquiries are made in private unless, perhaps upon the insistence of relatives, he is persuaded to hold a public inquiry. It is in general mandatory to hold a public fatal accident inquiry when the death has resulted from an accident in the course of employment or where the deceased was in legal custody or, if a child, in secure accommodation. But if a prosecution is contemplated, an inquiry is seldom held because the trial establishes the facts in public. There is a discretion to hold inquiries into a wide variety of sudden, suspicious or unexplained deaths, particularly where there is serious public concern. The inquiry is conducted by a sheriff sitting in a civil capacity. Evidence is led by the fiscal or occasionally by Crown counsel.

Further Reading

Carmichael, I. H. B. (2005) *Sudden Deaths and Fatal Accident Inquiries*, 3rd edn (Thomson W. Green).

Cooper, J. (2011) *Inquests* (Hart Publishing).

Dorries, P. (2014) *Coroners' Courts: A Guide to Law and Practice*, 3rd edn (Oxford University Press).

Holburn, C. (2018) 'Nobody's friend? The expert witness in the coroner's court', *Expert Witness Institute Member Newsletter* (summer), pp. 10–14.

Thomas, L., Straw, A., Machover, D. and Friedman, D. (2014) *Inquests: A Practitioner's Guide*, 3rd edn (Legal Action Group).

Chapter 16

How to Read an Expert Medical Report

Anthony Howard and Keith Rix

Expert opinion evidence may be rebutted by showing the incorrectness or inadequacy of the factual assumptions on which the opinion is based, the reasoning by which he progresses from his material to his conclusion, the interest or bias of the expert, inconsistencies or contradictions in his testimony as to material matters ... Also, in cases involving the opinions of medical experts, the probative force of that character of testimony is lessened where it is predicated on subjective symptoms, or where it is based on narrative statements to the expert as to past events not in evidence at the trial.

District Judge Brewster in *Mims v United States*, 375 F.2d 135 (5th Cir 1967)

For expert evidence to be tested, a thorough understanding of the evidence is critical. Experts are privileged in that they are able to give evidence, on more than what they have directly observed, and they have the power to influence a judicial decision. For an expert opinion to be successfully challenged, its weaknesses or flawed logic need to be identified, and a thorough understanding of the medical topic is required. Achieving this is not straightforward, as what is being said appears to be based on impenetrable material. The ability to read a medical report effectively is a skill that perhaps is only acquired through litigation experience, but the narrative below should help accelerate the acquisition of that skill by taking a step-wise approach to analysing the medical report.

The guiding rule should be that if you cannot understand the medical report and thus evidence, you will not be able successfully to challenge the content or be aware of how the evidence supports your position no matter how correct it is; or if you are the judge, you will be able to attach little weight, if any, to such evidence. This conundrum lies at the heart of expert evidence. Evidence from experts is required because the subject matter is beyond common knowledge of judges and juries, but it still needs to be comprehended, otherwise it will remain beyond their common knowledge.

Is This the Appropriate Expert?

A West Indian bus driver sought to explain to a judge that he always strived to live within his means. Asked by counsel whether he was an extravagant man, he replied, 'I never put my hat where I cannot reach it' (www.elitedaily.com/life/5-caribbean-proverbs/1184033). So, the maxim 'Only put your hat where you can reach it' is appropriate when considering the starting point of whether the appropriate expert has been appointed. This quote poetically makes the point that experts should only give evidence on points that are within their field of expertise. It is always surprising when taking an expert through their evidence, how often they express views on topics of which either they have no practical experience or it is experience that occurred so long ago as to make it invalid. Being able to read about a particular topic within their specialism does not make them an expert on that topic.

The fundamental starting point is having the appropriate expert. Guidance for advocates states: '[Q]ualifications should not be equated with experience. Advocates must satisfy themselves that an expert has the requisite experience, up-to-date knowledge and, where necessary, has carried out sufficient research to give evidence which is credible and reliable' (Inns of Court College of Advocacy 2019). This may seem obvious, but as medicine becomes increasingly specialised, do not make the assumption that a medical expert is able to provide an expert opinion on any topic within their speciality. Take a step beyond what an expert sounds or looks like. Often, superficially, because they are talking on a topic that is foreign to the recipient, it can give the impression of the perfect evidence. However, the starting point has to be whether they have the relevant experience in order to reach the conclusions that form their evidence. The rate of change in medicine is becoming increasingly fast, as new technologies, medications and procedures are adopted, thus the importance of understanding the time gap between when the medical expert practised in this field and when they are expressing an opinion. It is also speciality-specific, but the issue should be explored, along with the actual level and volume of experience. It will be obvious that a psychiatrist who dealt in passing with a branch of psychiatry, whilst training, and has since specialised in a completely different area, is unlikely to be a true expert on that branch of psychiatry. Although a medical CV can often be lengthy, an assessment of the expert experience should be performed. For example, confidence could be gained by knowing that the expert has served on professional bodies, as they are likely to have a greater appreciation of the privileged position of giving evidence as an expert witness and the responsibilities it carries. With experience comes knowledge of particular experts, those to recommend and those whose reports or court performance give concern. It is often helpful to ask colleagues if they have experience of a particular expert, and sometimes an internet search can reveal useful information. However, as one judge observed, the fact 'that the experts usually have impressive academic credentials and extensive experience may serve to lend an air of "mystic infallibility" to the evidence' (*R v Murrin* (1999) 181 DLR (4th) 320). So, it is important not to be too deferential to the expert's expertise and fail to evaluate their evidence (*Vadakathu v George* [2009] SGHC 79).

When reading two competing medical reports, there can be a temptation to adopt unreliable markers as to expertise – for example, international reputation or level of seniority. In *R v Cannings* [2004] EWCA Crim 1, the court recognised that in Professor Sir Roy Meadow it had 'an expert witness of great distinction, if not pre-eminence in this field', but found that 'even the most distinguished expert can be wrong'.

What Is the Basis of the Expert's Instructions?

This basic step is critical. You need to understand the nature of the instructions that have been given to the expert, and the documents/written evidence that have been provided. The starting point is that an expert's primary duty is to the court, rather than to the party instructing them, so both the instructions and the evidence supplied should be set out in the report in a transparent way. In a sense, it protects the expert, and informs those evaluating their evidence. Thus, if when the evaluation occurs, and there has been additional evidence that is relevant to the expert's consideration, which has not been seen by the expert, this needs to be remedied. In most cases, it is not reasonable to expect, or feasible for, the expert to list every single document or item of evidence they have seen, but, for example, in a criminal case, 'prosecution witness statements' begs the question as to which witness statements, and a reference to hospital or general practitioner records gives rise to uncertainty as to how up-to-date the records were. Most advocates will be able to give anecdotal instances where, mid-trial, it becomes apparent that the expert has not seen all the papers, and their view changes as a result of digesting the additional material.

Are There Any Terms within the Report that Are a Mystery?

As experience of reading increases, the language starts to make more sense, but it is critical, particularly at the start, to take time to understand the language being used. Those with knowledge of Latin will find the whole process less problematic. Take, for example, 'adduction' (movement towards the midline or another part of the body) and 'abduction' (movement away from the midline or another part of the body). These two descriptors of movement demonstrate further need to appreciate that one letter within a medical term can completely change the meaning. This is compounded when many terms are used to describe the same thing.

The medical expert is engaged in an exercise in communication with both a medical and legal audience, with the duty upon the expert to ensure that the report is drafted in manner that it comprehensible to a lay individual.

Unless the language is properly understood, lawyers are incapable of asking meaningful questions, comprehending the answers given by the expert and appreciating the errors in the expert evidence. The practical approach of looking up the meaning of terms and reading medical material around the topic has to be balanced against the need to engage the expert through a conference in order for all matters to be fully explained. Further, if the written report fails to satisfy GMP (see Chapter 6, 'The Report') or is simply difficult to follow, it should be redrafted; this does not infringe the expert's independence, but merely enables more effective and efficient forensic analysis.

Does the Report Sound Like the Expert Is a Hired Gun?

With the advent of the SJE, the issue of 'hired guns' is less of a problem, but in every expert report the opinion needs to be balanced and needs to be seen to be balanced. A one-sided report reflecting a siding with the instructing party is unlikely to be indicative of an opinion that will become balanced when explained in the witness box. In a recent case, an expert's evidence was rejected at trial for being too partisan; already in the early stages in Part 35 questions (see Chapter 2, 'Written Questions to Experts'), in rejecting one point put to him for comment, he asserted that his response was 'high school physics' and suggested that the other party's experts needed 'to take an undergraduate university course on vehicle dynamics to understand the assumptions and their relevance to the circumstances of the incident' (*Hatfield v Drax Power Ltd, Simon Gibson Transport Ltd* [2017] 8 WLUK 224). His Part 35 answers should have anticipated the almost inevitable conclusion that he was not adopting a balanced approach to his opinion; it should not have been necessary to wait for the trial judge to find that his evidence was 'shot through with breath taking arrogance' and observe that '[h]is stance throughout was that he was right and everybody else was wrong'.

Objectivity may be revealed by the expert's inclusion and discussion of counter-arguments, alternative opinions within the range of opinion and contrary sources of information.

Has the Expert Got a Good Grasp of the Factual Background?

It is often tempting to go straight to the conclusion of the report, questioning whether it gives the reasons that are required to establish the opinion upon which the party's case depends for its success. However, remember that the facts upon which the expert expresses their opinion have to be correct for their conclusion to be valid. 'Expert evidence should be tested against known facts, as it is the primary factual evidence which is of the greatest importance', those facts must be ones which are proved, exclusive of the evidence of the expert, to the satisfaction of the court according to the appropriate standard of proof and '[w]hether or not the expert believes in that substratum of facts or knows them to be true or is satisfied that they are true, is completely beside the point' (Bell 2010). As held in *R v Turner* [1975] QB 834: 'Before a court can assess the value of an opinion it must know the facts upon which it is based. If the expert has been misinformed about the facts or has taken irrelevant facts into consideration or has omitted relevant ones, the opinion is likely to be valueless.' Without proof of the facts underlying the opinion, the court is deprived 'of an important opportunity of testing the validity of the process by which the opinion was formed, and substantially reduces the value and cogency of the opinion evidence' (*Bell v F.S. & U. Industrial Benefit Society Ltd* (Supreme Court of New South Wales, unreported, 9 September 1987)). So, after the conclusion of the medical report has been read, the factual basis of the expert's understanding, as expressed in the report, needs to be considered. If analysis of the factual understanding is not correct and the report has not been disclosed, then the report needs to be reconsidered by the expert, and if necessary with a further consultation between the expert and the subject.

The examination of the factual background within the report needs to extend to ensuring that the expert's narrative or factual analysis is consistent with the medical records. Within medical reports, often the relevant excerpts from medical records are set out. Check these quoted passages to ensure they are consistent with the actual record; an inconsistency could fundamentally change the expert's conclusion. Within a healthcare environment, often different HCPs write in different types of records; for example, there may be separate folders to which nurses, doctors and physiotherapists enter a contemporaneous record of their activity. Thus, when checking the consistency of the expert's grasp of the factual background, the various different subsets of records all need to be reviewed. If the case involves imaging, ensure that these have been reviewed directly by the expert rather than indirectly through others' reports on the images.

Remember that there is a positive duty on the expert to ensure that at a basic level the information contained within their report is true. The GMC requires the following: 'You must make sure that any report you write, or evidence you give, is accurate and not misleading. This means you must take reasonable steps to check the accuracy of any information you give, and to make sure that you include all relevant information' (AWLP). In *Liverpool Victoria Insurance Co. Ltd v Khan* [2018] EWHC 2581 (QB), a medical report in which further details were added, at the suggestion of the instructing solicitor, attracted a finding of contempt against the doctor. The court concluded that 'he allowed the assertions referred to at paragraph 153 above to be included in the revised report, not caring whether they were true or false, and not caring whether or not the Court was misled as a result. Accordingly, he is, in those respects, guilty of contempt of court'.

Do I Understand How the Expert Reached Their Conclusion?

The methodology and the reasoning behind the expert's conclusion need to be fully set out in the report. The trial judge will have to consider whether the methodology is flawed and it perhaps goes without saying that confused, inconsistent, illogical, irrational (*Drake v Thos Agnew & Sons Ltd* [2002] EWHC 294 (QB)), speculative (*Gorelike v Holder*, 339 Fed. Appx 70 (2nd Cir 2009)) or internally contradictory reasoning risks being rejected ultimately by a court. The opinion should be examined 'in terms of its rationality and internal consistency in relation to all the evidence' (Bell 2010). The absence of reasoning places the party relying on the evidence at an automatic disadvantage, as happened in *Massey v Tameside and Glossop Acute Services NHS Trust* [2007] EWHC 317, where the court found that 'the detailed reasoning of the expert witnesses in reaching their conclusions was not set out in their reports . . . the absence of clear written explanations of how conclusions . . . were reached has added to the difficulty of resolving the differences of opinion between the experts'. The lay reader needs to fully understand the reasoning.

There are areas of medicine where the conclusion is more of an art than a science; the conclusion is based on 'feel' rather than logical steps of reasoning; however, predicting whether it will be accepted is more speculative. Just as in law, where there are cases that are persuasive of a certain construction to be placed on previous authorities or legislation but do not answer the point definitively, the same is true of medicine. From the outside, medicine has the appearance of being precise and backed by science to fortify that precision. However, a great deal of the time, medical practice is based on anecdotal evidence and on what medical personnel around the expert did rather than best clinical practice. This is a double-edged sword, as those experts who are honest about the reality of medical science may be perceived as giving less convincing evidence compared to those adopting a 'there is only one answer' approach. However, the reality is somewhere in the middle and this reality needs to be remembered when evaluating a medical report.

Is the Opinion Based on Crackpot Science?

The sharing of medical knowledge through peer-reviewed journals is prevalent and can often form the basis for reasoning, adopted by a medical expert, in reaching their conclusions. For the lay reader of a report that starts to quote medical literature, there can be a temptation to switch off and accept the premises that are being advanced by the expert. However, there is a need to ensure that the literature is quoted accurately. This was highlighted in *Re C (Welfare of Child: Immunisation)* [2003] EWCA Civ 1148, which concerned childhood immunisation and the risk of side effects. The Court of Appeal concluded that the trial judge had been presented with junk science, as when the medical literature was properly examined, despite the expert's evidence, it failed to support their position and showed the reverse position.

This highlights the difficulty for the lay reader in reading medical reports; there has to be acceptance of the expert's experience and integrity in producing the report and that it correctly reflects the current knowledge of science behind their opinion. However, as experience and cases demonstrate, when reading medical reports there is a need to ensure that the expert is quoting the medical literature in a balanced manner rather than engaging in intellectually dishonest cherry picking (see Chapter 6, 'The Facts and Assumed Facts/Factual Analysis') to bolster their weak opinion.

Conclusion

In AH's experience, by far the best way to understand the medical report is to sit across a conference table and discuss its contents in a critical fashion with the expert. As experience grows, the terms, language and some of the treatments will become more familiar, but until this point is reached, look up all the terms that are not understood, and read around the topic to ensure you have a grasp of what the medical report is stating. Furthermore, one of the most helpful resources is your own expert, both in terms of educating you about the topic that is the subject of the report, but also in identifying weaknesses in the evidence relied upon by the opposing expert.

Further Reading

Bell, E. (2010) 'Judicial assessment of expert evidence', *Judicial Studies Institute Journal*, 2, 55–96.

Inns of Court College of Advocacy (2019) *Guidance on the preparation, admission and examination of expert evidence* (Council of the Inns of Court).

Chapter 17

Going to Court

Keith Rix

[T]he jury should be asked to consider whether the expert has, in the course of his evidence, assumed the role of an advocate, whether he has stepped outside his area of expertise, whether he was able to point to a recognised peer – reviewed source for his opinion, and whether his clinical experience is up to date and equal to that of others whose opinions he seeks to contradict.

Lord Clarke in *Hainey v HM Advocate* [2013] HCJAC 47

Avoiding It

The best way to avoid going to court is to produce a report that enables the parties to settle the case or which is so straightforward that in a criminal case parts of it are read to the jury or it is read by the judge without your having to attend.

The Order of Proceedings

If you are a party-appointed expert, you will probably be called to give evidence by the party that has instructed you, but there is 'no property in a witness'. An expert may be called by any party to the proceedings notwithstanding that his original instructions came from another party (*Harmony Shipping Co. SA v Saudi Europe Line* [1979] 1 WLR 1380). This is particularly likely to happen if you have prepared a report for the CPS and upon which the CPS does not want to rely. It will have been disclosed to the defence, so you may be called by the defence.

It is usual for one party, such as the claimant in a civil case or the prosecution in a criminal case, to call all of its evidence and then for the other party, such as the defendant in a civil case or the defendant in a criminal case, to call its evidence and for its expert evidence to be heard in rebuttal. The expert evidence usually follows that of the party's lay witnesses. However, you may be called before or after the other side's expert ('back to back') so that all of the evidence from your medical speciality is heard at the same time and so that both, or all, experts have heard, or can be informed about, all of the factual evidence. Indeed, you may be asked to attend to hear some of the factual evidence because experts, unlike lay witnesses (other than in Ireland), are permitted to hear the evidence of other witnesses before they give their own evidence (*Tomlinson v Tomlinson* [1980] 1 WLR 322). So, beware the zealous usher who, having identified you as an expert witness, seeks to exclude you from the court until you are called to give evidence. Give them a copy of the *Tomlinson* judgment.

Concurrent Expert Evidence

A development to be watched is 'concurrent expert evidence', 'hot-tubbing' or what in Ireland is called a 'debate'. Now established in Australia and becoming established in the British Isles, this involves calling all the experts at the same time. One side's experts may be in the dock and the other side's experts in the jury benches. There may be an agenda based on the matters not agreed at the experts' meeting supplemented by any additional issues that have arisen in the trial thus far. Counsel may be invited to contribute to the agenda. At the hearing, the judge takes control of the proceedings, effectively acting as chairman. In relation to each issue, the judge asks each expert the same questions or asks each expert to give an outline of the agreed evidence followed by presentation of the evidence on which they are not agreed. Where there is disagreement, the experts are able to explain why. The experts may be encouraged to add to, or explain, their own or another's evidence and they may be invited to question each other so that a healthy debate or discussion ensues. This means that experts must be thoroughly familiar with the detail of the case, ready and able to question the other party's or parties' experts on the hoof and sufficiently intellectually agile to assess immediately changes in assumptions or the assumed facts – and all this with an audience of at least three lawyers who may be hanging on to their every word. Then the parties' representatives are given the opportunity to ask their questions, but only to test the correctness of an expert's view or clarify it. They should not cover ground already fully explored and in general a full cross-examination or re-examination is not appropriate and will only take place if deemed necessary by the judge. Finally, the judge may seek to summarise the experts' positions and ask them to confirm or correct the summary. Such an approach favours the well-prepared expert and the expert who prepares carefully their questions for the other experts, but it may require experts to learn some advocacy skills. Where concurrent evidence on a child's future care was given by two psychiatrists and a clinical psychologist in *Local Authority v A (No. 2)* [2011] EWHC 590 (Fam), the judge estimated that evidence which would have filled two days of court time was completed within four hours.

Preparation

The best preparation for going to court is to prepare a quality report that enables the parties and the court to narrow down your evidence to that which needs elucidation and which deals with as much as possible of what might be put to you in cross-examination.

You need to have a basic understanding of court procedures. This helps you coordinate optimally with your instructing solicitors or their counsel and engage effectively with the trial judge. If it is the first time you are going to court, it should not be. You certainly should not enter a courtroom for the first time in your life when you go to give expert evidence. Shadow another expert, sit in the public gallery in a few cases or ask your presiding judge if you can sit with a judge and benefit from her tuition. Otherwise, watch a few episodes of *Kavanagh QC* or *Judge Deed*, but not US crime dramas, and do not expect all judges to have such interesting private lives as Judge Deed. I have written two fully scripted 'teaching plays', one based on a homicide in a psychiatric hospital and the other based on an accident at work, which allow participants to dress up as policemen, barristers and judges and in other outrageous costumes, as barristers and judges do every day, and have fun as well as learn about court procedures. There are details of these on my website.

On the subject of judges, Bill Braithwaite QC recommends that you should ask *about* the judge, his or her foibles and professional background. Please note the word 'about' – although many judges joke about being the subject of a psychiatric report, they may not take too kindly to a formal psychiatric assessment before your examination in chief. Perhaps experts should contribute to a website devoted to judges' foibles. This might make as interesting reading as the files some barristers maintain on experts. If you know the judge, point this out as the judge will have to decide if there is a real possibility that they may be subconsciously biased as a result of your relationship.

Allow sufficient time to read not only your report, but also other expert reports, although *in Scotland* or *Ireland*, in a action where there is no prior exchange of reports, you may find yourself going into court without knowledge of your opposing expert's opinion because it is intended to lead only their oral testimony. You may need to read transcripts of the evidence of other witnesses. In *O'Driscoll (Minor) v Hurley* [2015] IECA 158, the Irish Court of Appeal rejected the assertion that giving an expert transcripts of the evidence of previous witnesses was unacceptable 'prepping'; it was not unusual and perfectly proper. Familiarise yourself again with the factual basis for your opinions. Remind yourself of, and annotate, key evidence in medical records, witness statements or documentary exhibits. If you are allowed to take your own files into the witness box, which is almost always allowed, use coloured marker tags and highlighting to make it easy to navigate your way around the important information. Anticipate questions and have coloured tags with the subject written on them. If you know your way around the documents, you will be a more confident and authoritative witness. If you have to fumble backwards and forwards through your files or retrieve scattered sheets of paper from the well of the court, your credibility may be damaged. But you need to ask counsel whether or not you can take annotated and marked files into the witness box.

If you are not going to be able to take your own files, because the court insists that you work from a 'clean copy', try to memorise a small number of key points and practise reducing your opinions into a few memorable bullet points, but it is preferable to have them written down. However, giving evidence should not be a memory test or game. Be that as it may, be clear about your main points before you give evidence and be able to define them succinctly. Do a 'dummy run' with your secretary or some other lay person, or even a teenager. Make a list of what you think are the questions that will be put to you in cross-examination and your answers.

Usually, there will be a trial bundle. Get this in advance and number the pages of your report to correspond to its page numbers in the trial bundle or put your copy of the report into the bundle, with corresponding numbering, so that you have everything at your fingertips. Familiarise yourself with the organisation and contents of the trial bundle and where your opinion relates to key passages in, for example, medical records, have these tagged so that you can refer to them quickly and be ahead of the game. Remember that sometimes pagination, especially of medical records, will differ from the pagination in the records as they were originally supplied, and you may even have to spend time changing all the page references in your report to correspond to the numbering in the trial bundle.

Performance on the day is proportional to preparation. As a final stage in preparation, remind yourself of the test which the judge will apply when evaluating your evidence (Box 17.1). As to demeanour in the witness box, you will be participating in a drama, probably a costume drama, and there may well be some repartee, but leave the theatrics to the lawyers and remember *Coughlan v Whelton* (High Court (Ireland), unreported, 22 January 1993),

Box 17.1 The Judge's Test of Oral Testimony

- the internal consistency and logic of the evidence;
- the care with which the expert has considered the subject and prepared his evidence;
- his precision and accuracy of thought as demonstrated by his answers;
- how he responds to searching and informed cross-examination;
- the extent to which the expert faces up to and accepts the logic of a proposition put in cross-examination or is prepared to concede points that are seen to be correct;
- the extent to which the expert has conceived an opinion and is reluctant to re-examine it in the light of later evidence, or demonstrates a flexibility of mind which may involve changing or modifying opinions previously held;
- whether or not the expert is biased or lacks independence;
- the demeanour of the expert in the witness box.

Stuart Smith LJ in *Loveday v Renton (No. 1)* [1990] 1 Med LR 117

where the court was more impressed with the defendant's experts than with the theatrical presentation of the plaintiff's.

When in Rome

Dress and behaviour should convey an appropriate professional demeanour. Be punctual. Nod or bow slightly in the direction of the judge when entering, leaving or moving about in court. If you need to speak to someone, keep your voice down. Do not speak or move about when a witness or juror is taking the oath or affirming or, if you are present, during the judge's summing-up.

Outside Court

A lot of time is spent outside the courtroom. Be careful to whom you speak. You can talk to those instructing you. Do not discuss your evidence with other witnesses, especially the witnesses for the other side, without permission. Do not talk to the other side's solicitor or barrister unless specifically instructed to do so. This does not mean that you cannot exchange greetings or other pleasantries. As long as the parties agree, there is usually no reason why you should not talk to your opposite number about matters unrelated to the case. Occasionally, experts are asked to confer on an issue, on a without-prejudice basis, and report back to their respective solicitor or barrister. This can assist the parties in narrowing issues further.

Forms of Address

Etiquette requires an appropriate form of address for the judge. Ask the barrister or solicitor how to address the judge. Some courtrooms have a notice outside that gives the form of address. You may have the opportunity to hear how the solicitors or barristers do so. If you are stuck, you may or may not want to apply the convention of calling every police constable 'sergeant', and although a circuit judge will not object to being 'My Lord' instead of 'Your Honour', you will only draw attention to your ignorance if 'Your Honour' comes out as 'Your Holiness' (as a coroner was recently addressed).

Giving Evidence

When you are called to give evidence, go to the witness box. The judge, jury and other side's counsel may be looking at you for the first time. First impressions! If you have not already been asked, whisper to the court usher and tell her whether you will take the oath, on an appropriate religious text, or make the affirmation.

Face the judge. If it is the oath, take the book in your right hand and hold it just below shoulder level with the elbow flexed at about 45 degrees (not with arm outstretched like a Nazi salute). Either repeat the oath after the usher or judge or read it from the card. If possible, wait for eye contact with the judge, but do not wait too long! If you make eye contact at this point, you are already establishing a rapport with the judge.

The judge may invite you to sit. Standing usually makes a better impression unless you cannot see to read. However, *in Ireland* witnesses sit. The judge and jury will scrutinise your body language closely. Remember that as the judge does not have to think about the next question to ask, he is well-placed to observe your non-verbal communication and body language as you respond to the questions.

If there is an adjournment during your evidence, do not talk to anyone about the case. The judge should remind you of this. *In Ireland* this only applies if you are under cross-examination at the time.

Evidence in Chief

Your counsel starts unless it is an inquest and the coroner calls you. You will be asked your full name, possibly your address and your appointment. Give your professional address. Keep your feet facing the judge and swivel to listen to counsel ('the turning technique'). Swivel back, if there is no jury, address your answer to the judge and, if there is a jury, still address the judge, but look at the furthermost juror and make sure your voice reaches him or her. Addressing the judge or judge and jury is courteous and it further assists with rapport building.

Keep your eye on the judge or she will tell you to watch her pen or her fingers. She will usually be writing or typing your evidence. If she is not, do not panic, but ask yourself why not. It might be a rare situation in which there is a computer link from the court stenographer to the judge's bench. Only when she has finished writing or typing, turn back slowly to face counsel and signal that you are ready for the next question. Keep control.

There will probably be a microphone. This is usually to record your evidence and not to amplify your voice. If you are repeatedly reminded to speak up, or more slowly, it will adversely affect the impression you make.

You will be asked to look at the signature page of your report, in the trial bundle, confirm that it is your report and signature, and confirm, or otherwise explain if not, that it continues to be your opinion. Correct any significant errors and indicate whether or not your opinion needs to be modified in the light of any evidence you have heard. Any other change of opinion should already have been communicated; if necessary, remind the court that you have done so.

In a criminal case, you may be asked for your qualifications. If you have set them out fully, in your report's Appendix 1, you may be asked to confirm 'x', 'y' and 'z'. Counsel should have advised you how much he wants to elicit. If given free rein, do not confuse the jury with letters of the alphabet in what they will see as random order. 'The basic qualification of a medical doctor' makes more sense than 'MB, BS' and even Latin scholars will not immediately understand 'MB, BChir'. In a civil or family case, you may be asked only to confirm that your qualifications are as set out in what should be Appendix 1 of your report. The judge will have read the report.

If there is a jury, remember that you must be understood by the least intelligent member and remember that few lawyers and, at the time of writing, no judges are medically qualified, although some medically qualified barristers sit as deputy high court judges and recorders. It is not enough to have a glossary of medical terms at the end of the report. You will have to communicate 'technical' information simply and clearly as you go along by either avoiding or explaining what will be seen as medical jargon.

A few weeks after I gave evidence about hyperventilation in a rape case, I was in the same court building and responded, with two or three pathologists, to a request for any doctor in the building to make their way to the jury waiting area. On the stairs, we met the court clerk, who had been in my previous case, and he told us that there was no hurry as it was just a case of hyperventilation and the juror was recovering with the aid of a paper bag. His diagnosis and treatment were correct.

This is your evidence in chief. Questioned by your counsel, in a criminal case, you will be taken over the key points in your report. Jurors are particularly likely to attend and understand when the facts of the case are woven into a comprehensive, unfolding story of the evidence. The longer this takes, the more your confidence grows. Try to recreate orally the structure of your written report with 'signposts' – for example: 'There are four groups of symptoms that are important. First . . .'. However, in a civil case, your report stands as your evidence in chief, so do not expect much more than a request to confirm that it remains your opinion, although some judges do like to hear the expert explain their relevant expertise and set out their key points.

If you want to refer to a document, suggest to the judge that it may be helpful to do so and indicate where it is to be found. Wait for the judge to find it. She will probably read it, or at least scan it, so wait until she looks up before making the point that arises from it. As you do so, you can use a change in the tone of voice and emphasise words like 'conclude' to focus attention on what you regard as the significance of the document.

Counsel may get you to expand on certain points or respond to questions based on evidence already given of which you are unaware or of which you were unaware when you prepared your report. But do not be tempted to moderate your opinion without good reason. In *England v Foster Wheeler* (Sheffield County Court, unreported, 14 August 2009), the judge preferred the evidence of the defendant's experts to that of the claimant's expert, as 'there seemed to be no new factor that Dr X brought into consideration in moderating his view . . . there was no real explanation for resiling from his view set out in the joint statement'.

It is important how you give your evidence – 'authoritative, careful and straightforward' (*Manning v King's College Hospital NHS Trust* [2008] EWHC 1838 (QB)). You have to appear, as you should be, the master of the facts and your opinion; you need to be convincing and authoritative. Make use of your voice and learn to vary the tone for effect, employing a persuasive tone where appropriate. The better structured your evidence is, the more convincing it will be, and it will be easier to follow if you explain the structure. If you are not convincing and authoritative, you will lose credibility with the judge, the jury or both. As Braithwaite and Waldron (2010) say: 'Part of the art of being a good witness, and therefore a good expert, is to be able to communicate opinions clearly, despite provocation from opposing counsel, to someone who seems ignorant of the basics.'

Cross-Examination

Then comes cross-examination. Remember to swivel back to face the judge and/or jury when you have heard the question. Keep calm as a change in demeanour can give the wrong impression. Not looking at your cross-examiner helps. Console yourself in the fact that you and the other experts know more than counsel or the judge does about the subject of your evidence. Barristers are not experts in your field, but they may try to give that impression. They have the advantage, however, of knowing what the next question will be; they are likely to have done extensive reading on your subject, with the help of other experts; and they may also have the advantage of being assisted by your opposite number, who will be furiously scribbling adhesive notes that your cross-examiner will line-up where you can see them in order to remind you who she thinks is in control.

The purpose of cross-examination is to weaken, qualify or destroy the other side's case. So, be prepared for an attack on your veracity, reputation and expertise. '[E]xperts must be prepared for everything they do and say to be the subject of challenge' (*County Council v SB*). Be able to explain why your qualifications and experience are relevant and why you should be regarded as at least comparable in qualifications, training and experience to the other side's expert. The bigger the case, the more likely it is that your cross-examiner will use your CV to persuade the judge that you are not qualified and use any other information, whether or not in the public domain, to discredit you. You may be asked about your fees, as if to suggest that the higher the fee, the greater the difficulty you have in being impartial, but in *O'Driscoll*, the Irish Court of Appeal held that there was no basis for a 'bald assertion' that a fee of €5,000 was likely to affect impartiality and such questioning challenging the expert's honesty, independence and integrity could not be put without any evidence to back it up. If it is suggested that your name is on a website devoted to judicial criticism of experts, you are entitled to ask for details, as this may be no more than 'dirty tricks'.

If you survive any attack on your credibility, cross-examination will then move on to the testing of the validity of your opinions and bringing out evidence that supports the other side's case.

Remember a Maudsley-style case conference where several professors and other psychiatrists question your opinion. Try to bear in mind, but you should have anticipated, the stimulating, helpful and clarifying points that you would make in response to their questions.

Do not be drawn into a contest or argument or try to evade the question. In *Siegel v Pummell*, a neuropsychiatrist called by the defendant was criticised by the judge because '[h]is evidence was combative' as well as 'dismissive of that of other medical professionals who were not in the same field as himself', this being a reference to the neurologist and neuropsychologist called by the claimant. In *R (PS) v G (Responsible Medical Officer)* [2003] EWHC 2335 (Admin), a psychiatrist was criticised for his 'evasive and overdefensive approach in answering questions when cross-examined'. Defensiveness may be interpreted as a sign of lack of objectivity.

You are there to assist the court. It is the lawyers who argue:

> While I am sure that both experts were trying to assist the Court, I found the evidence of Dr. (X) of more assistance than that of Dr. (Y). Although Dr. (X)'s measured and careful approach was more persuasive than Dr. (Y)'s more argumentative and didactic approach, it was not just the manner in which they gave their evidence. It seemed to me that the content of Dr. (Y)'s evidence was unconvincing: for example . . . (Simon J in *Rabone v Pennine Care NHS Trust* [2009] LS Law Med 503)

The judge wants to know your opinion not witness, or have to referee, an argument, a slanging match or even a joust. In *Qualcomm Inc. v Nokia Corp.* [2008] EWHC 329 (Pat), the judge considered that the expert was more interested in jousting with counsel, and scoring what he thought were points for his side, than in answering the technical questions put to him.

The case is not about you. As soon as you start arguing, you lose your objectivity and give the impression that you are not impartial. Remember that 'anything other than a courteous, moderated and seemingly impartial response to questioning in court will damage [your] credibility' (Lewis 2006). If your cross-examiner does engage in fencing, the judge may not like it.

According to expert witness folklore 'crafted in the wine bars of The Strand . . . [the cross examiner] has three minutes to unsettle the expert and consign the expert's opinion into the bin marked "Thank you very much for coming". If this is not achieved, it is said, the barrister's task will be that much harder' (Smethurst 2006).

So, keep calm. Do not rush into answering the question. This may allow time for your counsel to object or require clarification and it allows time for your considered response. But do not delay too long.

You may be asked a very technical/medical question at an early stage and your cross-examiner will be wanting to try and unsettle you with an impression that she has an immediate and full grasp of the medical issues (Smethurst 2006). Barristers are taught only to ask questions to which they know the answer. If you have to ask for clarification, it may be she who becomes unsettled. *In Scotland*, such questions may be put by reference to academic journal articles of which you have no forewarning as there is no requirement to lodge such documents or identify them in advance of the trial.

You will be asked 'yes'/'no' questions, but do not hesitate to add some important qualification if appropriate. If you do not, you will have forgotten it later or you will not see how to introduce it. If you think that an explanation is needed, give it. If you do not say all you need to say on an issue, you have only yourself to blame if it was your only opportunity. If necessary, appeal to the judge and make it clear that the answer depends on 'x' or 'y'.

Answer the question asked. It was a finding of the GMC in *Pool* that Dr Pool's evidence was 'very unclear and [he] often gave long, rambling answers that did not address the question'. It is not in your interests to answer, however well, anything other than the question you have been asked. In *Manning*, an expert was criticised because he often volunteered 'by way of addition, answers to questions which he had not been asked which appeared to support the Defendant's case'. Wait to answer the next question, even if you know what it is, and do not be evasive. If the question takes you outside your expertise, say so and, if necessary, appeal to the judge.

Do not hesitate to ask for a question to be repeated or clarified; but asking for too many questions to be repeated can give jurors a bad impression.

Do not be rushed. If it is a particularly difficult question, write it down and do not be afraid to ask for more time. The judge wants your carefully considered opinion and not the first thing that comes into your head.

Keep your answers to the point. Do not give a lecture. The longer the answer, the more cross-examination it generates.

If your cross-examiner creates a 'pregnant pause', beware filling it. If in doubt, it is even more important to keep answers brief; this is when you are most likely to fall into hidden traps.

If you are asked several questions in one, repeat the questions you remember, write them down, answer these and then ask to be reminded of the others. There is no reason why you should not write down even a single question in order to be sure that you understand it and answer it rather than another question. You will not be criticised for asking to be reminded of the questions, although counsel may be criticised for asking so many at once.

If you are interrupted – for example, with 'We'll come back to this point' – but perhaps because the cross-examiner does not want to hear what you have to say, politely insist on completing your answer.

If you are asked to make an assumption, do not be afraid to question it. If you do not, it might be assumed that you accept it. Even if you are not sure about its basis, it tips off your counsel, so, by the time you are re-examined, she may use your evidence to invalidate the assumption. Make it clear how your answer differs according to whether it is based on hypothesis or what appear to be the actual facts.

You may be told to respond to a question that relates to something in a document. Ask to be taken to the document. It gives you time to think, you can check exactly what is in the document, which may not be what was in the question, and you may want to draw attention to the context so that the reference is not taken in misleading isolation. Address the context before the question.

You may be asked if the opinion of the other side's expert is within the range of reasonable opinion. If you agree, say so, but say why you think that your opinion should be preferred.

Do not be afraid to make appropriate concessions where necessary and which on all of the evidence, perhaps now better clarified, it is reasonable to concede. It is not the same as wholesale surrender. You may impress the judge by your integrity in making appropriate concessions and this will add to your credibility. As Lord Justice McFarlane has observed, the most impressive and valuable experts are those who can accept parts of an alternative analysis whilst disagreeing with other parts, and who are not partisan or dogmatic (Keynote Address, Bond Solon Experts Conference 2018). You will gain no respect for sticking to your opinion through thick and thin and when forced into a corner if the evidence does not justify this. Doing so will risk creating the same impression as the expert who 'perhaps because he believed in the Defendant's case . . . was somewhat inflexible in his answers and reluctant to concede points which on their merits were persuasive' (*Manning*).

Be prepared for opinions that do not appear to survive cross-examination. Be careful not to appear to be scraping the bottom of the barrel. If an abandoned opinion can be salvaged, your counsel will return to it on re-examination.

You should be able to recognise when you are being led up the garden path and the end of the path is obvious. If there do not seem to be answers that can halt your passage, do not fear. If there was no alternative but to go to the end of the path, you will be credited for having gone there. If there was another path you ought to have taken, your own counsel will probably have seen it and will take you there in re-examination.

You may be asked questions which require some memory of the evidence. However well you have prepared, there will be some evidence that you will have forgotten. Do not answer if you do not remember the evidence. Ask to be reminded. Take time, but not too long, to look through your documents.

Cross-examination is meant to be conducted with courtesy. Occasionally, it is not. However unpleasant your cross-examiner is, remain calm and relentlessly polite. Do not lose your cool, get angry or flustered, or allow her to get under your skin. Avoid being defensive or argumentative. Do not descend into the arena and try to score points. Concentrate on the question and not how it is asked. If it appears that a question is based on a misunderstanding, answer in a way that implies counsel's misunderstanding rather than her total ignorance. Appeal to the judge more in sorrow than in anger. If it seems that your cross-examiner is trying to be really offensive, appeal to the judge, but with some restraint, suggesting that you have been misunderstood. The case is not about you; unless you have failed in your duties as an expert, you should not be subjected to personal attack. When the judge or jury retires, you may have made the better impression.

Watch out for questions that tempt you to give a different answer, perhaps disguised, to that already given in evidence or in your report. Just confirm what you have already said.

However well you think you have prepared and however good your report, you are bound to be asked something that you have not anticipated. Take your time. Remember that you are there to assist the court and it is not a contest between you and your cross-examiner. Give your answer after careful consideration. Give your opinion rather than an argument for one side or the other. Avoid being too definite. Avoid 'never' and 'always', but equally beware of 'possibly'. What should hopefully come across as an obviously genuine degree of uncertainty on one matter may make the court more likely to accept evidence you have given on another matter without such uncertainty.

If questioning appears to have blown a hole in your side's case, do not try to repair the damage unless you can do so as an expert. By the time you are re-examined, your counsel will have had time to think about this and, if you missed a defence of the case, you may be led to deliver it.

If you think that you have given an incorrect answer, say so as soon as possible, even if it means interrupting another line of enquiry. It will be useless writing three weeks later.

If the cross-examiner responds with a look of disbelief or puzzlement, do not worry. Like the pregnant pause, it may be intended to encourage you to say something you might not otherwise say. Wait for the actual question. There may not be one.

Do not be taken by surprise at the suddenness of the ending of the cross-examination, but, if your cross-examiner says that she has only a few more points, or it will not last much longer, do not lower your guard. However, cross-examination will come to an end.

This is the best time to turn to the judge, if appropriate, and ask to be allowed to make further points, if you think that the thrust of your evidence has not been taken on board. But be careful: (1) you should have got your message across already; (2) if permitted, it will inevitably invite further cross-examination; (3) you are about to be re-examined. Counsel should have picked up anything which needs rectifying or clarifying.

Throughout, remember that you are there to assist the court and not to support the side that has instructed you. For this reason, do not make non-verbal contact with those instructing you when under cross-examination; it will give the wrong impression. Assisting the court depends on your ability to connect with judge and/or jury and come across as likeable (friendly, respectful, kind, well-mannered, pleasant), confident or demonstrably self-assured, knowledgeable and trustworthy (Parrott *et al.* 2015). Contrast this with criticism of the expert in *Re U (Serious Injury: Standard of Proof)* [2004] EWCA Civ 567: 'The court must always be on guard against the over-dogmatic expert, the expert whose reputation or amour-propre is at stake, or the expert who has developed a scientific prejudice.'

Box 17.2 lists a number of 'don'ts' for experts.

Box 17.2 Don'ts for the Expert Witness

- act in a condescending manner;
- act pompous;
- pontificate;*
- appear egotistical;
- be pedantic;
- be dogmatic;*
- argue with counsel;
- praise oneself;
- be arrogant;
- be boring;
- be cute;
- be overconfident;
- be sharp;
- be evasive;*
- be verbose;
- change demeanour on cross-examination;
- answer the wrong question;*
- confuse the jury;
- patronise;
- engage in nervous habits;
- fumble for papers or documents;
- look or act anxious, nervous or worried;
- turn your back on the jury;
- overwhelm the jury.

*Added by the author.

Based on Babitsky *et al.* 2000

Re-examination

Now your re-examination. This is limited to the clarification of points made in cross-examination. It is not your opportunity to make any new points or get over what you have forgotten. Only with the leave of the court can new points be introduced. This is your counsel's opportunity to regain ground lost, or repair damage sustained, during your cross-examination. As you are there to assist the court, not those instructing you, resist the temptation to join battle. Just answer the question; keep it simple. Your credibility depends on the judge and/or jury seeing you as independent. Any other approach will undermine your evidence. Generally, no leading questions are allowed, lest they suggest an answer that is different to what you have given in cross-examination; so, re-examination may be limited or non-existent. This is the best time to turn to the judge, if it is appropriate, and ask to be allowed to make some further points. It may be your last chance to get your points across, but you are entering into highly fraught territory. There may be a profound heart-sink moment on one side, but likely apprehension all round. Be assured that more cross-examination is likely.

Remember:

> The way in which you give your evidence affects the weight of credibility attached to it. Imagine that, if your evidence is clear, succinct and truthful, it will weigh down heavily on the scales of justice . . . If, however, your evidence is confusing, and you are nervous, aggressive, pompous, rambling and inflexible, it will be given little or no weight. (Bond *et al.* 2007)

Psychiatrists will be relieved to know that the following judicial criticisms were not of a psychiatrist, but of a social work expert (*Re IA*):

> . . . quite extraordinarily uncompromising, interested only on repeating her own view and seemingly unwilling to countenance she may have misjudged anyone . . . quite arrogant . . . delivered her evidence at breakneck speed and could not be persuaded to slow down notwithstanding several reminders. She referred to the mother throughout as 'Mom' which seemed to me to be somewhat disrespectful.

Questions from the Judge

Even if the judge has already asked some questions, be prepared for more and remember that your counsel and your cross-examiner may want to clarify your answers.

Afterwards

The judge will probably thank you for your attendance. Reciprocate with a simple nod and, without grovelling, express appreciation, if appropriate, for accommodating your attendance to minimise interference with your professional duties or to allow you to go on that much deserved foreign holiday. However, if there is a jury, limit yourself to an appropriately formal response.

You may be released by the court, but your counsel may want you to assist in her cross-examination of the other side's expert (if you have not already done so). To do so, you will need to sit behind counsel and pass forward handwritten notes suggesting questions. For this, you need a pad of adhesive notes so that they can be attached to the back of the seat adjacent to her and then you need the confidence to tug at her gown, when it is necessary to draw attention to them, but also the skill to avoid distracting her from what she is saying. This is not so daunting in a case with leading and junior counsel, or if you are sitting next to the solicitor, as junior counsel or the solicitor can screen your notes and decide when to send them forward.

Afterwards, find out about the outcome. Do not be disheartened if the judge has not accepted your evidence. Judges are entitled to disagree with an expert witness, although to do so there must be a safe basis for the disagreement and as the judge will have to explain fully his reasons for rejecting expert evidence or for preferring the evidence of one expert to that of another, you may have something useful to learn from the judgment.

It matters not 'which side has won'. Has your testimony assisted in the delivery of justice?

Appendices

Specimen Reports

These two appendices are intended to illustrate how a criminal and a civil personal injury report should be set out – the structure, the content and the prose style. The constraints of space in reproducing an A4 sheet on a smaller page while trying to preserve legibility mean that the recommendations from Box 6.1 and elsewhere in this volume cannot be exactly followed.

Appendix A

IN THE CENTRAL CRIMINAL COURT

R v DANIEL MCNAUGHTAN

Case No. 20-6-1843

On the instructions of:	Monteith and Company, 15, Cheapside, London EC1
Who act on behalf of:	The Defendant
Their reference:	SM/BR
Subject matter:	Psychiatric assessment of the Defendant
Date of instruction:	11 February 1843
Date of report:	25 February 1843
Report reference:	ETM/XY/1
Dates of consultations:	18 and 20 February 1843
Place of consultation:	HMP Newgate, London
Consent:	Written

Report by
Dr. E. T. Monro,
BSc, MSc, MD, FRCPsych
Consultant Psychiatrist
499 Cleckheaton Street,
London W17 5OX

GMC No: 87654321

Tel: 020 999 1111 Fax: 020 999 6666
www.xxx.co.uk
ETMonro@499cleck.com

Report of: Dr. E.T. Monro
Specialism: Psychiatry
On the instructions of: Monteith and Company
Prepared for: The Central Criminal Court

CONTENTS[1]

[1] This report is based on the 'Model Form of Expert's Report' approved by the Judicial Committee of the Academy of Experts and on that of the Expert Witness Institute.

Report of: Dr. E.T. Monro
Specialism: Psychiatry
On the instructions of: Monteith and Company
Prepared for: The Central Criminal Court

Appendices

1. INTRODUCTION

1.1 The writer

1.1.1 I am Edward Thomas Monro, a licensed and registered medical practitioner approved under s 12 of the Mental Health Act 1983 (as amended by the Mental Health Act 2007) and registered with the General Medical Council as a specialist in general psychiatry according to the provisions of Schedule 2 of the European Specialist Medical Qualifications Order 1995. Full details of my qualifications and experience entitling me to give expert opinion evidence are in **Appendix 1**.

1.1.2 In my clinical practice I routinely have the care of adults with a range of mental disorders including the major mental illnesses, such as schizophrenia, bipolar disorder and depressive illness, organic disorders, such as dementia, less serious and less disabling mental disorders, including post-traumatic stress disorder and adjustment disorders, personality disorders, substance misuse disorders and intellectual (learning) disabilities. This case therefore falls within my area of expertise.

1.2 Synopsis

1.2.1 Daniel McNaughtan ('the Defendant') is indicted that on 20 January 1843, at the parish of St Martin's in the Fields, Middlesex, he murdered Mr Edward Drummond ('the Deceased'), the private secretary of Sir Robert Peel, the Prime Minister, against the peace of our Sovereign lady the Queen, Her Crown and Dignity, contrary to common law.

1.3 Instructions

1.3.1 I have been instructed by friends of the Defendant, through his solicitors, Monteith and Company, to visit him at Newgate and prepare a psychiatric report for his trial.

1.4 Disclosure of interests

1.4.1 The Defendant is not known to me professionally or personally. I do not know any of the parties involved. There are no conflicts of interest in respect to any of the identified parties but for the avoidance of doubt I am not a member of the Conservative Party or the Roman Catholic Church. I have no other interest which might cause a conflict based upon the nature of the case.

2. THE BACKGROUND TO THE CASE AND THE ISSUES

2.1 The relevant people

2.1.1 Henry C. Bell – Sheriff Depute of the County of Lanark
2.1.2 Sir James Campbell – The Lord Provost of Glasgow
2.1.3 Edward Drummond – The Deceased, Private Secretary to Sir Robert Peel
2.1.4 Mrs Dutton – The Defendant's London landlady

Report of: Dr. E.T. Monro
Specialism: Psychiatry
On the instructions of: Monteith and Company
Prepared for: The Central Criminal Court

2.1.5	William Gilchrist	– Glasgow printer with whom the Defendant lodged
2.1.6	John Gordon	– London acquaintance of the Defendant
2.1.7	John Hughes	– Tailor and the Defendant's Glasgow landlord
2.1.8	Alexander Johnston	– Member of Parliament
2.1.9	Alexander Martin	– Gunmaker, Paisley
2.1.10	Daniel McNaughtan	– The Defendant
2.1.11	Daniel McNaughtan (Sen)	– The Defendant's father
2.1.12	Sir Robert Peel	– The Prime Minister
2.1.13	James Silver	– Police Constable
2.1.14	John Tierney	– Police Inspector
2.1.15	Benjamin Weston	– Office Porter
2.1.16	Hugh Wilson	– Commissioner of Police for Glasgow

2.2 The assumed facts and substance of all material instructions

2.2.1 The Defendant is indicted that on 20 January 1843, at the parish of St Martin's in the Fields, Middlesex, he murdered Mr Edward Drummond, the private secretary of Sir Robert Peel, the Prime Minister. The Deceased was on terms of intimacy and friendship with the Prime Minister and occupied apartments in the official residence of the Prime Minister. He was in the constant habit of passing from those rooms to the Prime Minister's private residence in Whitehall Gardens.

2.2.2 There is evidence that the Defendant had been seen loitering about these spots for many days and watching the persons who went in and out of the public offices and the houses in Whitehall Gardens.

2.2.3 On Friday 20 January 1843, the Deceased left his apartments in Downing Street and went to the Treasury and thence to the Admiralty, from there he visited his bank in Charing Cross and on his return, near the 'Salopian' coffee house, it is alleged that the Defendant came behind him and discharged a pistol almost close to him. After discharging it, he drew another from his breast, presented it to the Deceased and was in the act of firing it when a policeman restrained him. Although the Deceased managed to walk back to his bank, he died from his injuries on 25 January 1843.

2.2.4 It is further the case for the Crown that, from the facts of the case, from the threats used by the Defendant before he committed his crime, and his declaration afterwards, it was not the life of the Deceased that he sought. It was the life of Sir Robert Peel that he desired to take, and it was his life that he believed he was destroying when he discharged the fatal pistol against the person of the Deceased.

2.2.5 The Defendant was initially arraigned at Bow Street on 21 January 1843 and he subsequently appeared before the Grand Jury on both 30 January and 2 February 1843 where he pleaded not guilty to murder.

2.2.6 I have included a brief chronology as **Appendix 6**.

2.3 The issues to be addressed

2.3.1 I have been asked:
(a) whether or not the Defendant was insane according to 'The M'Naghten Rules';
(b) whether or not the Defendant has a defence of 'diminished responsibility'; and
(c) whether or not the Defendant could have been feigning his delusions.

Report of: Dr. E.T. Monro
Specialism: Psychiatry
On the instructions of: Monteith and Company
Prepared for: The Central Criminal Court

2.4 The assumptions adopted

2.4.1 I regard what the Defendant and any informant has told me and what is contained in the medical records and other documents as 'assumed facts'. The only facts within my own knowledge are my findings on examination of the Defendant and as set out below in the section 'psychiatric examination' (4.7) and my knowledge of the practice of psychiatry.

2.4.2 Unless otherwise indicated I have assumed that:

2.4.2.1 What the Defendant and any informant have told me is true, but ultimately the truthfulness of the Defendant and any witnesses is a matter for the court;

2.4.2.2 The evidence of the prosecution witnesses is true;

2.4.2.3 The information contained in documentary sources of information is accurate.

2.4.3 Where there is a conflict between documentary evidence and the Defendant's evidence I have assumed that the Defendant's version of events is correct unless the same is so technically or manifestly incorrect in which case I will explain why I do not accept the Defendant's version of events.

3. INVESTIGATION OF FACTS AND ASSUMED FACTS[1]

3.1 Methodology

3.1.1 In compliance with CrPR 19.4(1)(h) and in order to assist the court in determining the reliability of my opinion, I have set out in **Appendix 2** the methodology that I have employed.

3.2 Interview and examination

3.2.1 I have interviewed and examined the Defendant twice (see **Appendix 3**). On 18 February 1843, I was accompanied by Sir Alexander Morison, my colleague at Bethlem and author of the celebrated work *The Physiognomy of Mental Disease* (1840). Also present were Mr William McClure, a surgeon residing at Harley Street, and other professional gentlemen. At the Gaol we met Dr A. J. Sutherland, Jnr, Physician to St Luke's Hospital, and Dr Bright who had been instructed by the Crown. I saw the defendant again on 20 February 1843 in the company of Dr Hutcheson and Dr Crawford. We all asked questions in turn. I did not make notes of the examination at the time, but did so afterwards at my rooms and they form the basis of this report.

3.2.2 We were able to discuss the Defendant's physical health with Dr Lavies, Physician to Newgate Gaol.

3.3 Documents

3.3.1 The documents made available or obtained are listed in **Appendix 4**.

3.3.2 There are no medical records for the Defendant. This is because he has not attended a doctor or hospital since he was a child.

[1] It is possible that some of the facts and assumed facts in this report are not true, but this may be for the court to decide. I have ended this report with the same declaration of truth as a witness statement made according to the provisions of the Criminal Justice Act 1967, the Magistrates' Courts Act 1980 and the Magistrates' Courts Rules 1981. Insofar as I have stated that the contents of this report are true, this must be taken to mean that it is true that the facts and assumed facts are as stated and not that each and every fact or assumed fact is in itself true.

Report of: Dr. E.T. Monro
Specialism: Psychiatry
On the instructions of: Monteith and Company
Prepared for: The Central Criminal Court

3.4 Medical terms and explanations

3.4.1 I have indicated any medical or related terms in **bold type**. I have defined these terms and included them in a glossary in **Appendix 5**.

4. FACTUAL ANALYSIS

4.1 Background history

4.1.1 In order to understand the Defendant as a person and consider how any mental disorder may have arisen, I followed normal psychiatric convention and I took an account from the Defendant of his background history. It is set out in **Appendix 3**.

4.1.2 So far as his personality is concerned, the Defendant has been described by a number of the witnesses in such terms as sullen, gloomy, reserved and unsocial and Mrs Dutton, with whom he lodged in London, said that he was not in the habit of looking people in the face. (It is not clear if these were his characteristics before he became ill (i.e. his premorbid personality) or the early signs of the illness – ETM.)

4.2 Self-reported medical history and background to the alleged offence

4.2.1 With regard to his physical health, the Defendant responded by saying that physicians could be of no service to him. He said that if he took a ton of drugs it would be of no service to him.

4.2.2 So far as his mental health is concerned, the Defendant referred to 'the persecution' and he referred to 'grinding of the mind'.

4.2.3 He spoke of people watching him in Glasgow, pointing to him and speaking of him, saying that he was a murderer and the worst of characters. In Edinburgh, he had seen a man on horseback watching him and another had nodded to him and said: 'That's he.'

4.2.4 He was critical of Sheriff Bell for not having put an end to 'the persecution' and said that if he had had a pistol in his possession he would have shot him dead. He said that Sheriff Bell, Sheriff Alison and Sir Robert Peel could have put a stop to the system of persecution if they had wanted to do so.

4.2.5 He referred to seeing a man with a bundle of straw under his arm and he knew well enough what that meant as everything was done by signs: the straw denoted that he should lie upon straw in an asylum.

4.2.6 He had seen paragraphs in *The Times* newspaper containing allusions directed at him and he complained that there had been articles in the *Glasgow Herald* which were beastly and atrocious and insinuated things which were untrue and insufferable of him.

4.2.7 He said that on one or two occasions pernicious things had been put in his food.

Report of: Dr. E.T. Monro
Specialism: Psychiatry
On the instructions of: Monteith and Company
Prepared for: The Central Criminal Court

4.3 Witness evidence as to the defendant's mental state

4.3.1 The Defendant's father, Daniel McNaughtan, says that about two years ago the Defendant had called at his house and begged him to speak to the authorities in town to have 'a stop put on them'. He said that he was being persecuted and followed day and night by spies. Although they never spoke to him, they laughed at him and shook their fists in his face and those who had sticks shook them at him. He said that one of them threw straws in his face. This he thought meant that he was to be reduced to a state of beggary. His father never went, as the Defendant wanted, to any of the civil authorities because he realised that he was 'labouring under some extraordinary delusion, and therefore considered it quite unnecessary'. He did not consult any medical gentleman because he thought that the delusions would eventually pass away.

4.3.2 William Gilchrist, with whom the Defendant lodged in the Gorbals, sleeping in the same bed, said that the Defendant frequently used to get up in the night and walk about the room uttering incoherent sentences and making use of ejaculations such as 'By Jove' and 'My God'. On occasions, he burst out into immoderate fits of laughter without any cause whatsoever. At other times, he would moan. He said that the Defendant had told him about a visit to the House of Commons and how he was highly delighted at having heard Sir Robert Peel. However, he said that he had never heard the Defendant speak of Sir Robert Peel's political character nor heard him make use of any threat towards him. When he last saw the Defendant in July 1842, his conversation was not so connected as formerly.

4.3.3 John Hughes, the landlord of the house, in which the Defendant and William Gilchrist had lodged, confirmed the evidence of William Gilchrist and said that in consequence of the Defendant's strange manner he asked him to leave.

4.3.4 Henry Bell, one of the sheriffs depute of the county of Lanark, said that the Defendant had been to see him and complained about being harassed to death by a system of persecution. He said that the Defendant gave a long, rambling, unintelligible statement from which it appeared that he believed that he was constantly beset by spies and considered that his life and property were in danger.

4.3.5 Similar evidence has been given by Alexander Johnston, MP, whom the Defendant had consulted. The Defendant had told him that he was also being attacked through the newspapers.

4.3.6 Sir James Campbell, the Lord Provost of Glasgow, says that the Defendant had been to complain to him as well. He told him that he was compelled to sleep in the fields in the suburbs of the town to evade his persecutors.

4.3.7 Hugh Wilson, the Commissioner of Police for Glasgow, says that the Defendant had told him that he thought that the persecution proceeded from the priests at the Catholic chapel in Clyde Street, who were assisted by a parcel of Jesuits. Two or three days later, he returned and said that the Tories had joined the Catholics. He mentioned how, when he had fled to France, as soon as he landed at Boulogne, he had seen one of the spies peep from behind the watch-box on the Custom House Quay.

4.3.8 John Gordon, who had known the Defendant for six years, said that he had never seen anything particular about his conduct. However, in November 1842, when the Defendant was in search of employment, they walked past Sir Robert Peel's house and the Defendant said: 'Damn him, sink him.' When they passed the Treasury, he said: 'Look across the street, there is where all the treasure and worth of the world is.'

Report of: Dr. E.T. Monro
Specialism: Psychiatry
On the instructions of: Monteith and Company
Prepared for: The Central Criminal Court

4.4 Transcript of the Defendant's statement at Bow Street Police Court

4.4.1 When the Defendant appeared before Bow Street Police Court he made the following statement to the magistrate:

4.4.2 The Tories in my native city have compelled me to do this. They follow and persecute me wherever I go, and have entirely destroyed my peace of mind. They followed me to France, into Scotland, and all over England; in fact they follow me wherever I go. I can get no rest from them night or day. I cannot sleep at night in consequence of the course they pursue towards me. I believe they have driven me into a consumption. I am sure I shall never be the man I formerly was. I used to have good health and strength, but I have not now. They have accused me of crimes of which I am not guilty; they do everything in their power to harass and persecute me; in fact, they wish to murder me. It can be proved by evidence; that's all I have to say.

4.5 Defendant's account of the alleged offence[1]

4.5.1 We asked the Defendant more than once if he knew it was Sir Robert Peel he shot at. The Defendant hesitated and paused and at length said that he was not sure whether it was Sir Robert Peel or not.

4.5.2 The Defendant said that the person at whom he fired had given him a scowling look as he passed. He said that he was one of the crew that was destroying his health. At that moment, all the feelings of the months and years rushed into his mind and he thought that he could only obtain peace by shooting him.

4.5.3 He went on to say that he imagined that the person at whom he fired at Charing Cross was 'one of the crew – a part of the system that was destroying his health' and 'every feeling of suffering which he had endured for months and years rose up at once on his mind, and that he conceived that he should gain peace by killing him'.

4.6 Evidence of witnesses concerning the alleged offence

4.6.1 Benjamin Weston said that the Defendant had drawn his pistol 'very deliberately, but at the same time very quickly . . . a very cool, deliberate act'.

4.6.2 James Silver, a police constable, witnessed the shooting and restrained the Defendant. On the way to the police station the Defendant 'either said "he" or "she" (he could not recollect) shall not break my peace of mind any longer'.

4.6.3 Police Inspector, John Turney, who had custody of the Defendant after his arrest, says that the Defendant spoke about being the object of persecution by the Tories. Inspector Tierney said to him: 'I suppose you are aware who the gentleman is you shot at?' The Defendant replied: 'It is Sir Robert Peel, is it not?'

4.7 Psychiatric examination on 18 and 20 February 1843[2]

4.7.1 In accordance with normal psychiatric practice I made an examination of the Defendant's mental state. By this I mean that I used my powers of observation and clinical skills objectively to evaluate the Defendant's appearance, behaviour, mood, form of talk, content of thought, abnormal beliefs and experiences, cognition and insight. A full account of the mental state examination is set out at **Appendix 3**.

[1] I have assumed that there is no truth in the allegations made by the Defendant and I have assumed that he did not hear what he reported hearing said about him.
[2] These are the only facts within my own knowledge.

Report of: Dr. E.T. Monro
Specialism: Psychiatry
On the instructions of: Monteith and Company
Prepared for: The Central Criminal Court

4.7.2 I noted the following abnormalities.

4.7.3 He seemed tired and his features were somewhat drawn as if from lack of sleep. Eye contact was maintained only sporadically at best, the Defendant shifting his gaze at various points in the interview.

4.7.4 A faint smile was observed on several occasions when giving consideration to matters of apparent and professed seriousness and import.

4.7.5 I noted hesitancy when discussing the character of his delusions.

4.7.6 The content of his thought appeared to be dominated by a great fear that he is 'continuously dogged about' by what he described as a 'spy system' or 'crew' at Glasgow, Edinburgh, Liverpool, London and Boulogne which intended to ruin his good name. He complained that 'go where I will, they watch over me and see me home to my lodgings and watch out for me again'. He said that he had seen in *The Times* and *The Glasgow Herald* newspapers paragraphs containing 'beastly and atrocious' allegations directed at him. On occasions, he has observed men pointing at him on the street and he said that he was afraid to go out at night for fear of being assassinated. He described himself as being 'like a cork tossed on the sea'.

4.7.7 He expressed his beliefs with great conviction and when it was put to him that medical treatment might be of benefit, he said that a ton of drugs could not relieve him of his fears.

5. OPINION

5.1 Evaluation of the evidence and the defendant's clinical plausibility

5.1.1 In this case, in order to give opinions on the issues that have been identified, I am reliant on documentary evidence and my assessment of the Defendant.

5.1.2 The important documentary evidence is the transcript of the Defendant's evidence at the police court and the statements of the witnesses.

5.1.3 My assessment of the Defendant has two components: history and examination.

5.1.4 The Defendant gave his history in a straightforward manner. He unhesitatingly answered all of our questions apart from those relating to the character of his delusions. He did not otherwise appear defensive or evasive. His responses seemed proportionate. He did not describe any unexpected or bizarre symptoms or experiences that might have been out of keeping with the rest of his presentation. He did not report what might have been an excessive number of symptoms or a lot of symptoms of extreme severity. The history that he gave had a 'face validity' that was similar to that which I have encountered in patients with a similar condition seen outside the forensic context. The findings on examination of his mental state were consistent with the history that he gave and with the evidence of the witnesses. There were no unusual or unexpected findings on examination. Overall, there was a consistency between the evidence of the lay witnesses, the Defendant's history and the examination findings. I concluded that the level of clinical plausibility was high.

5.1.5 Having regard to my evaluation of the evidence available to me at this time, I am sufficiently confident to set out my opinions, on the balance of probabilities, on the identified issues. I accept that I may need to reconsider my opinions in the light of any further documentary evidence, and if there is any evidence that calls into question the reliability of the Defendant.

R v DANIEL MCNAUGHTAN *9*
Report of Dr. E.T. Monro concerning Daniel McNaughtan **25 February 1843**

5.1.6 This report contains conclusions based on the Defendant's account of the alleged offence. If he is pleading not guilty or if this account of the alleged offence is at variance with that given to his solicitors, it may be appropriate to delay disclosure of this report pending clarification of his instructions.

5.2 Diagnosis

5.2.1 In my opinion, the Defendant is suffering from a mental disorder within the meaning of the Mental Health Act 1983 (as amended by the Mental Health Act 2007). It is probable that it is the mental illness known as **schizophrenia** or another **psychotic** illness so like schizophrenia that it makes no difference exactly what it is called.

5.2.2 I make this diagnosis because the Defendant has a history of the following: (a) persecutory **delusions**, (b) **delusions of reference**, (c) what were probably auditory **hallucinations** in that he heard people referring to him in the third person, (d) what were probably gustatory hallucinations insofar as he thought that something had been put in his food, although this could have been a belief rather than a hallucination, (e) inappropriate **affect** and (f) what is probably schizophrenic **thought disorder** (as evidenced by his disconnected and incoherent speech). There seems to have been a history of personality change, in particular a tendency to social withdrawal, which is consistent with this diagnosis and it is also relevant that his illness has begun in relative youth which is when schizophrenia usually has its onset.

5.2.3 There is a range of opinion. Although delusions can occur in severe depressive illness there is little or nothing to suggest this diagnosis. I cannot rule out a physical cause for his mental illness on the information available but if there is such a cause it must be an obscure one in view of the fact that it was not detected by Dr Lavies or any of the distinguished medical and surgical gentlemen who accompanied me. Given the evidence that the Defendant was a person of sober habits, it is unlikely that his condition is a result of the use of alcohol or other substances.

5.3 Insanity

5.3.1 According to The M'Naghten Rules, 'to establish a defence on the ground of insanity, it must be clearly proved, that at the time of the committing of the act, the party accused was labouring under such a defect of reason, from disease of the mind, as not to know the nature and quality of the act he was doing; or, if he did know it, that he did not know he was doing what was wrong'.

5.3.2 It is more probable than not that the Defendant was suffering from a disease of the mind at the material time, but whether it is a disease of the mind is ultimately for the court to decide. There is a clear history of delusions prior to the alleged offence, there has been evidence of delusions when he has been medically examined since the alleged offence and his account of the alleged offence suggests that he was deluded at the time.

5.3.3 Insofar as the Defendant came to believe that the only way that he could obtain peace from all of the suffering of the previous months and years was to shoot Mr Drummond, this makes it more probable than not that the defect of reasoning, due to his schizophrenia, which led him to believe falsely that he was subject to persecution by the Tories and the Jesuits, also led him to the false belief that he would obtain peace from the persecution by shooting Mr Drummond. In relation to this point it does not matter whether he thought that it was Sir Robert Peel or not.

Report of: Dr. E.T. Monro
Specialism: Psychiatry
On the instructions of: Monteith and Company
Prepared for: The Central Criminal Court

5.3.4 Although it does not appear that the Defendant was questioned in depth about what he believed that he was doing, it does not appear that there is evidence which would convince a jury, on balance of probability, that he was unaware of the nature and quality of his action. Furthermore, what evidence there is suggests that he was aware of what he was doing when he shot Mr Drummond. This is also true if it is the case that he thought that he was shooting Sir Robert Peel.

5.3.5 Likewise, there is nothing to indicate that the Defendant did not know that what he was doing was wrong.

5.3 6 I therefore conclude that the Defendant does not have a defence of insanity.

5.4 Diminished responsibility

5.4.1 In order to establish a defence of 'diminished responsibility', the Defendant has to satisfy the court that he was suffering from an abnormality of mental functioning such that his ability to understand his own conduct, form a rational judgment or exercise self-control was substantially impaired. Further, if the jury finds that the Defendant was suffering from an abnormality of mental functioning, they have to be satisfied that it was due to a recognised medical condition and that the abnormality of mental functioning explains the killing.

5.4.2 I am not aware of a legal definition of 'abnormality of mental functioning', but I am aware of the legal definition of 'abnormality of mind'. Having regard to the clear evidence of serious mental illness in this case I am of the opinion that the Defendant has a basis for this defence insofar as he had, at the material time, an abnormality of mental functioning.

5.4.3 Schizophrenia, and its related disorders, are widely accepted as mental diseases or disorders and in this case I would expect that medical evidence would be unanimous to the effect that the Defendant's abnormality of mental functioning was caused by a recognised medical condition.

5.4.4 The matter of substantial impairment of ability is ultimately for the jury. However, I am mindful of the usual practice of the courts in admitting medical evidence on this issue to assist the jury and of the recent case law to the effect that the psychiatrist should give an opinion on all components of 'diminished responsibility'.

5.4.5 My opinion is that the Defendant's ability was impaired and in my opinion that impairment was substantial. I am mindful that he was, and still is, suffering from a severe mental illness. It was not of his own making. He appears to have been in a state of steadily growing fear for his safety, albeit an irrational fear. He had no insight into the fact that he was ill, and for which reason he had not sought medical help. Thus, in his deeply distressed state he is likely to have reacted without the rational judgement which he might have applied if his mind had been functioning normally.

5.4.6 Having regard to the other aspects of his ability, it appears to me to be the evidence that he did understand his own conduct and he was capable of exercising self-control at the material time.

5.4.7 It is my opinion that the Defendant's mental illness, specifically his psychotic illness, provides an explanation for the killing of Edward Drummond.

5.4.8 Therefore, I conclude that there is a medical basis for a defence of 'diminished responsibility' on the basis that the Defendant had an abnormality of mental functioning that was caused by a recognised medical condition, as a result of which he did not form a rational judgement, and his abnormality of mental functioning provides an explanation for the killing.

Report of: Dr. E.T. Monro
Specialism: Psychiatry
On the instructions of: Monteith and Company
Prepared for: The Central Criminal Court

5.5 Feigned delusions

5.5.1 It seems improbable to me that the Defendant's delusions should be feigned. They had been present for months, indeed years, before the alleged offence when there is no sensible reason for the Defendant feigning mental illness. The delusions he has reported are typical of those which occur in schizophrenia and related illnesses and, although, it is possible that he might have read sufficient about diseases of the mind in the library to which he had access at the Glasgow Mechanics' Institution, his account has a sophistication which I would not credit to him, having regard to his background, and again there is the question of why he should go to such lengths to present himself as mentally ill.

5.5.2 In addition, and more importantly, to seemingly uninterested observers, he has displayed what are probably objective manifestations of schizophrenia and its prodromal decline, specifically social withdrawal, inappropriate affect and thought disorder.

5.5.3 I therefore conclude that on balance the Defendant is not feigning mental illness. However, I do acknowledge that ultimately the genuineness of the Defendant is a matter for the learned judge and jury.

6. SUMMARY OF CONCLUSIONS

6.1 Overall, there was a consistency between the evidence of the lay witnesses, the Defendant's history and the examination findings so I concluded that the level of clinical plausibility was high.

6.2 Having regard to my evaluation of the evidence available to me at this time, I am sufficiently confident to set out my opinions, on the balance of probabilities, on the identified issues.

6.3 The Defendant is suffering from a mental disorder within the meaning of the Mental Health Act 1983 (as amended by the Mental Health Act 2007); it is probable that it is the mental illness known as schizophrenia.

6.4 It is more probable than not that the Defendant was suffering from a disease of the mind at the material time.

6.5 The defect of reasoning, due to his schizophrenia, which led him to believe falsely that he was subject to persecution by the Tories and the Jesuits, also led him to the false belief that he would obtain peace from the persecution by shooting Mr Drummond.

6.6 It does not appear that there is evidence which would convince a jury, on balance of probability, that he was unaware of the nature and quality of his action; what evidence there is suggests that he was aware of what he was doing when he shot Mr Drummond.

6.7 There is nothing to indicate that the Defendant did not know that what he was doing was wrong.

6.8 I therefore conclude that the Defendant does not have a defence of insanity.

6.9 The Defendant has a basis for the defence of diminished responsibility insofar as he had, at the material time, an abnormality of mental functioning.

R v DANIEL MCNAUGHTAN *12*
Report of Dr. E.T. Monro concerning Daniel McNaughtan **25 February 1843**

Report of: Dr. E.T. Monro
Specialism: Psychiatry
On the instructions of: Monteith and Company
Prepared for: The Central Criminal Court

6.10 I would expect that medical evidence would be unanimous to the effect that the Defendant's abnormality of mental functioning was caused by a recognised medical condition, namely schizophrenia.

6.11 The Defendant's ability was impaired and in my opinion that impairment was substantial because he is likely to have reacted without the rational judgement which he might have applied if his mind had been functioning normally.

6.12 He did understand his own conduct and he was capable of exercising self-control at the material time.

6.13 The Defendant's mental illness, specifically his psychotic illness, provides an explanation for the killing of Edward Drummond.

6.14 I conclude that the Defendant had an abnormality of mental functioning, which was caused by a recognised medical condition, as a result of which he did not form a rational judgement and his abnormality of mental functioning provides an explanation for the killing.

6.15 It seems improbable to me that the Defendant's delusions should be feigned.

6.16 In addition, and more importantly, to seemingly uninterested observers, he has displayed what are probably objective manifestations of schizophrenia and its prodromal decline.

6.17 I therefore conclude that on balance the Defendant is not feigning mental illness; however, I do acknowledge that ultimately the genuineness of the Defendant is a matter for the jury.

7. DECLARATION

1. I understand that my duty is to help the court to achieve the overriding objective by giving assistance by way of objective, unbiased opinion on matters within my area of expertise, both in preparing reports and giving oral evidence. I understand that this duty overrides any obligation to the party by whom I am engaged or the person who has paid or is liable to pay me. I confirm that I have complied with and will continue to comply with that duty.

2. I confirm that I have not entered into any arrangement where the amount or payment of my fees is in any way dependent on the outcome of the case.

3. I know of no conflict of interest of any kind, other than any which I have disclosed in this report.

4. I do not consider that any interest which I have disclosed affects my suitability as an expert witness on any issues on which I have given evidence.

5. I have shown the sources of all information I have used.

6. I have set out in my report what I understand from those instructing me to be the questions in respect of which my opinion as an expert is required. All of the matters on which I have expressed an opinion lie within my field of expertise.

7. I have exercised reasonable care and skill in order to be accurate and complete in preparing this report. I have covered all relevant issues concerning the matters stated which I have been asked to address. Absence of any comment in this report does not indicate that I have no opinion on a matter. I may not have been asked to deal with it.

Report of: Dr. E.T. Monro
Specialism: Psychiatry
On the instructions of: Monteith and Company
Prepared for: The Central Criminal Court

8. I have endeavoured to include in my report those matters, of which I have knowledge or of which I have been made aware, that might adversely affect the validity of my opinion. I have clearly stated any qualifications to my opinion.

9. Where, in my view, there is a range of reasonable opinion, I have indicated the extent of that range in the report and given reasons for my own opinion.

10. I have not, without forming an independent view, included or excluded anything which has been suggested to me by others including my instructing lawyers.

11. At the time of signing the report I consider that it is complete and accurate. I will notify those instructing me immediately, and confirm in writing if for any reason I subsequently consider that the report requires any correction or qualification or if between the date of this report and the trial there is any change in circumstances which affect my declarations at 3 and 4 above.

12. I understand that:

(a) my report, subject to any corrections before swearing as to its correctness, will form the evidence to be given under oath;
(b) the court may at any stage direct a discussion to take place between the experts;
(c) the court may direct that, following a discussion between the experts, a statement should be prepared showing those issues which are agreed and those issues which are not agreed, together with a summary of the reasons for disagreeing;
(d) I may be required to attend court to be cross-examined on my report by a cross-examiner assisted by an expert;
(e) I am likely to be the subject of public adverse criticism by the judge if the court concludes that I have not taken reasonable care in trying to meet the standards set out above.

13. This report is provided to those instructing me with the sole purpose of assisting the court in this particular case. It may not be used for any other purpose, nor may it be disclosed to any third party, other than the National Probation Service, without my express written authority or that of the court.

14. I have read Part 19 of the Criminal Procedure Rules and the accompanying Practice Direction and I have complied with their requirements.

15. I confirm that I have acted in accordance with, the Royal College of Psychiatrists' College Report CR193 *Responsibilities of psychiatrists who provide expert opinion to courts and tribunals* by Keith Rix, Nigel Eastman and Gwen Adshead (2015) and the General Medical Council's *Good Medical Practice*, which includes 'Giving evidence as an expert witness'.

8. STATEMENT OF TRUTH

I confirm that the contents of this report (consisting of 22 pages) are true to the best of my knowledge and belief and that I make this report knowing that, if it is tendered in evidence, I would be liable to prosecution if I have wilfully stated anything which I know to be false or that I do not believe to be true.

E. T. Monro,
BSc, MSc, MD, FRCPsych,
Consultant Psychiatrist.

25 February 1843

R v DANIEL MCNAUGHTAN *14*
Report of Dr. E.T. Monro concerning Daniel McNaughtan **25 February 1843**

Report of: **Dr. E.T. Monro**
Specialism: **Psychiatry**
On the instructions of: **Monteith and Company**
Prepared for: **The Central Criminal Court**

APPENDIX 1

QUALIFICATIONS, TRAINING AND EXPERIENCE

Qualifications

I am a medical graduate of the University of London where I obtained an intercalated **Bachelor of Science (Honours)** degree in neuropathology in 1802 and qualified **Bachelor of Medicine and Bachelor of Surgery** in 1805. I have obtained higher degrees of **Master of Science** (Manchester) and **Doctor of Medicine** (London) following study and research in psychiatry. I obtained the **Membership of the Royal College of Psychiatrists** in 1809 and was elected to the **Fellowship** in 1821. In 1825, I became a **Member of the Academy of Experts.** In 1825, I also became a **Member of the Expert Witness Institute** and in 1830 I was elected **Fellow.**

Clinical training and experience

My general professional training in psychiatry was as **Senior House Officer** and **Registrar in Psychiatry** in Manchester from 1806 to 1809. I undertook higher training as **Lecturer in Psychiatry** and **Honorary Senior Registrar** at Edinburgh University from 1809 to 1813. From 1813 to 1820, I was **Senior Lecturer and Consultant Psychiatrist** at the Royal Edinburgh Hospital and **Visiting Consultant Psychiatrist** at HMP Saughton, Edinburgh. Since 1820, I have been **Consultant Psychiatrist** at the Bethlem Hospital, **Honorary Senior Lecturer in Psychiatry** in the University of London and a **Visiting Consultant Psychiatrist** at HMP Newgate. I am responsible for the Bow Street Police Court Mental Health Assessment and Diversion Scheme. I am a subscribing **Member of the British Academy of Forensic Sciences** and a subscribing **Member and Past President of the Medico-Legal Society of London**. I am a **Member of the Parole Board** for England and Wales. I am in good standing for CPD with the Royal College of Psychiatrists.

Expert witness training and experience

I have 18 years' experience of preparing expert reports, about 60 per cent for the defence and about 40 per cent for the prosecution. I undertook expert witness training at the Royal College of Psychiatrists in 1825. I refresh this training every four years. I attend The Grange Annual Conference to keep up to date with practice as an expert witness and to learn more about issues on the interface between psychiatry and the law.

Research and publications

I am the author of books on the classification of psychoses. My research includes studies of mentally disordered offenders in a London police court, psychiatric disorder in prison (for my MSc dissertation), a study of patients detained in Broadmoor Hospital upon conviction of diminished responsibility manslaughter and the symptomatology of schizophrenia (based on research for my MD). My published case reports include one on the insanity defence.

Report of: Dr. E.T. Monro
Specialism: Psychiatry
On the instructions of: Monteith and Company
Prepared for: The Central Criminal Court

APPENDIX 2

THE PROCESS OF PSYCHIATRIC ASSESSMENT

1. Psychiatrists, as doctors, employ the time-honoured processes of history-taking and examination in order to achieve a formulation of the subject that encompasses diagnosis, aetiology (causation), treatment recommendations and prognosis. Examination may and often does include physical examination, but examination of the mental state is an important psychiatric skill.

2. The history is particularly important in the case of many psychiatric disorders because diagnosis depends largely, and in some cases entirely, on self-reported symptoms and if, for whatever reason, the Defendant is unreliable in their report of the nature, duration, severity or effects of their symptoms, this can affect the validity of any diagnosis reached and the conclusions as to the impact of their condition. I recognise, of course, that the reliability of the Defendant is an ultimate issue for the court, but in a forensic assessment I have to decide whether or not to accept at face value what the Defendant has reported to me and what he has reported to other experts in this case. In this regard, I am mindful of the observation of HHJ Seymour QC in *Turner v Jordan* [2010] EWHC 1508 (QB), albeit in a civil case, but an observation in my view as readily applicable to a criminal case:

> A consequence of the fact that diagnosis in a psychiatric case depends on assessment of what is reported by the patient is the necessity for the psychiatrist confronted by a patient to consider whether or not to accept at face value what the patient reports. Inevitably there is a disposition on the part of the psychiatrist to take as genuine what the patient reports, because otherwise it is difficult to consider the issue of diagnosis.

3. Psychiatric examination of the Defendant, or what psychiatrists describe as the mental state examination, is my professional analysis of the Defendant's appearance, behaviour, mood, form of talk, thought content, unusual or abnormal beliefs or experiences, cognitive functioning and insight. It may take into account my reaction to the Defendant.

4. My approach to the process of differential diagnosis is based on normal clinical practice and a hierarchical system of psychiatric classification. By this I mean that I have considered diagnosis in the order in which mental disorders appear section by section in *The ICD-10 Classification of Mental and Behavioural Disorders* (Geneva: World Health Organization, 1992): organic, including symptomatic, mental disorders; mental and behavioural disorders due to substance misuse (including alcohol); schizophrenia and related disorders; mood disorders; neurotic, stress-related and somatoform disorders; personality and related disorders; and learning disabilities. At each level, I have considered the evidence for and against the diagnosis of a mental disorder at that level and then I have proceeded to the next level. This accords approximately with the logical ordering of sections in ICD-10. I have highlighted, if there are any, factual assumptions, deductions from factual assumptions, and any unusual, contradictory or inconsistent features of the case.

5. My approach to aetiology has been to apply to the defendant's case my knowledge of the causes of psychiatric disorder in order to be able to give an opinion as to how the psychiatric disorder came about or why it ran the course it did.

Report of: Dr. E.T. Monro
Specialism: Psychiatry
On the instructions of: Monteith and Company
Prepared for: The Central Criminal Court

6. Where I have made recommendations for treatment, or commented on treatment already given, I have relied on approaches that have wide acceptance by psychiatrists and, if possible, given weight to treatments for which there is the strongest evidence base with regard to effectiveness and safety. However, as in medicine in general, there are many treatments that are accepted as effective but for which there have not been trials that satisfy the most stringent criteria of evidence based medicine.

7. So far as prognosis is concerned, I have applied my knowledge of the course and outcome of psychiatric disorders to the features of this individual case. My approach to risk assessment is based on structured clinical judgement. By this, I mean that I have used my training, experience and skill to relate what is known about the prognoses of mental disorders in general to the specific features of the subject's case, endeavouring to make predictions about identified risks with which I would expect other psychiatrists to concur. It is important to realise that the value of predictions diminishes rapidly with time and this is probably because with time circumstances change so much.

8. Clinical practice, including psychiatric practice, depends in part on knowledge for which there is a sound evidence base and partly on experience-based knowledge which has stood the test of time, but lacks a robust foundation in the rigorous research that now forms the basis of 'evidence-based medicine'. In relying on both categories of knowledge, I have done so in accordance with what I would regard as a responsible body of psychiatric practice and I therefore regard my methodology as sufficiently reliable for the court's purposes.

Report of: Dr. E.T. Monro
Specialism: Psychiatry
On the instructions of: Monteith and Company
Prepared for: The Central Criminal Court

APPENDIX 3

HISTORY AND EXAMINATION

History

1. The Defendant was born in Glasgow in 1813. His father was a wood turner. The Defendant was his apprentice for four and a half years, living in his father's house, and then he worked for him as a journeyman for three years, but living away from home in lodgings.

2. Then the Defendant set up business on his own in 1835, as he was dissatisfied that his father would not let him have a share in his business. This was because his father wanted to provide for the Defendant's younger siblings.

3. By the time he left the business in 1840, the Defendant had saved a considerable amount of money. It had been a prosperous and thriving business. In July 1842, he responded to an advertisement in a London newspaper, *The Spectator*. It was for a partnership 'in a very genteel business in London' and with a view to succeeding to the whole business. Any gentleman having £1,000 was invited to apply. The Defendant did not have the exact amount of money specified, but wrote in response to say that he had been engaged in business on his own account for a few years, was under 30 years of age and was very active and of sober habits.

4. The Defendant had first come to London in July 1841 and stayed in lodgings with a Mrs Dutton. Before doing so, he opened a deposit account with the Bank of Scotland and then shifted it to the London Joint Stock Bank.

5. In his spare time in Glasgow, the Defendant attended lectures on natural philosophy[1] at the Glasgow Mechanics' Institution. He took an active part in various alterations which were made to the rules of the Institution and also in the arrangement of the rooms and conveniences of the building. He was in the habit of getting books from the library; he was known to all the persons who frequented that institution and he attended lectures on anatomy, including attending the dissecting room every day.

6. The Defendant described himself as a person of sober habits.

7. At the time of the alleged offence, the Defendant was lodging at 7 Poplar Row, Newington, with Mrs Dutton again. He had returned to London again in July 1842.

Examination

8. On examination, the Defendant presented as a young, Caucasian male, clean-shaven and of a mild and prepossessing appearance. He was tidily, if somewhat shabbily, dressed in thin overcoat, waistcoat and plain trousers. His linen was over-darned, but clean. He seemed tired and his features were somewhat drawn as if from lack of sleep.

9. Eye contact was maintained only sporadically at best, the Defendant shifting his gaze at various points in the interview.

10. His manner was initially placid and contented. There was later evidence of discomfort at being interviewed, although he continued to respond thoughtfully and with unerring politeness to all the questions put to him.

[1] In Scotland, physics is known as natural philosophy.

Report of: Dr. E.T. Monro
Specialism: Psychiatry
On the instructions of: Monteith and Company
Prepared for: The Central Criminal Court

11. A faint smile was observed on several occasions when giving consideration to matters of apparent and professed seriousness and import.

12. His speech was mild and not at all distracted. I noted hesitancy when discussing the character of his delusions.

13. The content of his thought appeared to be dominated by a great fear that he is 'continuously dogged about' by a 'spy system' or 'crew' at Glasgow, Edinburgh, Liverpool, London and Boulogne which intended to ruin his good name. 'Go where I will, they watch over me and see me home to my lodgings and watch out for me again.' He said that he had seen in *The Times* and *The Glasgow Herald* newspapers paragraphs containing 'beastly and atrocious' allegations directed at him. On occasions, he said that he had left his lodgings and remained out all night with only a fishing rod and line with which to procure food. On other occasions, he has observed men pointing at him on the street and he said that he was afraid to go out at night for fear of being assassinated. He described himself as being 'like a cork tossed on the sea'.

14. His higher faculties appeared to be intact and the overall impression imparted was that of superior intelligence.

15. He expressed his beliefs with great conviction and when it was put to him that medical treatment might be of benefit, he said that a ton of drugs could not relieve him of his fears.

16. He was in apparent good physical health and this was confirmed by Dr Lavies, Physician to Newgate Gaol.

R v DANIEL MCNAUGHTAN *19*
Report of Dr. E.T. Monro concerning Daniel McNaughtan **25 February 1843**

Report of: Dr. E.T. Monro
Specialism: Psychiatry
On the instructions of: Monteith and Company
Prepared for: The Central Criminal Court

APPENDIX 4

DOCUMENTS STUDIED

Indictment
Bow Street Police Court depositions
Prosecution witness statements

- Henry C. Bell
- Sir James Campbell
- Mrs Dutton
- William Gilchrist
- John Gordon
- John Hughes
- Alexander Johnston
- Alexander Martin
- Daniel McNaughtan (Sen)
- James Silver
- John Tierney
- Benjamin Weston
- Hugh Wilson

Report of: Dr. E.T. Monro
Specialism: Psychiatry
On the instructions of: Monteith and Company
Prepared for: The Central Criminal Court

APPENDIX 5

GLOSSARY OF MEDICAL AND OTHER TERMS

affect – Synonymous with mood, the patient's emotional state. It has a subjective component which takes the form of feelings which each person can describe or recognise in himself (e.g. unhappiness) and an objective component which is the outward manifestation of the feelings (e.g. sad facial expression; dejected posture) (K. J. B. Rix, *A Handbook for Trainee Psychiatrists* (London: Baillière Tindall, 1987)).

delusion – A delusion is a false belief held with total conviction and inappropriate to the patient's intelligence, social background and subcultural beliefs (K. J. B. Rix, op. cit.).

delusion of reference – A delusion of reference occurs when a normal perception is interpreted with delusional meaning of usually overwhelming personal significance to the patient, i.e. the normal perception refers to the patient.

hallucination – A false perception lacking an adequate basis in external stimuli (K. J. B. Rix, op. cit.). Hallucinations can occur in all of the sensory modalities. Auditory hallucinations commonly take the form of 'voices', but sounds of music and machinery can occur. Visual, gustatory (taste), olfactory (smell) and tactile (touch) hallucinations can also occur.

schizophrenia – Schizophrenia is a serious mental illness characterised in general by fundamental distortions of thinking and perception and by inappropriate or blunted affect. Thus, typical symptoms include: (a) disorders of the possession of thought, such as the subjective experience of thoughts being withdrawn, inserted or broadcast to others; (b) delusions, for example, of being controlled, influenced or persecuted or that unconnected events or circumstances relate to the patient; (c) hallucinations, particularly in the form of voices which give a running commentary on the patient's behaviour, refer to the patient in the third person; (d) persistent grandiose delusions, including religious delusions – for example, being able to control the weather or being the Virgin Mary; (e) disorders of the form of thought (thought disorder); (f) catatonic behaviour, such as excitement, mutism and stupor; (g) negative symptoms in the form of apathy, poverty of speech, blunting of emotional responses. It can occur as a single episode, as a recurrent disorder or as a chronic, progressive disorder without full recovery between episodes. When chronic, there is usually a disintegration of the personality with coarsening and loss of identifying personality characteristics (*The ICD-10 Classification of Mental and Behavioural Disorders: Clinical Descriptions and Diagnostic Guidelines* (Geneva: World Health Organization, 1992)).

thought disorder – This is a term usually employed in relation to disturbances in the process of thinking as found in **schizophrenia (q.v.)**. Such disorder can take a number of forms and there are a number of approaches to their classification. One of the most widely accepted identifies the following forms of thought disorder: muddling; snapping-off; fusion or literally melting of thoughts; and derailment. Careful observation and analysis of the patient's speech is necessary to classify as well as recognise these forms of thought disorder.

Report of: Dr. E.T. Monro
Specialism: Psychiatry
On the instructions of: Monteith and Company
Prepared for: The Central Criminal Court

APPENDIX 6

CHRONOLOGY

1813	Daniel McNaughtan born
1828	Apprenticed to father as a wood turner
1832	Completed apprenticeship and started working for father
1835	Set up his own business
1840/1841	Sold his business
1841	Visited father and expressed concerns about persecution
July 1841	First visit to London
Early 1842	Expressed concerns to Commissioner of Police, Glasgow
July 1842	Purchased pistols
	Returned to London
November 1842	Walked past Sir Robert Peel's house, said 'Damn him, sink him'
20 January 1843	Shot Edward Drummond
25 January 1843	Edward Drummond died
18 February 1843	Examined in Newgate Prison
20 February 1843	Re-examined in Newgate Prison

Appendix B

IN THE CITY OF LONDON AND MAYOR'S COURT **Claim No.:**

BETWEEN:

CHARLES JOHN HUFFAM DICKENS

Claimant

and

SOUTH-EASTERN AND CHATHAM RAILWAY COMPANY

Defendant

On the instructions of:	Ouvry, Solicitors, Lincoln's Inn Fields, London
Acting on behalf of:	The Claimant
Their reference:	FO/BC
For the attention of:	Frederic Ouvry
Subject matter:	Psychiatric assessment of the Claimant
Date of consultation:	9th June 1869
Place of consultation:	10 Harley Street, London
Date of report:	10th June 1869
Status of report:	Provisional
Report reference number:	HM/EML/W
Consent:	Written

Provisional Report
of
Professor Henry Maudsley
MB, MD, Hon LLD, MRMPA, FRCP,
Consultant Physician
The West London Hospital
Queen Street
Hammersmith
London W6
DX 12345 Hammersmith
Tel.: 0200 878604 Fax: 0200 869898
henrymaudsley@drmaudsley.co.uk

Report of: Professor Henry Maudsley
Specialism: Psychiatry
On the instructions of: Ouvry & Co
Prepared for: The City of London and Mayor's Court

CONTENTS[1]

[1] This report is based on the 'Model Form of Expert's Report' prepared by the Judicial Committee of the Academy of Experts and by the Expert Witness Institute.

Report of: Professor Henry Maudsley
Specialism: Psychiatry
On the instructions of: Ouvry & Co
Prepared for: The City of London and Mayor's Court

Appendices

1. INTRODUCTION

1.1 The writer

1.1.1 I am Henry Maudsley, a licensed and registered medical practitioner approved under s 12 of the Mental Health Act 1983 and registered with the General Medical Council as a specialist in general psychiatry and forensic psychiatry according to the provisions of Schedule 2 of the European Specialist Medical Qualifications Order 1995. Full details of my qualifications and experience entitling me to give expert opinion evidence are in **Appendix 1**.

1.1.2 In both general adult and forensic psychiatry I have routinely had the care of adults with a range of mental disorders including the major mental illnesses, such as schizophrenia, bipolar disorder and depressive illness, organic disorders, such as dementia, less serious and less disabling mental disorders, including post-traumatic stress disorder and adjustment disorders, personality disorders, substance misuse disorders and intellectual (learning) disabilities. I continue to encounter patients with a range of mental disorders in my in-patient unit, my out-patient clinic and in my capacity as a s 12 approved doctor called upon, usually in situations of urgency, to assess people in contemplation of admission to, or detention in, hospital under the Mental Health Act 1983. This case therefore falls within my area of expertise.

1.2 Synopsis

1.2.1 My instructing solicitors act for Charles Dickens ('the Claimant'), the well-known author and playwright, in connection with a claim for damages arising out of an accident which took place on 9 June 1865.

Provisional report of Prof H. Maudsley concerning Charles Dickens 10 June 1869 *3*
CHARLES DICKENS (Claimant) v SOUTH-EASTERN AND CHATHAM RAILWAY COMPANY (Defendant)

Report of: Professor Henry Maudsley
Specialism: Psychiatry
On the instructions of: Ouvry & Co
Prepared for: The City of London and Mayor's Court

1.3 Instructions

1.3.1 I have been instructed to examine the Claimant and thereafter provide my instructing solicitors with a full medico-legal report dealing with the matters set out at 2.3 below.

1.4 Disclosure of interests

1.4.1 I do not know the Claimant professionally or personally. I do not know any of the parties involved. There are no conflicts of interest in respect to any of the identified parties. I have no other interest which might cause a conflict based upon the nature of the dispute.

2. THE BACKGROUND TO THE CASE AND THE ISSUES

2.1 The relevant people

2.1.1 Charles Dickens – the Claimant
2.1.2 Ellen Ternan – friend and travelling companion
2.1.3 Frances Ternan – mother of Ellen Ternan and travelling companion

2.2 The assumed facts and substance of all material instructions[1]

2.2.1 The Claimant alleges personal injury sustained in an accident on a train whilst returning from a short holiday in Paris. He alleges that for a period following the accident he was in a state of distress. He is nervous about travelling in trains and now prefers slow trains.

2.2.2 In **Appendix 2** I have set out my full instructions.

2.3 The issues to be addressed[2]

2.3.1 I have been instructed to examine the Claimant and provide a full and detailed report dealing with any relevant pre-accident medical history, the injuries sustained, treatment received and present condition, dealing in particular with the capacity for work and prognosis. Since it is central to the assessment of the Claimant's injuries to establish the extent and duration of any continuing disability, in the prognosis section I have been asked to comment specifically on any areas of continuing complaint or disability or impact on daily living. If there is such continuing disability I have been asked to comment upon the level of suffering or inconvenience caused and, if I am able, give my view as to when or if the complaint or disability is likely to resolve.

[1] This summary is based on my instructions. The facts set out in this section and Appendix 2 may differ from the facts as related to me by the Claimant and any informant and as established by me from my own analysis of the documents and records in the case. This section should be read in conjunction with 'Issues to be addressed' which sets out the issues I have been instructed to address.
[2] Unless I have indicated otherwise, these are the only matters I have been asked to address. The absence of an opinion on a particular issue does not mean that I have no opinion on the issue. It means only that I have not been asked to address the issue.

Provisional report of Prof H. Maudsley concerning Charles Dickens **10 June 1869** *4*
CHARLES DICKENS (Claimant) v SOUTH-EASTERN AND CHATHAM RAILWAY COMPANY (Defendant)

Report of: Professor Henry Maudsley
Specialism: Psychiatry
On the instructions of: Ouvry & Co
Prepared for: The City of London and Mayor's Court

2.4 The assumptions adopted

2.4.1 I regard what the Claimant and any informant has told me and what is contained in the medical records and other documents as 'assumed facts'. The only facts within my own knowledge are my findings on examination of the Claimant and as set out below in the section 'Psychiatric examination'.

2.4.2 Where there is a conflict between the records and the Claimant's evidence, I have assumed that the Claimant's version of events is correct unless the same is so technically or manifestly incorrect in which case I will explain why I do not accept the Claimant's version of events.

2.4.3 Unless I have indicated otherwise, I regard the information contained in documentary sources of information as accurate.

3. INVESTIGATION OF FACTS AND ASSUMED FACTS

3.1 Methodology

3.1.1 In **Appendix 3**, I have described the process of psychiatric assessment which I have employed in my investigation of this case.

3.2 Interview and examination

3.2.1 I have interviewed and examined the Claimant. Information attributed to the Claimant in the next section was provided by the Claimant at the consultation unless otherwise indicated.

3.2.2 The Claimant was unaccompanied. I saw him on his own. There was no informant for me to interview.

3.2.3 I have set out details of the Claimant's self-reported history, including his account of the accident, and my examination findings in Section 4. It also includes his medical history prior to the accident. As I have not yet been provided with copies of his medical records, I am unable to set out his medical history as based on documented sources.

3.2.4 The only facts within my own knowledge are my findings on examination of the Claimant's mental state ('psychiatric examination') and my knowledge of the practice of psychiatry.

3.2.5 The details of the Claimant's history and the examination findings in Section 4 are taken from my consultation notes, which I have retained and which can be made available to the parties or the court on request.

Report of: Professor Henry Maudsley
Specialism: Psychiatry
On the instructions of: Ouvry & Co
Prepared for: The City of London and Mayor's Court

3.3 Documents

3.3.1 The documents made available or obtained are listed in **Appendix 4**.

3.3.2 I do not intend to keep copies of the Claimant's medical records for any longer than is necessary for the purposes of this claim or any subsequent claim or complaint relating to it. It is my intention to destroy copies of the Claimant's medical records seven years after the Claimant's case is discontinued or settled. Please advise me when the Claimant's case is discontinued or settled.

3.4 Medical terms and explanations

3.4.1 I have indicated any medical or related terms in **bold type**. I have defined these terms and included them in a glossary in **Appendix 5**. Where I have tried to define and explain terms outside the speciality of psychiatry, the definitions should not be regarded as having the same authority as those given by experts from the relevant speciality, but in most cases they should be sufficient for the lay reader of this report to understand the report.

3.5 Comments

3.5.1 If it seems helpful for me to comment on facts or assumed facts, my comments are in brackets followed by my initials – HM.

4. FACTUAL ANALYSIS

4.1 Family background

4.1.1 The Claimant's mother developed senility and had **delusions** of grandeur in old age. There is otherwise no family history of mental disorder.

4.1.2 The Claimant and a younger sister, now a widow living in poor circumstances, are the only survivors of a sibship of five. One brother, who was always 'sponging' off the Claimant, and whose estranged wife the Claimant supported, died six months prior to our consultation. The Claimant also supported the abandoned wife of his now deceased youngest brother and said that, when he went on tour in the USA, he had to avoid Chicago as a result of hostility arising from the fact that when his brother died there, he left his common-law wife and three children without support.

4.2 Childhood and education

4.2.1 Although the Claimant looks back on his early childhood years in Chatham as the golden age of his childhood, a period of relative prosperity when family fortunes were at their peak and a period of which he has a number of fond memories, he felt somewhat in want of love and care from his parents and so he grew up with feelings of emotional uncertainty and a sense of neglect. At school, which the Claimant liked and where he enjoyed friendships, he was not robust enough to join in games and preferred to watch others at play, something which led to him feeling somewhat detached.

Report of: Professor Henry Maudsley
Specialism: Psychiatry
On the instructions of: Ouvry & Co
Prepared for: The City of London and Mayor's Court

4.2.2 Just before he was 11 years old, the family moved back to London. It was an upsetting time. The family slipped into debt and he described it as a cruel sacrifice having to sell his treasured books, his sister Harriet died and he was kept at home helping with housework and looking after the younger children. Then on his 12th birthday he was shocked to find that he was starting work two days later. Shortly after this, his father was committed to a debtors' prison and he was sent to live with a family acquaintance who took in homeless boys. The sense of abandonment hurt him, the loss of his childhood was traumatic and he felt prematurely cast into adulthood.

4.2.3 In the meantime, the Claimant felt that his father seemed to have utterly lost the idea of educating him. Eventually, at the age of about 18 years, after six years of menial factory work and an improvement in his father's financial circumstances, he resumed his education. He said that he did not distinguish himself particularly, but he was awarded the Latin prize and he was first boy by the time he left three years later. However, he had to leave before the end of the summer term as his father was unable to pay the school fees.

4.3 Adult employment

4.3.1 On leaving school, the Claimant went to work as a clerk to a firm of solicitors. He disliked this work, but he had already started writing small news items when he was at school and he was soon supplementing his income with earnings from reporting. Then freelance reporting of Parliament led to employment as a parliamentary shorthand writer and freelance journalism. Within a short time, he was able to give up shorthand writing and devote himself completely to journalism and then the writing of novels and plays which has made him a household name.

4.4 Relationships, marriage and children

4.4.1 The Claimant has been married for twenty years, but looking back he believes that he made a terrible mistake. He said that it was a good marriage until after the birth of their second child. Then his wife's personality changed, and they grew apart both emotionally and physically, and lived unhappily together. In time, the state of his marriage became a skeleton in his cupboard, although some report of their domestic troubles did spread through London society.

4.4.2 Ten years ago, the Claimant met Ellen Ternan. She is twenty-seven years his junior and comes from a theatrical family. He said no more about their relationship than to indicate that he paid the rent for her cottage and he hinted that they had a child who died.

4.4.3 The Claimant and his wife have had eight children. His oldest son, Charley, has an office job that the Claimant got for him at *All the Year Round*, having previously refused to bail him out when his paper mill venture failed. He has a daughter who is married to Wilkie Collins's younger brother and the Claimant spoke somewhat disparagingly of his son-in-law and his Anglo-Catholic views. Their fourth child, Walter, an army officer who had become burdened with debts, died in Calcutta from an **aneurysm** as he was in the process of being invalided home. This was about eighteen months before the Claimant's accident. The Claimant said that he had not been able to share his grief with his wife. Fifth is a son who had caused the Claimant some anxiety some years ago with his stammer, recurrent deafness and sleep-walking, but he is now a commissioned officer in the Bengal police. He described the sixth son, Sydney, as a spendthrift, but he spoke about him with pride as he is the youngest to have been promoted to second lieutenant in the Army.

Provisional report of Prof H. Maudsley concerning Charles Dickens 10 June 1869 *7*
CHARLES DICKENS (Claimant) v SOUTH-EASTERN AND CHATHAM RAILWAY COMPANY (Defendant)

4.5 Interests, recreation, alcohol and substance use

4.5.1 As well as enjoying the theatre and socialising with friends, the Claimant is involved in a great deal of philanthropic work and is constantly in demand from charities.

4.5.2 Although the Claimant reported occasional drunkenness as a young man and a difficulty resisting the temptations of porter and other malt liquor, in recent years he has drunk only the occasional glass of gin punch. He smokes the occasional cigar, but has no history of other substance use.

4.6 Personality

4.6.1 Although the Claimant described himself as a child as having been delicate and easily hurt both bodily and mentally, he described himself in adulthood as being of resilient temper and able to use work to achieve a cheerful mood even when weary and unwell.

4.7 Medical history

4.7.1 As a child, the Claimant was plagued by bouts of **renal colic** and **migraine**-like attacks when he was particularly anxious, and he recalled being chagrined and depressed when the family moved back to London and he was briefly left in Chatham until the end of the school term. The following year, when the family fell into debt, he recalled having a fresh bout of his 'feverish spasms'. He said that long before adulthood he slipped into the family habit of self-centred complaint.

4.7.2 When he was 29 years old, the Claimant had surgery for an **anal fistula**, which he described as 'a disease caused by working over much'.

4.7.3 A few months before the accident, the Claimant developed a painful swelling in his left foot and the doctor said that it was gout, but the Claimant thought that it was frostbite from walking continually in the snow.

4.8 Recent history

4.8.1 Eighteen months before the accident, the Claimant's son Walter died. Subsequently, he found it hard to settle to his new story, *Our Mutual Friend*. When he did work on it, he found that he was writing in a rather dull, slow way. He felt very unwell and out of sorts after completing the first instalment. He described finding writing an effort. Then, in October 1864, he suffered a great shock when an old friend died, and he felt that he was losing his resilience.

4.8.2 In spite of the **gout** with which he was diagnosed earlier in 1865, by March the Claimant was 'working like a dragon' and sufficiently recovered physically to be walking ten miles a day. But with *Our Mutual Friend* almost complete, he felt that 'work and worry, without exercise, would soon make an end of me'. He had therefore resolved to go to Paris for a short holiday. He said: 'If I were not going away now, I should break down. No one knows as I know today how near it I have been.'

Report of: Professor Henry Maudsley
Specialism: Psychiatry
On the instructions of: Ouvry & Co
Prepared for: The City of London and Mayor's Court

4.9 The accident

4.9.1 The accident occurred on the Claimant's return from Paris in the company of Mrs Frances Ternan and her daughter, Ellen Ternan. He describes being suddenly aware of the train being off the rail and their carriage beating the ground like a half-emptied balloon might do. His travelling companions cried out and screamed and the Claimant caught hold of both of them and he reassured them before asking them to remain where they were while he climbed out of the window.

4.9.2 Once out of the carriage, the Claimant was struck by an unimaginable scene of ruined carriages, of people trapped beneath them and of people twisted up among iron, wood, mud and water. With the assistance of a workman he then assisted his travelling companions from their carriage. In her scramble to escape, Miss Ternan lost her gold watch-chain, some trinkets and a seal with her name engraved on it. Later, the Claimant had to write to the station master at Charing Cross to ask if these items had been found.

4.9.3 The Claimant then went to assist the casualties. They included a man who had such a frightful cut across his skull that he could not bear to look at him, although he did pour some water over his face, gave him a brandy and laid him down on the grass. Once the immediate shock had worn off, the Claimant realised that that he had left behind the manuscript of *Our Mutual Friend*, so he scrambled back into the wreckage to retrieve it. He then spent the next two or three hours rendering assistance to the injured and dying. He said that the sights were terrific, and he noticed that his hand had become unsteady.

4.10 History since the accident

4.10.1 The Claimant began his report of the effects of the accident by saying that it was an emotional shock as it had broken open his secret life. There was a risk of all that he had so carefully hidden becoming public knowledge. By this, he implied his relationship with Miss Ternan.

4.10.2 Although the Claimant said that within twenty days of the accident he was able to thank God that he felt all right again, he then went on to say that for some time he was in a state of distress, he felt curiously weak and even his watch had palpitations for six months after the accident. He clarified that he felt that the effect of the accident had been delayed, he did not feel quite right within and he was affected more and more by the accident rather than less and less as he had expected. Nevertheless, he was writing again by the summer and by September 1865 he had finished *Our Mutual Friend*.

4.10.3 The Claimant described how he had become nervous travelling in trains and how any unusual movement upset him. For a while, he avoided rail travel; he still avoids express trains. He described how one day when driving to Rochester he had felt more shaken than at any time since the accident. He said that the physical sensation of the crash seemed to have fused with a debility that was beginning to affect the left side of his body. He described how, with anything like speed, he experienced 'a perfect conviction, against the senses, that the carriage is down one side', an experience that he found inexpressibly distressing. He pointed out that curiously his experience was generally of the carriage being on its left side, which was not the side on which it really went over in the accident.

Report of: Professor Henry Maudsley
Specialism: Psychiatry
On the instructions of: Ouvry & Co
Prepared for: The City of London and Mayor's Court

4.10.4 Other symptoms he described included feeling curiously weak and, after writing half a dozen notes, feeling faint and sick. However, his appetite and sleep were not affected.

4.10.5 In January 1866, the Claimant noticed that his pulse was irregular and he obtained a prescription for **iron**, **quinine** and **digitalis**. At this time, he realised that he lacked his usual buoyancy and hopefulness.

4.10.6 The Claimant went on tour in May 1866 and towards the end he found this a strain. He related how, one evening, when he was billed to read the trial from *Pickwick*, instead he read from *Nickleby*. He took a break in the country at the end of the tour, worried about his health and concerned that doing five readings a week was affecting his health. He said that he developed pains in his left eye, a persistent cold and severe digestive discomfort. Twice in one week he said that he was seized in a most distressing manner, apparently in the heart, but he realised that it was his nervous system that was affected.

4.10.7 In 1867, the Claimant went on another tour and soon felt the strain so much that he had to take a rest from reading. He was fainter at night. This caused him to dash back to London, but the shaking of the train upset him and he had a curious feeling of soreness all around his body. He lost a lot of blood when his piles played up, but in spite of all of this, he remained cheerful and good-humoured. However, he soon noticed that he was so tired that he could not undress himself at night.

4.10.8 The Claimant went on tour again in October 1868. Although the first evenings went well, he quickly felt the strain and within three weeks he felt unwell with a heavy tiredness. It was not long after this that he heard of the death of his only surviving brother. He reflected on his brother's rather wasted life. He had been a poorly paid clerk in the Treasury and separated from his wife. Then, his health and spirits flagged further, he had trouble sleeping and he was troubled with nausea.

4.10.9 Although the Claimant had managed to complete *Our Mutual Friend*, he had trouble applying himself to another novel. He did not manage to produce *The Mystery of Edwin Drood* for four years. It had hurt him when Wilkie Collins called it 'the work of a worn out brain', but he seemed to accept that to some extent his brain was indeed worn out.

4.11 Psychiatric examination

4.11.1 On examination, the Claimant looked desperately aged and worn. He gazed ahead, making little eye contact and wearing a worried frown. The lines in his cheeks and around his eyes were deeply furrowed. There was a weariness in his gaze and a general air of fatigue and depression. He described his mood as 'tired'. He was clearly uncomfortable and even with my explanation about confidentiality he was only a little reassured; he was concerned that if the case went to court his relationship with Miss Ternan would become more widely known. A recurring comment was how the accident was 'a dreadful significance' for him. At several points in the consultation, he became more distressed: when talking about the deaths of his mother, his son, his brother and his old friend John Leech; when talking about having to write to the station master about Miss Ternan's lost belongings; when talking about the symptoms affecting the left side of his body; and when talking about how he is nervous travelling by train.

Report of: Professor Henry Maudsley
Specialism: Psychiatry
On the instructions of: Ouvry & Co
Prepared for: The City of London and Mayor's Court

5. OPINION

5.1 Clinical plausibility

5.1.1 In this case, in order to give opinions on the issues that have been identified, I am usually reliant on documentary evidence in addition to my assessment of the Claimant. The important documentary evidence is what is contained in the Claimant's general practitioner records. My assessment of the Claimant has two components: history and examination.

5.1.2 As far as the Claimant's medical records are concerned, those have so far not been disclosed. When they are, I will have to take into account whether they appear to be complete, whether handwritten records are legible and have regard to the possible significance of any redactions.

5.1.3 The Claimant gave his history in a straightforward manner. He unhesitatingly answered all of my questions. He did not appear defensive or evasive except when talking about his relationship with Miss Ternan; whereas he appeared to have been quite frank about the painful details of his marriage, he seemed to want to say as little as possible about his relationship with Miss Ternan, disclosing only a little more than has been the subject of rumour in London society. His responses seemed proportionate. He did not describe any unexpected or bizarre symptoms or experiences that might have been out of keeping with the rest of his presentation. He did not report what might have been an excessive number of symptoms or a lot of symptoms of extreme severity, which seemed a little surprising given that he described himself as having adopted the family habit of self-centred complaint. The history that he gave had a 'face validity' that was similar to that which I have encountered in patients with a similar condition seen outside the forensic context. The findings on examination of his mental state were consistent with the history that he gave. There were no unusual or unexpected findings on examination. However, without his medical records and with no history from an informant, I am unable to comment on the consistency between the documentary evidence, the Claimant's history, the history from any informant and the examination findings.

5.1.4 Having regard to my evaluation of the evidence available to me at this time, I am sufficiently confident to set out my opinions, on the balance of probabilities, on the identified issues. I accept that I may need to reconsider my opinions in the light of documentary evidence, in particular his medical records, and if there is any evidence that calls into question the reliability of the Claimant.

5.2 Any relevant pre-accident medical history

5.2.1 The Claimant might have been what is sometimes termed 'a delicate child', but not to any great extent and only his migraine-like attacks brought on by anxiety suggest any childhood tendency to psychosomatic complaint.

5.2.2 As an adult, the Claimant appears to have been free of frank psychiatric illness or psychosomatic complaint. Indeed, he appears to have been a person of customary phlegm and normal fortitude. Neither his unhappy marriage nor the considerable financial demands made by his close family, his extended family and various charities have had any obvious effect on his mental health.

5.2.3 The accident did occur at a time when the Claimant's mental health seems to have been compromised. He himself recognised that he had been on the verge of some sort of nervous or mental breakdown and indeed this was the reason why he had gone to Paris for a holiday.

Report of: Professor Henry Maudsley
Specialism: Psychiatry
On the instructions of: Ouvry & Co
Prepared for: The City of London and Mayor's Court

5.2.4 Not long before this holiday, the Claimant had been finding writing an effort and he had been unusually slow at writing. Also, he had been physically unwell. Therefore, notwithstanding the likely restorative effect of the holiday in Paris, it is reasonable to regard the Claimant as having been vulnerable to psychiatric disorder at this time.

5.2.5 It is probable that this precarious state of his mental health had something to do with the various bereavements that had occurred and the strain of leading a double life in that he tried to represent his marriage as having the semblance of normality, but at the same time he was in what seems to have been a clandestine relationship with Miss Ternan.

5.3 The nature of any injuries sustained

5.3.1 The symptoms the Claimant has experienced since the accident fall into three categories: post-traumatic stress symptoms, physical symptoms and phobic symptoms.

5.3.2 The Claimant describes an experience in which he relives the accident, with some attendant distress, he is nervous about rail travel and he is upset by any unusual movement. However, he does not report nightmares of the accident, he does not avoid rail travel now, although he did for a while and he still avoids express trains, he does not describe any other avoidance phenomena, he does not describe any loss of interest or numbing of emotional responsiveness and he does not describe a sense of a foreshortened future. Although he described being upset by any unusual movement, he does not otherwise report or exhibit an increased startle response and he does not have any other symptoms of persistently increased arousal. He has had some insomnia, but not the sort of insomnia that is a manifestation of persistently increased arousal following trauma. Therefore, although he has some symptoms found in post-traumatic stress disorder, he is not suffering from a post-traumatic stress disorder as such.

5.3.3 I do need to point out that some clinicians would make a diagnosis of a form of non-specific adjustment disorder and this is a positive and recognisable form of psychiatric illness. However, strictly speaking, his symptoms have lasted for too long to meet the strict criteria for an adjustment disorder and, as they are distressing but do not affect his functioning, it is arguable whether or not they are an actual mental disorder. I make this point in order to cover what I regard as a reasonable range of opinion on this aspect of diagnosis.

5.3.4 The Claimant reports physical symptoms in the form of weakness, feelings of faintness, sickness, dyspepsia and what seem to be widespread muscular aches and pains. It is probable that these symptoms represent what is known as neurasthenia. This is a form of neurosis. He reports the typical complaint of increased fatigue and weakness after both mental and physical effort along with worries about decreased mental and bodily functioning. He has had typical accompanying symptoms in the form of muscular aches and pains and dyspepsia. In order to make this diagnosis, any depressive symptoms must not be sufficiently persistent and severe to fulfil the criteria for an actual depressive disorder. This appears to be the case here. The Claimant reports a lack of his usual buoyancy and cheerfulness and he does look depressed, but he does not report any actual depression of mood and it should be noted that his sleep and appetite have been normal except that he has had some trouble sleeping since his brother's death.

5.3.5 The Claimant reports feeling nervous when travelling by train and being upset by unusual movements. Initially, he avoided rail travel completely and he still avoids express trains. Although he does not meet the criteria for a phobia of rail travel in general, he does have a specific phobia of express train travel.

Report of: Professor Henry Maudsley
Specialism: Psychiatry
On the instructions of: Ouvry & Co
Prepared for: The City of London and Mayor's Court

5.3.6 Although he reported feeling shocked, the Claimant does not seem to have had any of the symptoms of an acute stress reaction.

5.4 Causation

5.4.1 There does not seem to be any explanation for the Claimant's nervousness about rail travel, his re-experiencing of the accident and his tendency to be upset by sudden movements other than the accident. However, these symptoms do not add up to any recognised mental disorder and in themselves, although distressing, they are not associated with any impairment of functioning. I therefore conclude that, insofar as they do not amount to a positive and recognisable psychiatric illness, they cannot be regarded as a psychiatric injury attributable to the rail crash.

5.4.2 There is no explanation for the Claimant's phobia of express train travel but the accident. Therefore, the Claimant's phobia of express train travel amounts to a psychiatric injury attributable to the accident.

5.4.3 The causation of the Claimant's neurasthenia is problematic. It appears that it had been developing before the accident. I do not recall that I have previously encountered neurasthenia as a psychiatric disorder brought about by traumata such as road, industrial or railway accidents. For these two reasons, I do not think that it could be proved on a balance of probability that the Claimant's neurasthenia has been caused by the accident, but it is fair to say that its causation is often obscure.

5.4.4 I note that when asked to tell me about the psychological and emotional effects of the accident, the Claimant immediately began to tell me about his worry about the public learning of his relationship with Miss Ternan. This is why the accident seems to have had deep significance for him. If the accident has made a contribution to his neurasthenia, it has probably been mediated through the worry about people learning of the true state of his marriage and his relationship with Miss Ternan rather than the emotional trauma of the accident itself.

5.4.5 I note that although he described himself as shocked by his experience, he was able to act responsibly with regard to his fellow passengers and was not deterred from climbing back into the precariously balanced carriage to retrieve his manuscript. I do not think that he would have done this if he had been acutely traumatised by the accident as such. Thus, not only does it appear that he did not have an acute stress reaction, but also it appears that at the time there is no evidence of any acute mental disturbance.

5.4.6 I have taken into account the Claimant's more recent bereavement, through the loss of his brother, but that has been too recent to account for his symptoms.

5.4.7 Within a range of reasonable opinion, some clinicians would credit that the accident did result in a period of worsening of his neurasthenia or had the effect of hastening its development. It is not possible to say to what extent it was made worse or to what extent the development of the condition has been accelerated.

Report of: Professor Henry Maudsley
Specialism: Psychiatry
On the instructions of: Ouvry & Co
Prepared for: The City of London and Mayor's Court

5.5 Treatment received

5.5.1 The Claimant has not received any treatment apart from some medication which has probably been of little or no value in his condition.

5.6 Present condition

5.6.1 I rate the Claimant's condition as one of moderate degree. It is clear that he has not been able to apply himself to his writing as assiduously as he used to do. His performance on his promotional tours has been affected and he is unable to travel by express train.

5.7 Prognosis

5.7.1 The Claimant's condition has been present for four years at least. It has run a fairly chronic, that is continuous, course. It is my experience that in people of his age, this condition tends not to remit spontaneously or respond to any drug or psychological therapy. I anticipate that his condition will continue indefinitely and will probably get worse.

5.7.2 I am concerned that this litigation will in itself make the Claimant's condition worse as he is bound to worry about the publicity that even a county court case will attract.

5.7.3 No other serious or delayed long-term psychiatric sequelae of the accident are expected. I have no reason to believe that his life expectancy has been affected.

6. SUMMARY OF CONCLUSIONS

6.1 Only the Claimant's migraine-like attacks brought on by anxiety suggest any childhood tendency to psychosomatic complaint.

6.2 As an adult, the Claimant appears to have been a person of customary phlegm and fortitude.

6.3 However, it is reasonable to regard the Claimant as having been vulnerable to psychiatric disorder at the time of the accident.

6.4 The symptoms the Claimant has experienced since the accident fall into three categories: post-traumatic stress symptoms, physical symptoms and phobic symptoms.

6.5 Although he has some symptoms found in post-traumatic stress disorder, he is not suffering from a post-traumatic stress disorder as such.

6.6 Some clinicians would make a diagnosis of a form of non-specific adjustment disorder and this is a positive and recognisable form of psychiatric illness.

6.7 It is probable that his physical symptoms represent what is known as neurasthenia, which is a form of neurosis.

6.8 Although he does not meet the criteria for a phobia of rail travel in general, he does have a specific phobia of express train travel.

Report of: Professor Henry Maudsley
Specialism: Psychiatry
On the instructions of: Ouvry & Co
Prepared for: The City of London and Mayor's Court

6.9 The Claimant does not seem to have had any of the symptoms of an acute stress reaction.

6.10 Insofar as the Claimant's post-traumatic stress symptoms do not amount to a positive and recognisable psychiatric illness, they cannot be regarded as a psychiatric injury attributable to the rail crash.

6.11 The Claimant's phobia of express train travel amounts to a psychiatric injury attributable to the accident.

6.12 The causation of the Claimant's neurasthenia is problematic.

6.13 I do not think that it could be proved on a balance of probability that the Claimant's neurasthenia has been caused by the accident.

6.14 If the accident has made a contribution to his neurasthenia, it has probably been mediated through the worry about people learning of the true state of his marriage and his relationship with Miss Ternan rather than the emotional trauma of the accident itself.

6.15 Within a range of reasonable opinion, some clinicians would credit that the accident did result in a period of worsening of his neurasthenia or had the effect of hastening its development.

6.16 The Claimant has not received any treatment apart from some medication which has probably been of little or no value in his condition.

6.17 I rate the Claimant's condition as one of moderate degree.

6.18 I anticipate that his condition will continue indefinitely and will probably get worse.

6.19 I am concerned that this litigation will in itself make the Claimant's condition worse.

6.20 No other serious or delayed long-term psychiatric sequelae of the accident are expected.

6.21 I have no reason to believe that his life expectancy has been affected.

7. DECLARATION

1. I understand that my duty is to help the court to achieve the overriding objective by giving assistance by way of objective, unbiased opinion on matters within my area of expertise, both in preparing reports and giving oral evidence. I understand that this duty overrides any obligation to the party by whom I am engaged or the person who has paid or is liable to pay me. I confirm that I have complied with and will continue to comply with that duty.

2. I confirm that I have not entered into any arrangement where the amount or payment of my fees is in any way dependent on the outcome of the case.

3. I know of no conflict of interest of any kind, other than any which I have disclosed in this report.

4. I do not consider that any interest which I have disclosed affects my suitability as an expert witness on any issues on which I have given evidence.

Provisional report of Prof H. Maudsley concerning Charles Dickens 10 June 1869 *15*
CHARLES DICKENS (Claimant) v SOUTH-EASTERN AND CHATHAM RAILWAY COMPANY (Defendant)

Report of: Professor Henry Maudsley
Specialism: Psychiatry
On the instructions of: Ouvry & Co
Prepared for: The City of London and Mayor's Court

5. I have shown the sources of all information I have used.

6. I have set out in my report what I understand from those instructing me to be the questions in respect of which my opinion as an expert is required. All of the matters on which I have expressed an opinion lie within my field of expertise.

7. I have exercised reasonable care and skill in order to be accurate and complete in preparing this report. I have covered all relevant issues concerning the matters stated which I have been asked to address. Absence of any comment in this report does not indicate that I have no opinion on a matter. I may not have been asked to deal with it.

8. I have endeavoured to include in my report those matters, of which I have knowledge or of which I have been made aware, that might adversely affect the validity of my opinion. I have clearly stated any qualifications to my opinion.

9. Where, in my view, there is a range of reasonable opinion, I have indicated the extent of that range in the report and given reasons for my own opinion.

10. I have not, without forming an independent view, included or excluded anything which has been suggested to me by others, including my instructing lawyers.

11. At the time of signing the report, I consider that it is complete and accurate. I will notify those instructing me immediately, and confirm in writing if for any reason I subsequently consider that the report requires any correction or qualification or if between the date of this report and the trial there is any change in circumstances which affect my declarations at 3 and 4 above.

12. I understand that:
(a) my report, subject to any corrections before swearing as to its correctness, will form the evidence to be given under oath;
(b) the court may at any stage direct a discussion to take place between the experts;
(c) the court may direct that, following a discussion between the experts, a statement should be prepared showing those issues which are agreed and those issues which are not agreed, together with a summary of the reasons for disagreeing;
(d) I may be required to attend court to be cross-examined on my report by a cross-examiner assisted by an expert;
(e) I am likely to be the subject of public adverse criticism by the judge if the court concludes that I have not taken reasonable care in trying to meet the standards set out above.

13. This report is provided to those instructing me with the sole purpose of assisting the court in this particular case. It may not be used for any other purpose, nor may it be disclosed to any third party without my express written authority or that of the court.

14. I am aware of the requirements of Part 35 and Practice Direction 35, the *Guidance for the Instruction of Experts to give evidence in civil claims* and the Practice Direction for pre-action conduct. I have obtained The Bond Solon Civil Procedure Rules for Expert Witnesses Certificate as evidence of my understanding and compliance with the above requirements.

15. I confirm that I have acted in accordance with the Royal College of Psychiatrists' College Report CR193, *Responsibilities of psychiatrists who provide expert opinion to courts and tribunals*, by Keith Rix, Nigel Eastman and Gwen Adshead (2015) and the General Medical Council's *Good Medical Practice*, which includes 'Giving evidence as an expert witness'.

Report of: Professor Henry Maudsley
Specialism: Psychiatry
On the instructions of: Ouvry & Co
Prepared for: The City of London and Mayor's Court

8. STATEMENT OF TRUTH

I confirm that the contents of this report are true to the best of my knowledge and belief and that I make this report knowing that, if it is tendered in evidence, I would be liable to prosecution if I have wilfully stated anything which I know to be false or that I do not believe to be true.

Henry Maudsley, MB, MD, Hon LLD, MRMPA, FRCP,
Consultant Physician,
Professor of Medical Jurisprudence.

10 June 1869

Report of: Professor Henry Maudsley
Specialism: Psychiatry
On the instructions of: Ouvry & Co
Prepared for: The City of London and Mayor's Court

APPENDIX 1

QUALIFICATIONS AND EXPERIENCE

Qualifications

I am a medical graduate of University College London where I qualified **Bachelor of Medicine** in 1856. I subsequently obtained the higher degree of **Doctor of Medicine** following study and research in mental science. I am a **Member of the Royal Medico-Psychological Association**. I was elected **Fellow of the Royal College of Physicians** in 1869. I have been awarded the honorary degree of **Doctor of Laws** by the University of Edinburgh.

Clinical training and experience

Following **House Physician** and **House Surgeon** appointments at University College Hospital London, I undertook my general professional training as a **Registrar in Psychiatry** at the West Riding Lunatic Asylum, Wakefield, from 1856 to 1858 and my higher training as a **Specialty Registrar in Psychiatry** at the Essex County Asylum, Brentwood, from 1858 to 1859. In 1859, I was appointed **Physician Superintendent** of the Manchester Royal Lunatic Asylum (Cheadle Royal). In 1862, I moved to London, where I was in independent practice until my appointment as **Physician** to the West London Hospital in 1865. I am now also **Professor of Medical Jurisprudence** at University College London, and I run Lawn House, a private mental asylum established by Dr John Connolly. I am a co-editor of the *Journal of Mental Science.* I will be the next **Gulstonian Lecturer of the Royal College of Physicians**. I will deliver a series of lectures on 'Body and mind'.

Research and publications

I am the author of *The Physiology and Pathology of Mind* (1867) and I have been commissioned by Macmillan to write *Body and Mind: An Inquiry into Their Connection and Mutual Influence* and *Mental Responsibility in Health and Disease*. I am the author of papers on delusions, the causes of insanity and the treatment of insanity.

Report of: Professor Henry Maudsley
Specialism: Psychiatry
On the instructions of: Ouvry & Co
Prepared for: The City of London and Mayor's Court

APPENDIX 2

THE SUBSTANCE OF ALL MATERIAL INSTRUCTIONS

The Claimant was returning from a short holiday in Paris and was a passenger on the Folkestone Boat Express (the 'tidal' train) when it was derailed at Staplehurst. It was known as the 'tidal train' because, as the Channel packet docked at the top of the tide, the train's departure time changed from day to day.

On the long straight stretch between Headcorn and Staplehurst, the foreman of a gang of platelayers had miscalculated the alteration in time and the leading carpenter, who had also been issued with a copy of the timetable, had dropped his on the rail, where it had been destroyed by a passing train, so he could not correct the foreman's error. As the train approached, almost fifty feet of track were out of place. A platelayer's labourer was protecting the up line just 554 yards from the viaduct. He had been issued with only two detonators (fog signals) and told not to use them unless it was foggy. It was a bright and sunny afternoon. He should have placed six fog signals at strategic positions and he should have been positioned with his flag 1,000 yards from the viaduct.

The driver could do nothing to avoid a wreck. The express was travelling at 50 miles an hour. Her driver acted promptly as soon as he saw the platelayer's red flag, but in so short a distance he could not hope to bring his train of thirteen vehicles to a halt. The leading van and the first two coaches were fitted with Cremar's patent brakes, but unfortunately the guard in charge did not himself see the platelayer's frantic signal and in response to the brake signal he applied only his ordinary screw brake. Not until half the critical distance had been covered did he realise the urgency and apply the patent brakes. By that time, the locomotive was practically upon the bridge. This was a very modest structure that carried the line a mere ten feet above a muddy stream.

The locomotive, its tender and the leading brake van actually succeeded in crossing the rail-less gap on the timber baulks, but the following train was less fortunate. The first coach, in which the Claimant was travelling, came to rest at a perilous angle, supported by the van coupling, and hung over the ruined bridgework. The next five coaches fell through the gap into the muddy bed of the stream, where they lay in a confusion of splintered wreckage. Ten passengers in these coaches were killed and forty-nine injured.

The Claimant was able to climb out of his compartment through a window and with the assistance of a workman he rescued his travelling companions from their precarious perch. When the immediate shock wore off, the Claimant realised that he had left the manuscript for the next part of *Our Mutual Friend* in the compartment and he managed to get back into the wreckage and retrieve it. Although his clothing was soiled, the Claimant was physically unhurt. For a period following the accident, the Claimant was in a state of distress. He is nervous about travelling in trains and now prefers slow trains.

Report of: Professor Henry Maudsley
Specialism: Psychiatry
On the instructions of: Ouvry & Co
Prepared for: The City of London and Mayor's Court

APPENDIX 3

THE PROCESS OF PSYCHIATRIC ASSESSMENT

1. Psychiatrists, as doctors, employ the time-honoured processes of history-taking and examination in order to achieve a formulation of the subject that encompasses diagnosis, aetiology (causation), treatment recommendations and prognosis. Examination may and often does include physical examination, but examination of the mental state is an important psychiatric skill.

2. The history is particularly important in the case of many psychiatric disorders because diagnosis depends largely, and in some cases entirely, on self-reported symptoms and if, for whatever reason, the Claimant is unreliable in their report of the nature, duration, severity or effects of their symptoms, this can affect the validity of any diagnosis reached and the conclusions as to the impact of their condition. I recognise, of course, that the reliability of the Claimant is an ultimate issue for the court, but in a forensic assessment I have to decide whether or not to accept at face value what the Defendant has reported to me and what he has reported to other experts in this case. In this regard, I am mindful of the observation of HHJ Seymour QC in *Turner v Jordan* [2010] EWHC 1508 (QB)

> A consequence of the fact that diagnosis in a psychiatric case depends on assessment of what is reported by the patient is the necessity for the psychiatrist confronted by a patient to consider whether or not to accept at face value what the patient reports. Inevitably there is a disposition on the part of the psychiatrist to take as genuine what the patient reports, because otherwise it is difficult to consider the issue of diagnosis.

3. Psychiatric examination of the Claimant, or what psychiatrists describe as the mental state examination, is my professional analysis of the Claimant's appearance, behaviour, mood, form of talk, thought content, unusual or abnormal beliefs or experiences, cognitive functioning and insight. It may take into account my reaction to the Claimant.

4. My approach to the process of differential diagnosis is based on normal clinical practice and a hierarchical system of psychiatric classification. By this, I mean that I have considered diagnosis in the order in which mental disorders appear section by section in *The ICD-10 Classification of Mental and Behavioural Disorders* (Geneva: World Health Organization, 1992): organic, including symptomatic, mental disorders; mental and behavioural disorders due to substance misuse (including alcohol); schizophrenia and related disorders; mood disorders; neurotic, stress-related and somatoform disorders; personality and related disorders; and learning disabilities. At each level, I have considered the evidence for and against the diagnosis of a mental disorder at that level and then I have proceeded to the next level. This accords approximately with the logical ordering of sections in ICD-10. I have highlighted, if there are any, factual assumptions, deductions from factual assumptions, and any unusual, contradictory or inconsistent features of the case.

Report of: Professor Henry Maudsley
Specialism: Psychiatry
On the instructions of: Ouvry & Co
Prepared for: The City of London and Mayor's Court

5. My approach to aetiology has been to apply to the defendant's case my knowledge of the causes of psychiatric disorder in order to be able to give an opinion as to how the psychiatric disorder came about or why it ran the course it did.

6. Where I have made recommendations for treatment, or commented on treatment already given, I have relied on approaches that have wide acceptance by psychiatrists and, if possible, given weight to treatments for which there is the strongest evidence base with regard to effectiveness and safety. However, as in medicine in general, there are many treatments that are accepted as effective, but for which there have not been trials that satisfy the most stringent criteria of evidence-based medicine.

7. So far as prognosis is concerned, I have applied my knowledge of the course and outcome of psychiatric disorders to the features of this individual case. My approach to risk assessment is based on structured clinical judgement. By this, I mean that I have used my training, experience and skill to relate what is known about the prognoses of mental disorders in general to the specific features of the subject's case, endeavouring to make predictions about identified risks with which I would expect other psychiatrists to concur. It is important to realise that the value of predictions diminishes rapidly with time and this is probably because with time circumstances change so much.

8. Clinical practice, including psychiatric practice, depends in part on knowledge for which there is a sound evidence base and partly on experience-based knowledge which has stood the test of time, but lacks a robust foundation in the rigorous research that now forms the basis of 'evidence-based medicine'. In relying on both categories of knowledge, I have done so in accordance with what I would regard as a responsible body of psychiatric practice and I therefore regard my methodology as sufficiently reliable for the court's purposes.

Provisional report of Prof H. Maudsley concerning Charles Dickens **10 June 1869** *21*
CHARLES DICKENS (Claimant) v SOUTH-EASTERN AND CHATHAM RAILWAY COMPANY (Defendant)

Report of: Professor Henry Maudsley
Specialism: Psychiatry
On the instructions of: Ouvry & Co
Prepared for: The City of London and Mayor's Court

APPENDIX 4

DOCUMENTS STUDIED

MacKenzie, N. and MacKenzie, J. (1979) *Dickens – A Life*. (Oxford University Press).

[KR fully acknowledges his heavy reliance on this biography for almost all of the factual content of this report. The opinion is entirely that of KR and perhaps not consistent with the accepted view that Dickens was badly affected by the accident, he did not recover from its effects and when he died prematurely five years to the day after the accident it was as a result of the accident that he died so prematurely.]

Rolt, L. T. C. (1966) *Red for Danger* (Pan Books).

Trimble, M.R. (1981) *Post-Traumatic Neurosis – From Railway Spine to the Whiplash* (John Wiley).

Report of: Professor Henry Maudsley
Specialism: Psychiatry
On the instructions of: Ouvry & Co
Prepared for: The City of London and Mayor's Court

APPENDIX 5

GLOSSARY

anal fistula – A fistula is an abnormal communication between two surfaces. In this case, it is the channel that communicates between the inner surface of the anus (back passage) and the skin of the buttocks. It gives rise to local irritation and pain. There is a risk of infection.

aneurysm – An aneurysm is a defect in the lining of the wall of a blood vessel. It may not manifest in any symptoms, although this does depend on the location of the blood vessel. If it bursts, there may be such massive blood loss that death occurs.

delusion – A delusion is a false belief held with total conviction and inappropriate to the patient's intelligence, social background and subcultural beliefs (K. J. B. Rix, *A Handbook for Trainee Psychiatrists* (Baillière Tindall, 1987)).

digitalis – Digitalis is a drug derived from the fox-glove plant. It strengthens the pumping of the heart and can regulate some irregularities of heart rhythm.

gout – Gout is a disorder of metabolism. It occurs when the metabolism of the nitrogen-based constituent of many foods, purine, goes wrong and the end-product of the metabolic process, uric acid, crystallises as monosodium urate in joints and tendons, characteristically at the base of the big toe, causing swelling, pain and redness.

iron – Iron is used in the treatment of some forms of anaemia

migraine – Migrainous headaches have their onset usually in puberty or the second and third decades of life and occur intermittently, although with decreasing frequency and severity with advancing years. They seem to be caused by the constriction and then the dilatation of branches of the external carotid artery. There are various precipitants, including fatigue, hunger, bright lights, excitement, alcoholic beverages, certain foods and oral contraceptives. Typically, there is an aura or prodromal phase with depression, irritability and restlessness which may be accompanied by transient neurological symptoms such as flashes of light, bright spots, impaired vision, etc. Minutes or hours later comes the increasingly severe and intense headache. However, there is considerable variability of symptoms.

quinine – Quinine is a naturally occurring substance found in the bark of the *Cinchona* tree. It has anti-malarial properties and is also a treatment for shivering, rigors and diarrhea.

renal colic – Renal colic is the pain caused by a stone that has formed in the collecting system of the kidney where urine is concentrated before making its way to the bladder through the urethra. It is usually a severe and debilitating pain.

References

Advocate's Gateway (2014) General principles when questioning witnesses and defendants with mental disorder. Toolkit 12.

Allen, D. (2014) *Business for Medics: How to Set Up and Run a Medical Practice* (Kindle Direct Publishing).

American Psychiatric Association (2013) *Diagnostic and Statistical Manual of Mental Disorders*, 5th edn (American Psychiatric Association).

Anon (2018) *The Secret Barrister: Stories of the Law and How It's Broken* (Macmillan).

Ashton, G., Letts, P., Oates, L. and Terrell, M. (2006) *Mental Capacity: The New Law* (Jordans), p. 84.

Babitsky, S., Mangravati, Jr, J. J. and Todd, C. J. (2000) *The Comprehensive Forensic Services Manual: The Essential Resources for All Experts* (SEAK).

Bell, E. (2010) 'Judicial assessment of expert evidence', *Judicial Studies Institute Journal*, **2**, 55–96.

Bluglass, R. (1990) 'Infanticide and filicide' in R. Bluglass and P. Bowden (eds), *Principles and Practice of Forensic Psychiatry* (Churchill Livingstone), pp. 523–8.

Bond, C., Solon, M., Harper, P. and Davies, G. (2007) *The Expert Witness: A Practical Guide*, 3rd edn (Shaw & Sons).

Booth, T., Booth, W. and McConnell, D. (2004) 'Parents with learning difficulties, care proceedings and the family courts: threshold decisions and the moral matrix', *Child and Family Law Quarterly*, **16**, 409–21.

Bourne, T., Wynants, L., Peters, M., Van Audenhove, C., Timmerman, D., Van Calster, B. and Jalmbrant, M. (2015) 'The impact of complaints procedures on the welfare, health and clinical practise of 7926 doctors in the UK: a cross-sectional study', *BMJ Open*, **4**, e006687.

Bowers, L., Gournay, K. and Duffy, D. (2000) 'Suicide and self-harm in inpatient psychiatric units: a national survey of observation policies', *Journal of Advanced Nursing*, **33**, 437–44.

Boyle, D. (2016) *On Experts: CPR35 for Lawyers and Experts* (Law Brief Publishing).

Bradley, K. (2009) *People with Mental Health Problems or Learning Disabilities in the Criminal Justice System* (Home Office).

Braithwaite, B. and Waldron, W. (2010) *Brain and Spine Injuries: The Fight for Justice* (Exchange Information).

British Medical Association and the Law Society (2015) *Assessment of Mental Capacity: A Practical Guide for Doctors and Lawyers*, 4th edn (Law Society).

Buchan, A. (gen. ed) (2019) *Lewis and Buchan: Clinical Negligence. A Practical Guide*, 8th edn (Bloomsbury Professional).

Butler-Sloss, E. and Hall, A. (2002) 'Expert witnesses, courts and the law', *Journal of the Royal Society of Medicine*, **95**, 431–4.

Charleton, P., McDermott, P. and Bolger, M. (1999) *Criminal Law* (Bloomsbury).

Civil Justice Council (2011) *Access to Justice for Litigants in Person (or self-represented litigants).*

Civil Justice Council (2014) *Guidance for the instruction of experts in civil claims.*

Clough, A. J. (2015) 'Mercy killing: three's a crowd?' *Criminal Law Review*, **79**, 358–72.

Cooper, P. (2006) 'Training' in L. Blom-Cooper (ed), *Experts in the Civil Courts (Expert Witness Institute)* (Oxford University Press).

Cooper, P. and Grace, J. (2016) 'Vulnerable patients going to court: a psychiatrist's guide to special measures', *BJPsych Bulletin*, **40**, 220–2.

Crichton, J. (2014) 'Civil issues' in L. Thomson and J. Cherry (eds), *Mental Health & Scots Law in Practice*, 2nd edn (W. Green), pp. 192–209.

Cromwell, T. A. (2011) *Macfadyen Lecture: 'The Challenges of Scientific Evidence'* (Scottish Council of Law Reporting).

Curtice, M. and Kelson, A. (2011) 'The Sexual Offences Act 2003 and people with mental disorders', *The Psychiatrist*, **35**, 261–5.

Dimopoulos, A. (2009) 'Intellectually disabled parents before the European Court of Human Rights and English courts', *European Human Rights Law Review*, **1**, 70–83.

d'Orbán, P. (1979) 'Women who kill their children', *British Journal of Psychiatry*, **134**, 560–71.

Dorries, P. (2014) *Coroners' Courts: A Guide to Law and Practice*, 3rd edn (Oxford University Press).

Duncan, A., Snr (1795) *Heads of Lectures on Medical Jurisprudence* (G. Mudie & Son).

Ebrahim, I. O. and Fenwick, P. (2008) 'Sleep-related automatism and the law', *Medicine, Science and the Law*, **48**, 124–36.

Ellis, P. *Clinical practice guidelines and the law* (Lamb Chambers).

Eyre, G. and Alexander, L. (2015) *Writing Medico-Legal Reports in Civil Claims: An Essential Guide* (Professional Solutions Publications).

Faculty of Occupational Medicine (2018) *Ethics Guidance for Occupational Health Practice.*

Fenwick, P. (1990) 'Automatism' in R. Bluglass and P. Bowden (eds), *Principles and Practice of Forensic Psychiatry* (Churchill Livingstone), pp. 271–85.

Gerada, C. (2019) 'The GMC is no longer a bogeyman to fear', *British Medical Journal*, **368**, m647.

Grubin, D. H. (1996) 'Silence in court: psychiatry and the Criminal Justice and Public Order Act 1994', *Journal of Forensic Psychiatry*, **7**, 647–52.

Gudjonsson, G. H. (2003) *The Psychology of Interrogations and Confessions: A Handbook* (Wiley).

Gudjonsson, G. H., Clare, I. C. H., Rutter, S. and Pearse, J. (1993) *Persons at Risk During Interviews in Police Custody: the Identification of Vulnerabilities* (Royal Commission on Criminal Justice, HMSO).

Gunn, J. and Taylor, P. J. (eds) (1993) *Forensic Psychiatry, Clinical, Legal and Ethical Issues* (Butterworth-Heinemann).

Hagan, L. D. and Guilmette, T. J. (2015) 'DSM5: challenging diagnostic testimony', *International Journal of Law and Psychiatry*, **42–3**, 128–34.

Hallett, N. (2020) 'To what extent should expert psychiatric witnesses comment on criminal culpability?', *Medicine, Science and the Law*, **60**, 67–74.

Handford, P. (2006) *Mullany & Handford's Tort Liability for Psychiatric Damage*, 2nd edn (Lawbook Co.).

Hershman, D., McFarlane, A. and Ward, A. (1991) *Children, Law and Practice* (Update 42) (Jordan Publishing).

Hodgkinson, T. and James, M. (2015) *Expert Evidence: Law and Practice*, 4th edn (Sweet & Maxwell).

Horsfall, S. (2014) *Doctors Who Commit Suicide while under GMC Fitness to Practise Investigation: Internal Review* (General Medical Council).

Horwath, J. and Morrison, T. (2001) 'Assessment of parental motivation to change' in J. Horwath (ed), *The Child's World: Assessing Children in Need* (Jessica Kingsley).

Inns of Court College of Advocacy (2019) *Guidance on the Preparation, Admission and Examination of Expert Evidence* (The Council of the Inns of Court).

Jackson, E. (2019) *Medical Law: Text, Cases and Materials*, 5th edn (Oxford University Press).

Jackson, J. and Johnstone, J. (2005) 'The reasonable time requirement: an independent and meaningful right?', *Criminal Law Review*, January, 3–23.

Kloss, D. (2015) 'Consent to occupational health reports', *Occupational Medicine*, **65**, 700–3.

Langbein, J. H. (1985) 'The German advantage in civil litigation', *University of Chicago Law Review*, **52**, 823–66.

Law Commission (2011) *Expert Evidence in Criminal Proceedings in England and Wales* (Law Com. No. 325) (Law Commission).

Law Commission (2013) *Criminal Liability: Insanity and Automatism. A Discussion Paper.*

Law Society of Ireland (2016) *Criminal Litigation* (Oxford University Press).

Lewis, C. J. (2006) *Clinical Negligence*, 6th edn (Wiley-Blackwell).

Linden, M. (2003) 'Posttraumatic embitterment disorder', *Psychotherapy and Psychosomatics*, **72**, 195–202.

Lockwood, G., Henderson, C. and Thornicroft, G. (2012) 'The Equality Act 2010 and mental health', *British Journal of Psychiatry*, **200**, 182–3.

Mackay, R. D. (1993) 'The consequences of killing very young children', *Criminal Law Review*, 21.

Mackay, R. (1995) *Mental Condition Defences in the Criminal Law* (Oxford University Press).

Mackay, R. (2010a) 'The Coroners and Justice Act 2009 – partial defences to murder: (2) the new diminished responsibility plea', *Criminal Law Review*, 290.

Mackay, R. (2010b) 'Mental disability at the time of the offence' in L. Gostin, P. Bartlett, P. Fennell, J. McHale and R. Mackay (eds), *Principles of Mental Health Law and Policy* (Oxford University Press), pp. 721–55.

Mackay, R. and Mitchell, B. (2017) 'The new diminished responsibility plea in operation – some initial findings', *Criminal Law Review*, 18.

Malek, H. M. (ed) (2013) *Phipson on Evidence*, 18th edn (Sweet & Maxwell).

Marks, P. (1995) 'Drink-driving legislation: medicine and the law', *Medico-Legal Journal*, **63**, 119–27.

Marshall D., Kennedy J. and Azib, R. (2012) *Litigating Psychiatric Injury Claims* (Bloomsbury).

McFarlane, Lord Justice (2018) Keynote Address, Bond Solon Experts Conference.

Mirfield, P. (1997) *Silence, Confessions and Improperly Obtained Evidence* (Clarendon Press).

Munby, J. (2013) 'View from the president's chambers: expert evidence', *Family Law*, **43**, 816–20.

Murphy, P. (ed in chief) (1999) *Blackstone's Criminal Practice* (Blackstone Press).

Nathan, R. and Medland, S. (2016) 'Psychiatric expert evidence and the new partial defences of diminished responsibility and loss of control', *BJPsych Advances*, **22**, 277–84.

Norrie, A. (2010) 'The Coroners and Justice Act 2009 – partial defences to murder: (1) loss of control', *Criminal Law Review*, 275.

Northern Ireland Law Commission (2013) *Report on Unfitness to Plead* (NILC 16).

Ormerod, D. (2011) *Smith and Hogan's Criminal Law*, 13th edn (Oxford University Press).

Ormerod, D. and Perry, D. (gen. eds) (2019) *Blackstone's Criminal Practice* (Oxford University Press).

Parrott, C. T., Neal, T. M., Wilson, J. K. and Brodsky, S. L. (2015) 'Differences in expert witness knowledge: do mock jurors notice and does it matter?' *Journal of the American Academy of Psychiatry and Law*, **43**, 69–81.

Percival, T. (1803) *Medical Ethics or a Code of Institutes and Precepts Adapted to the Professional Conduct of Physicians and Surgeons* (S. Russell).

Piper, A. and Merskey, H. (2004) 'The persistence of folly: critical examination of dissociative personality disorder. Part II. The defence and decline of multiple personality or dissociative identity disorder', *Canadian Journal of Psychiatry*, **49**, 678–83.

Quick, O. (2006) 'Outing medical errors: questions of trust and responsibility', *Medical Law Review*, **14**, 22.

Rix, K. J. B. (1996a) 'Psychiatric reports for criminal proceedings in England and Wales', *Hospital Update*, **22**, 240–4, 282–6.

Rix, K. J. B. (1996b) 'Blood or needle phobia as a defence under the Road Traffic Act 1988', *Journal of Clinical Forensic Medicine*, **3**, 173–7.

Rix, K. J. B. (1998) 'Silence in interview: psychiatry and the Argent conditions', *Journal of Clinical Forensic Medicine*, **5**, 199–205.

Rix, K. J. B. (1999) 'Capacity to manage property and affairs: old case, new law', *Journal of Forensic Psychiatry*, **10**, 436–44.

Rix, K. J. B. (2001) 'Provocation and the "battered woman syndrome": two women with something more in common', *Journal of Forensic Psychiatry*, **12**, 131–49.

Rix, K. J. B. (2006) 'Mental capacity', *Solicitors Journal*, **150**, 1370–1.

Rix, K. J. B. (2011a) 'Medico-legal work of psychiatrists: direction, not drift. Commentary on . . . "You are instructed to prepare an expert report"', *The Psychiatrist*, **35**, 272–4.

Rix, K. J. B. (2011b) *Expert Psychiatric Evidence* (RCPsych Publications).

Rix, K. J. B. (2012) 'Fitness to plead and stand trial – then, now and in the future', *The Expert and Dispute Resolver*, **17**, 16–20.

Rix, K. J. B (2015a) 'The common law defence of automatism: a quagmire for the psychiatrist', *BJPsych Advances*, **21**, 242–50.

Rix, K. J. B. (2015b) 'Prizing open the door to justice: reforming the "wrongfulness limb" of the M'Naghten Rules' in N. Wake, A. Reed and B. Livings (eds), *Mental Condition Defences and the Criminal Justice System: Perspectives from Law and Medicine* (Cambridge Scholars), pp. 105–29.

Rix, K. J. B. (2016) 'Towards a more just insanity defence: recovering moral wrongfulness in the M'Naghten Rules', *BJPsych Advances*, **22**, 44–52.

Rix, K. J. B. (2018) 'Adjustment disorders in legal settings' in P. Casey (ed), *Adjustment Disorders: From Controversy to Clinical Practice* (Oxford University Press), pp. 189–205.

Rix, K. J. B. and Agarwal, M. (1999) 'Risk of serious harm or a serious risk of harm? A trap for judges', *Journal of Forensic Psychiatry*, **10**, 187–96.

Rix, K. J. B. and Clarkson, A. (1994) 'Depersonalisation and intent', *Journal of Forensic Psychiatry*, **5**, 405–19.

Rix, K. J. B. and Cory-Wright, C. (2018) 'How shocking: compensating secondary victims for psychiatric injury', *BJPsych Advances*, **24**, 110–22.

Rix, K. J. B., Eastman, N. and Adshead, G. (2015) *Responsibilities of Psychiatrists Providing Expert Evidence to Courts and Tribunals*, College Report CR193 (Royal College of Psychiatrists).

Rix, K. J. B., Eastman, N. and Haycroft, A. (2017) 'After *Pool*: good practice guidelines for expert psychiatric witnesses', *BJPsych Advances*, **23**, 385–94.

Rix, K. J. B., Haycroft, A. and Eastman, N. (2017) 'Danger in deep water or just ripples in the pool: has the *Pool* judgment changed the law on expert evidence?', *BJPsych Advances*, **23**, 347–57.

Rix, K. J. B., Thorn, S. and Neville, W. (1997) 'Medical evidence concerning the suitability to succeed to the tenancy of a farm: "the case of Toad of Toad Hall"', *Journal of Clinical Forensic Medicine*, **4**, 25–32.

Rix, K. J. B. and Tracy, D. (2017) 'Malingering mental disorders 2: medicolegal reporting', *BJPsych Advances*, **23**, 115–22.

Rogers, R. (ed) (2008) *Clinical Assessment of Malingering and Deception*, 3rd edn (Guilford Press).

Royal College of Psychiatrists (1978) *Infanticide: Report to the Criminal Law Revision Committee* (Chairman: R. Bluglass) (Royal College of Psychiatrists).

Royal College of Psychiatrists (2004) *The Impact of Extended Sentencing on the Ethical Framework of Psychiatry* (College Report CR 147) (Royal College of Psychiatrists).

Royal College of Psychiatrists (2008) *Rethinking Risk to Others in Mental Health Services* (College Report CR150) (Royal College of Psychiatrists).

Royal College of Psychiatrists (2010) A Competency Based Curriculum for Specialist Training in Psychiatry: Specialists in Forensic Psychiatry (update approved 2 October 2014, revised March 2016 and May 2017), www.rcpsych.ac.uk/docs/default-source/training/curricula-and-guidance/curricula-tw-tr-forensic-psychiatry-curriculum-august-2017.pdf?sfvrsn=833f68e5_2 (Royal College of Psychiatrists).

Rutherford, J., Chalmers, J., Zigmond, A. and Burn, W. (2015) *Guidance for Detaining Authorities and Tribunal Panels about Medical Evidence for First Tier Tribunal – Mental Health* (Royal College of Psychiatrists/Tribunals Judiciary).

Sayles, G. O. (1936) *Select Cases in the Court of King's Bench under Edward I* (Bernard Quaritsch).

Shapiro, C. M., Trajonovic, N. N. and Fedoroff, J. P. (2003) 'Sexsomnia – a new parasomnia', *Canadian Journal of Psychiatry*, **48**, 311–17.

Shapiro, F. R. (1993) *The Oxford Dictionary of American Legal Quotations* (Oxford University Press).

Smethurst, P. D. (2006) 'Giving evidence – the expert view on examination', *Barrister Expert Witness*, suppl., 12–13.

Tamin, J. (2010) 'GMC guidance on confidentiality: is it ethical?' *Occupational Medicine*, **60**, 6–7.

Taylor, C. and Krish, J. (2010) *Advising Mentally Disordered Offenders: A Practical Guide*, 2nd edn (Law Society).

Ventress, M. A., Rix, K. J. B. and Kent, J. H. (2008) 'Keeping PACE: fitness to be interviewed by the police', *Advances in Psychiatric Treatment*, **14**, 369–81.

Vos, G. (2019) *The White Book 2019* (Sweet & Maxwell).

Wall, N. (2007) *A Handbook for Expert Witnesses in Children Act Cases* (Jordan Publishing).

Weiss, K. J. and Westphal, A. R. N. (2015) 'Autistic spectrum disorders and criminal justice' in K. J. Weiss and C. Watson (eds), *Psychiatric Expert Testimony* (Oxford University Press), pp. 67–83.

Williams, G. (1983) *Textbook of Criminal Law*, 2nd edn (Stevens).

Wong, M. G. P. and Choong, K. A. (2013) 'The GMC and access to occupational health reports: issues and challenges', *European Journal of Current Legal Issues*, **19**.

Wood, H. and Rix, K. J. B. (2016) 'Common psychiatric and psychological disorders explained and examined' in P. Radcliffe, G. Gudjonsson, A. Heaton-Armstrong and D. Wolchover (eds), *Witness Testimony in Sexual Cases: Evidential, Investigative and Scientific Perspectives* (Oxford University Press), pp. 309–324.

World Health Organization (1992) *The ICD-10 Classification of Mental and Behavioural Disorders* (World Health Organization).

World Health Organization (2018) *ICD-11 for Mortality and Morbidity Statistics* (World Health Organization).

Yannoulidis, S. (2012) *Mental State Defences in Criminal Law* (Ashgate).

Index